Health Policy and Systems Responses to Forced Migration

Kayvan Bozorgmehr • Bayard Roberts
Oliver Razum • Louise Biddle
Editors

Health Policy and Systems Responses to Forced Migration

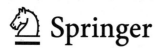 Springer

Editors
Kayvan Bozorgmehr
Department of Population Medicine
and Health Services Research
School of Public Health
Bielefeld University
Bielefeld, Nordrhein-Westfalen, Germany

Department of General Practice and Health
Services Research
University Hospital Heidelberg
Heidelberg, Baden-Württemberg, Germany

Oliver Razum
Department of Epidemiology
and International Public Health
School of Public Health
Bielefeld University
Bielefeld, Nordrhein-Westfalen, Germany

Bayard Roberts
Department of Health Services Research
and Policy
London School of Hygiene and Tropical
Medicine
London, UK

Louise Biddle
Department of General Practice and Health
Services Research
University Hospital Heidelberg
Heidelberg, Baden-Württemberg, Germany

ISBN 978-3-030-33814-5   ISBN 978-3-030-33812-1   (eBook)
https://doi.org/10.1007/978-3-030-33812-1

This Springer imprint is published by the registered company Springer Nature Switzerland AG
The registered company address is: Gewerbestrasse 11, 6330 Cham, Switzerland

Preface

Forced migration is on the increase, and it poses challenges to the health systems of most countries. The health of forced migrants has, to date, mostly been analysed with a focus on specific conditions, most notably infectious diseases and mental health. In this book, we attempt to fill a gap by applying a health policy and systems perspective on forced migration to identify areas of interaction. We determine relationships between elements of health systems and health needs of displaced populations, analyse tensions between policy areas and sectors, and shed light on potential synergies to inform system-level approaches aimed at improving health system responses to forced migration. In doing so, we aim to create a platform and basis to bring together research communities from the fields of political science, epidemiology, health sciences, economics, and sociology that have largely worked separately on *either* forced migration *or* health policy and systems research.

The book brings together for the first time the existing knowledge on health systems and health policy responses to forced migration with a focus on asylum seekers, refugees, and internally displaced people. Additionally, it contributes to advancing knowledge on forced migration towards health policy and system-level approaches, reforms, and interventions. The perspectives taken by this volume are local, national, international, and/or global, and authors use a range of spatial scales as necessary to address the relevant aspects and issues of concern. While we place a specific focus on European countries, we also highlight lessons learnt from countries in neighbouring regions hosting the highest numbers of forced migrants globally, such as Lebanon and Jordan.

By bringing together knowledge which is often scant, as well as scattered across several journals and disciplines, the book aims to be of use to policymakers and analysts, international organisations, front-line practitioners in the field, scholars in academia, think tanks, and students.

This book is intended to stimulate reflections, further research, political discourse, and eventually health systems and policy reforms. Through this process, we hope to contribute to the global efforts to improve the health of displaced populations, ultimately benefitting society as a whole. We wish to thank all authors for their expert contributions, as well as our readers for their interest in the topics of this book.

Bielefeld, Germany	Kayvan Bozorgmehr
London, UK	Bayard Roberts
Bielefeld, Germany	Oliver Razum
Heidelberg, Germany	Louise Biddle

Acknowledgements

We want to thank Janet Kim for her excellent guidance in getting this book published. We also thank Maren Hintermeier for her technical assistance in pulling elements of this book together.

Contents

Contributors

Dina Balabanova, PhD Associate Professor, London School of Hygiene & Tropical Medicine, London, UK; research focus: health systems, health policy, rapid appraisal methodology, sociology, qualitative research.

Louise Biddle, MSc Research Fellow in the Department of General Practice and Health Services Research at the University Hospital Heidelberg, Heidelberg, Germany; research focus: health systems research, health financing, health monitoring, social determinants of health, medical sociology.

Karl Blanchet, PhD London School of Hygiene & Tropical Medicine, Associate Professor in Health Systems Research and Codirector of the Health in Humanitarian Crises Centre; research focus: resilience in global health, specifically in post-conflict and conflict-affected countries.

Kayvan Bozorgmehr, MD, MSc Professor for public health, Head of Department of Population Medicine and Health Services Research, School of Public Health, Bielefeld University, Bielefeld, Germany, and Head of Social Determinants, Equity & Migration Group, Department of General Practice and Health Services Research at the University Hospital Heidelberg, Heidelberg, Germany; research focus: health services, social epidemiology, forced migration, global health, health policy and systems.

Rebecca Chanis, MSPH/MA Affiliate, Johns Hopkins Center for Humanitarian Health, Baltimore, MD, USA; research focus: health services research, health financing, maternal health.

Antonio Chiarenza Head of Research and Innovation Unit at the Azienda Unità Sanitaria Locale (Local Health Unit)—IRCCS of Reggio Emilia, Reggio Emilia, Italy; research focus: health services, health promotion, migrant health.

Valentina Chiesa, MD Specialist in Public Health at Local Health Unit of Reggio Emilia (Italy) and MSc student in Global Health Policy at the London School of Hygiene & Tropical Medicine, London (UK); research focus: global health policies, migrant health, public health.

Canan Coşkan Associated Scientist, Institute for Interdisciplinary Research on Conflict and Violence, Bielefeld University, Bielefeld, Germany//Based in Turkey; research focus: collective action, identity, intergroup conflict, immigration, acculturation, cultural differences.

Anne de Graaff, MSc Research Fellow, Department of Clinical, Neuro and Developmental Psychology, Public Health Research Institute, Vrije Universiteit Amsterdam, Amsterdam, The Netherlands; research focus: common mental disorders, trauma, brief psychological interventions, trials.

Jocelyn DeJong, MPhil, PhD Professor and Associate Dean, Faculty of Health Sciences, American University of Beirut, Beirut, Lebanon; research focus: sexual and reproductive health with a focus on the Middle East and conflict-affected populations, adolescent health and early marriage among Syrian refugees.

Karin Diaconu, PhD Research Fellow, Institute for Global Health and Development, Queen Margaret University, Edinburgh, UK; research focus: health systems research, systems dynamics methods, resilience, complex intervention evaluation (e.g., pay for performance), health technology assessment and priority-setting.

Antonia Dingle, PhD Research Fellow in Health Financing, Department of Global Health and Development, London School of Hygiene and & Tropical Medicine, London, UK; research focus: financing of reproductive, maternal, newborn, and child health, aid tracking.

Daniela C. Fuhr, DrPH Assistant Professor in Mental Health Systems, London School of Hygiene & Tropical Medicine, London, UK; research focus: mental health of refugees, migrants, and vulnerable populations, common mental disorders, low-intensity psychological intervention, trials.

Chuck Hui, MD, FRCPC Associate Professor, University of Ottawa, Chief of Infectious Diseases, Immunology and Allergy, Children's Hospital of Eastern Ontario, Ottawa, ON, USA; research focus: migration health, migrant health guidelines, migration health policy, migration health knowledge translation, immunizations of migrants, child migrant health, migration health international research network.

Alexandra Kaasch, PhD Assistant Professor in the Faculty of Sociology, Bielefeld University, Bielefeld, Germany; research focus: global social policy, global health policy, international organizations, global governance.

Philipa Mladovsky, PhD Assistant Professor in International Development, London School of Economics and Political Science, London, UK; research focus: global health, health systems, health financing, migrant and ethnic minority health.

Sara Barragán Montes, MA, MSc Freelance Writer and Editor; research focus: migration and health, health equity, social determinants of health, health governance, health emergencies.

Sandra Mounier-Jack, Msc, MBA Associate Professor in Health Policy, Department of Global Health Development, Faculty of Public Health and Policy, London School of Hygiene & Tropical Medicine, London, UK; research focus: health systems research, health financing, health service research, integrated care, immunization.

Ghina R. Mumtaz, PhD Assistant Research Professor at the Department of Epidemiology and Population Health at the Faculty of Health Sciences at the American University of Beirut, Beirut, Lebanon; research focus: infectious disease epidemiology, HIV, sexually transmitted infections, viral hepatitis, vulnerable populations.

Yudit Namer Bielefeld University, School of Public Health, Department of Epidemiology and International Public Health, Bielefeld, Germany; research focus: public mental health, migration and health, sexual orientation, gender identity.

Catherine Pitt, MSc Assistant Professor of Health Economics in the Department of Global Health and Development at the London School of Hygiene & Tropical Medicine, London, UK; research focus: health financing; economic evaluation; reproductive, maternal, newborn, and child health; malaria; neglected tropical diseases.

Kevin Pottie, MD, MClSc Full Professor and Clinician-Investigator, Department of Family Medicine, Bruyère Research Institute, Ottawa, ON, USA. School of Epidemiology, Public Health and Preventive Medicine, University of Ottawa, Ottawa, ON, USA; research focus: homeless health guidelines, WHO home based records, systematic review series on ID and migrants IJERPH

Oliver Razum Professor and Dean, School of Public Health, Department of Epidemiology and International Public Health, Bielefeld, Germany; research focus: social inequalities in health, migration and health.

Bernd Rechel Researcher at the European Observatory on Health Systems and Policies, London School of Hygiene & Tropical Medicine, London, UK; research focus: health systems, health policies, migrant health, public health.

Bayard Roberts, PhD Professor in Health Systems and Policy, London School of Hygiene & Tropical Medicine, London, UK; research focus: conflict-affected populations, non-communicable diseases, mental health, health systems and policy.

Alia H. Sabra Researcher at the Social Justice Section in the Social Development Division at UNESCWA and Consultant at the Department of Epidemiology and Population Health (EPH) at the Faculty of Health Sciences at the American University of Beirut, Beirut, Lebanon; research focus: public health, monitoring and evaluation, humanitarian and relief, health financing, social development.

Thea Scognamiglio, MD/MPH Faculty Affiliate at the Johns Hopkins Center for Humanitarian Health, Baltimore, MD, USA; research focus: health in conflict, trauma and mental health in forcibly displaced population, health monitoring.

Abla M. Sibai, PhD Professor of Epidemiology and Population Health, Faculty of Health Sciences, American University of Beirut, Beirut, Lebanon; research focus: aging, non-communicable diseases, social gerontology, Health in Humanitarian Crises.

Marit Sijbrandij, PhD Associate Professor, Department of Clinical, Neuro and Developmental Psychology, Public Health Research Institute, Vrije Universiteit Amsterdam, Amsterdam, The Netherlands; research focus: common mental disorders, trauma, brief psychological interventions, trials.

Neha S. Singh, PhD, MPH Assistant Professor in the Department of Global Health and Development, and Deputy Director of the Health in Humanitarian Crises Centre at the London School of Hygiene & Tropical Medicine, London, UK; research focus: health systems research, sexual and reproductive health, maternal health, adolescent health, research in conflict-affected settings.

Egbert Sondorp, PhD Researcher, KIT Royal Tropical Institute, Amsterdam, The Netherlands; research focus: health in fragile and conflict-affected areas, health policy and planning, health systems, disease control.

Paul Spiegel, MD, MPH Professor of Practice, Department of International Health, Johns Hopkins Bloomberg School of Public Health, Director, Johns Hopkins Center for Humanitarian Health, Baltimore, MD, USA; research focus: humanitarian emergencies, migration, health systems.

Antonio Trujillo, PhD Associate Professor; Baltimore, MD, USA; research focus: economics of chronic conditions; access to drugs; program impact evaluation.

Ursula Trummer, PhD, Mag rer. soc.oec., MSc Director at the Center for Health and Migration, Vienna, Austria (www.c-hm.com); research focus: migration governance and health, ethics and economics, vulnerable migrant groups, family solidarity and migration.

Maike Voss, MPH Researcher at Global Issues Division, German Institute for International and Security Affairs, Berlin, Germany; research focus: global health governance, health security, political determinants of health, development policy.

Katharina Wahedi, MD at the Department of General Practice and Health Services Research at the University Hospital Heidelberg, Heidelberg, Germany; research focus: health systems research, health services research, social determinants of health, infectious disease, health financing.

Kolitha Wickramage, Dr Global Migration Health Research and Epidemiology Coordinator, International Organization for Migration, Global Support Centre, Manila, Philippines; research focus: migration health, refugee health, health of internally displaced persons, health of migrant workers and their families in low to middle income countries, migration health policy, health systems, health diplomacy, global health emergencies in relation to cross-border disease transmission.

Sophie Witter, PhD Professor of International Health Financing and Health Systems, Institute for Global Health and Development, Queen Margaret University, Edinburgh, UK; research focus: health systems research, health financing, fragile and conflict-affected settings, resilience, evaluation of complex interventions, getting research into practice.

Aniek Woodward, MSc Research Fellow, KIT Royal Tropical Institute, Amsterdam, The Netherlands; research focus: refugee and migrant health, health systems, qualitative research.

Dominik Zenner, Dr Senior Regional Migration Health Adviser, Migration Health Division, Regional Office for the EEA, the EU and NATO, International Organization for Migration, Brussels, Belgium; research focus: migration health, TB epidemiology, TB screening, HIV, infectious disease epidemiology, migration health policy.

About the Editors

Kayvan Bozorgmehr, MD, MSc is full professor for public health. He heads the Department for Population Medicine and Health Services Research at Bielefeld University, and the Social Determinants, Equity and Migration Group at Heidelberg University Hospital in Germany. He trained as a medical doctor and social epidemiologist.

Bayard Roberts, PhD, MPH is Professor of Health Systems and Policy and Head of the Department of Health Services Research and Policy at the London School of Hygiene and Tropical Medicine in the United Kingdom.

Oliver Razum, MD, MSc is Dean of Bielefeld School of Public Health in Bielefeld, Germany. He is full professor and heads the Department of Epidemiology and International Public Health. He trained as a medical doctor and epidemiologist.

Louise Biddle, MSc is a social scientist and research fellow at the Social Determinants, Equity and Migration Group at Heidelberg University Hospital in Germany.

Chapter 1
Health Policy and Systems Responses to Forced Migration: An Introduction

Kayvan Bozorgmehr, Louise Biddle, Oliver Razum, and Bayard Roberts

Abbreviations

UCL   University College London
WHO   World Health Organisation

Introduction

Forced migration has become one of the defining political features of our time. Much of the discourse and research has, however, failed to engage in health system implications. The aim of this book is to overcome this gap and address the phenomenon of forced migration from a health policy and systems perspective.

Forced migration refers to a migratory movement in which "[..] an element of coercion exists, including threats to life and livelihood, whether arising from natural

---

K. Bozorgmehr (✉)
Department of Population Medicine and Health Services Research, School of Public Health, Bielefeld University, Bielefeld, Germany

Department of General Practice and Health Services Research, University Hospital Heidelberg, Heidelberg, Germany
e-mail: kayvan.bozorgmehr@uni-bielefeld.de

L. Biddle
Department of General Practice and Health Services Research, University Hospital Heidelberg, Heidelberg, Germany
e-mail: louise.biddle@med.uni-heidelberg.de

O. Razum
Department of Epidemiology and International Public Health, School of Public Health, Bielefeld University, Bielefeld, Germany
e-mail: oliver.razum@uni-bielefeld.de

B. Roberts
Health Systems and Policy, London School of Hygiene and Tropical Medicine, London, UK
e-mail: bayard.roberts@lshtm.ac.uk

© Springer Nature Switzerland AG 2020
K. Bozorgmehr et al. (eds.), *Health Policy and Systems Responses to Forced Migration*, https://doi.org/10.1007/978-3-030-33812-1_1

or man-made causes [..]" (IOM 2004). This includes movements of refugees and internally displaced persons (IDPs) as well as people displaced by natural or environmental disasters, chemical or nuclear disasters, famine, or development projects (IOM 2004). The number of forcibly displaced individuals rose by 65% in the last decade: from about 42.7 million in 2007 to a high of almost 70.8 million individuals by the end of 2018—the highest number of forced migrants ever recorded (UNHCR 2019). This figure corresponds to about nine in 1000 individuals worldwide who were forcibly displaced in 2018 (UNHCR 2019). Of the globally displaced population, about 60% (41.3 million) were IDPs, and 40% crossed international borders as refugees (25.9 million) and asylum seekers (3.5 million) (UNHCR 2019).

Migration trajectories are dynamic and complex, and individuals may shift between the migrant categories (Box 1.1) as they move within or between countries. Different motivations for migration add to this complexity, and recent population movements are increasingly characterised by "mixed movements" (UNHCR 2016), referring to movements driven by a complex array of factors and consisting of diverse, forced as well as voluntary, migrant groups such as refugees, asylum seekers, labour and economic migrants, unaccompanied minors, victims of human trafficking, and others (UNHCR 2016; IOM 2019). This entails varying needs of health and humanitarian profiles of those on the move, and entails challenges for systems responding to those movements (UNHCR 2016).

Box 1.1 Overview of Definitions of Migrant Groups

Migrant
"Persons who are moving or have moved across an international border or within a State away from their habitual place of residence, regardless of (1) the person's legal status, (2) whether the movement is voluntary or involuntary, (3) what the causes for the movement are, or (4) what length of the stay is" (IOM 2019).

Forced displacement (or displacement)[1]
"The involuntary movement, individually or collectively, of persons from their country or community, notably for reasons of armed conflict, civil unrest, or natural or man-made catastrophes".

Internally displaced person
"Internally displaced persons are people or groups of people who have been forced to leave their homes or places of habitual residence, in particular as a result of or in order to avoid the effects of armed conflict, situations of generalized violence, violations of human rights, or natural or man-made disasters, and who have not crossed an international border" (UNHCR 2019).

---

[1] Definitions taken from IOM Glossary on International Migration Law (IOM 2004).

Refugee (as defined by international law)[1]
"A person who, "owing to a well-founded fear of persecution for reasons of race, religion, nationality, membership of a particular social group or political opinions, is outside the country of his nationality and is unable or, owing to such fear, is unwilling to avail himself of the protection of that country". (Art. 1(A) (2), Convention relating to the Status of Refugees, 1951 as modified by the 1967 Protocol)

Refugee (as umbrella term)
In the colloquial sense often used as umbrella term for a wide range of individuals with different residence statuses (asylum seekers, rejected asylum seekers, irregular migrants, and detainees), even if this is incorrect from an international legal perspective.

Asylum-seeker[1]
"A person who seeks safety from persecution or serious harm in a country other than his or her own and awaits a decision on the application for refugee status under relevant international and national instruments. In case of a negative decision, the person must leave the country and may be expelled, as may any non-national in an irregular or unlawful situation, unless permission to stay is provided on humanitarian or other related grounds".

Mixed migration (or mixed movements)
"A movement in which a number of people are travelling together, generally in an irregular manner, using the same routes and means of transport, but for different reasons. People travelling as part of mixed movements have varying needs and profiles and may include asylum seekers, refugees, trafficked persons, unaccompanied/separated children, and migrants in an irregular situation" (UNHCR 2016).

Pre-, peri-, and post-migration factors (Zimmerman et al. 2011), such as political instability, unsafe travel routes, and living situations in host countries, affect the health and humanitarian needs of forcibly displaced populations. The health needs comprise (amongst other aspects) mental health, infectious diseases, sexual and reproductive health, nutrition, as well as chronic physical conditions (Abubakar et al. 2018). Among the forcibly displaced, victims of trauma and violence, victims of trafficking, pregnant women, children, people with disabilities, and the elderly constitute particularly vulnerable groups (European Commission 2013). The rising number, intensity, duration, and heterogeneity of contemporary migration movements create challenges for health systems in arrival, transit, and receiving countries. Pre-existing and generic weaknesses of national and regional health systems, such as poor health information systems, fragmented health care delivery, health workforce shortages, and an underdeveloped organisational infrastructure, are amplified in the context of forced migration. Language barriers, cultural differences, and legal barriers to health care contribute to existing weaknesses in many countries, limiting the ability of national health systems to adequately address the health needs of heterogeneous migrant populations (Rechel et al. 2013). The provision of good access to effective, efficient, and equitable health care services, including primary care and specialist services in countries of arrival, transit, or destination, is at the heart of this challenge. This ambition requires functional and strong health systems which are responsive to the underlying needs of the population they serve (WHO 2009). This includes transient, dynamic population groups, irrespective of their residence status or reason for migration, as well as populations in situations of protracted displacement.

The Health System: A Blind Spot in the Context of Forced Migration

Until now, however, health research in the field of forced migration has focused mainly on individual migrants and their medical needs. The majority of health research is disease-centred and predominantly focuses on biomedical and epidemiological aspects of infectious diseases and mental health (Sweileh 2017; Sweileh et al. 2018). Policy aspects, if considered at all, are often studied with the lens of legal entitlements to health care for specific migrant groups (IOM 2016; Norredam et al. 2006; Biswas et al. 2012; Stubbe Østergaard et al. 2017). While entitlements are an essential aspect for the study of access to health care, only considering legal policies is not sufficient to fully understand the complex interplay of factors which determine access to, quality of, and outcomes of health care as parts of a broader health system response.

This narrow perspective—on individuals, selected medical needs, and entitlements—has resulted in a limited understanding of the interplay between policies, health system responses, and health outcomes in the context of forced migration (Bozorgmehr and Jahn 2019). This, in turn, leads to limited knowledge on system-level interventions and policies to improve health system performance to the benefit of forced migrants and accommodating societies alike. The UCL-Lancet Commission on Migration and Health likewise notes that mainstream perspectives on health systems and migration are mostly concerned with service delivery in the boundaries of national or geopolitical jurisdictions, and less with the question of "how we can make existing real-world health systems more responsive to human mobility" (Abubakar et al. 2018) as a systemic phenomenon.

Health systems, however, include more than only service delivery and consist of "all organizations, people and actions whose primary intent is to promote health" (WHO 2007). According to the framework of the World Health Organization (WHO), a health system consists of six distinct, but interrelated, system "building blocks": (1) service delivery, (2) health workforce, (3) health information, (4) medical products, vaccines, and technologies, (5) financing, and (6) leadership and governance (WHO 2007). The building blocks can be considered as the elements of any health system, each providing a useful way of outlining the desirable functions of a health system as a whole (see Box 1.2).

However, as de Savigny and Adam (2009) note, "the building blocks alone do not constitute a system, any more than a pile of bricks constitutes a functioning building". Applying a health policy and systems perspective, Sheikh and colleagues

Box 1.2 Definitions, Aims, and Desirable Attributes of the Six Health System Building Blocks (as Outlined in WHO 2007)

(1) **Service delivery**:

"is concerned with how inputs and services are organized and managed, to ensure access, quality, safety and continuity of care across health conditions, across different locations and over time". Good services are "those which deliver effective, safe, quality personal and non-personal health interventions to those who need them, when and where needed, with minimum waste of resources".

(2) **Health workforce**:

"Health workers are all people engaged in actions whose primary intent is to protect and improve health. A country's health workforce consists broadly of health service providers and health management and support workers. This includes: private as well as public sector health workers; unpaid and paid workers; lay and professional cadres". "A well-performing health workforce is one which works in ways that are responsive, fair and efficient to achieve the best health outcomes possible, given available resources and circumstances. I.e. there are sufficient numbers and mix of staff, fairly distributed; they are competent, responsive and productive".

(3) **Health information**:

"ensures the production, analysis, dissemination and use of reliable and timely health information by decision-makers at different levels of the health system, both on a regular basis and in emergencies. It involves three domains of health information: on health determinants; on health systems performance; and on health status".

(4) **Medical products, vaccines, and technologies**:

"including medical products, vaccines and other technologies of assured quality, safety, efficacy and cost-effectiveness, and their scientifically sound and cost-effective use."

(5) **Financing**:

"raising adequate funds for health in ways that ensure people can use needed services, and are protected from financial catastrophe or impoverishment associated with having to pay for them. It provides incentives for providers and users to be efficient".

(6) **Leadership/governance**:

"ensuring strategic policy frameworks combined with effective oversight, coalition building, accountability, regulations, incentives and attention to system design".

supplement the WHO concept: while the building blocks can be regarded as system "hardware" (i.e. elements which can be found in any health system), the way the system and these elements work together strongly depend on the system "software", which is understood as ideas, interests, relationships, networks, and formal or informal power, as well as values and norms of individuals and groups within the health system (Sheikh et al. 2011).Thus, people are the central component of any health system (WHO 2009). Health systems are not static, but linked to each other through system characteristics, and as such are self-organising, constantly changing, tightly linked, non-linear, and governed through (negative) feedback loops (De Savigny and Adam 2009).

The way the building blocks interact with each other determines the overall design and functioning of a health system. Thereby, the dynamic architecture and interrelatedness of the system building blocks affects the extent to which the overall goals and outcomes of a health system, i.e. responsiveness, financial protection, improved health, health equity, as well as efficiency, are achieved (De Savigny and Adam 2009). Additionally, social, political, and historical, as well as regional, national, and international factors affect the achievement of these goals and overall health system performance, making health systems socially constructed, complex adaptive systems (Sheikh et al. 2011). As complex adaptive systems, health systems are history dependent and counter-intuitive, that is, they are non-linear and unpredictable with respect to the relations of their system blocks, or regarding the mechanisms and effects of interventions and reforms which may entail unintended consequences (De Savigny and Adam 2009). Despite being constantly changing and adaptive, health systems are—very often—resistant to change from above, as structures and actors in the system may have their own competing or conflicting agendas (De Savigny and Adam 2009).

Understanding the Health Policy and Systems Perspective

The health policy and systems perspective seeks to understand how "societies organize themselves in achieving collective health goals, and how different actors interact in the policy and implementation processes to contribute to policy outcomes" (Gilson 2013). The perspective roots in an interdisciplinary understanding of health systems, and builds on a blend of sociology, economics, political science, anthropology, as well as public health and epidemiology (Gilson et al. 2011; Gilson 2013). Health policy hereby refers to the "courses of action (and inaction) that affect the sets of institutions, organizations, services and funding arrangements of the health system" (Buse et al. 2005). This includes not only formal rules and laws or regulations but also de facto practices and actions taken by actors of the health system. Health policy is a process, and its content is defined, formally or informally, by individuals and groups who act in a specific context (Walt and Gilson 1994). This process is highly political, and understanding the actors and interests driving the process is of crucial importance to identify entry points for policy change and system-level interventions to strengthen health systems. From a systems perspective, health policy does not occur in isolation, but its implementation requires understanding of organisational dynamics of health systems, and its interaction with other societal sectors (economy, labour market, education) and systems (ecosystem, financial system).

Yet, health policy and systems considerations have not embraced forced migration to a sufficient extent despite substantial links, connections, reciprocal relationships, and interactions between the two areas.

A Health Policy and Systems Perspective on Forced Migration

In this book we apply a health policy and systems perspective on forced migration to identify such areas of interaction. We determine relationships, analyse tensions between policy areas, and shed light on potential synergies to inform system-level approaches aimed at improving health system responses. In doing so, we aim to create a platform and basis to bring together research communities from the fields of political science, epidemiology, health sciences, economics, and sociology, who have so far largely worked separately on either forced migration or on health policy and systems research.

The book gathers, synthesises, and integrates the existing knowledge on health systems and policy responses to forced migration with a focus on asylum seekers, refugees, and internally displaced people. In particular, it contributes to advancing knowledge on forced migration through its analytical perspective on health policy and system-level approaches, reforms, and interventions. As the first book in the health sciences field taking such a perspective on forced migration, and due to the previous neglect of these aspects in migration health research, we acknowledge that the evidence-base in some areas is fragmented, and that some discussions and debates are still at an early stage. However, we take this book as a starting point to frame the potential routes, priorities, and areas for further research in this field.

As outlined above, health policies and systems are embedded in socio-political, legal, and economic structures, norms, and values. These structures, which distribute power within and between countries, affect the causes and consequences of forced migration, as well as the responses to it. Among the causes or contributing factors of forced migration are war and conflict, arms exports, economic regimes, and trade agreements, as well as excessive exploitation of the world's natural resources by transnational and national industries. The world order in the aftermath of the 2008 financial crisis is currently in an "interregnum", i.e. a period in which the previous order (defined by expanding liberalisation of trade and finances, as well as institutional multilateralism) has been worn out, but a new order—both institutionally and geopolitically—has not yet been achieved (Stahl 2019). This transition is characterised by a rise in nationalism, both with respect to geopolitical, economic, and social policies (Mulvey and Davidson 2019). In this political environment, migration is often securitised, i.e. framed as a threat (Lazaridis and Wadia

2015). We face chronic tragedies of refugees and migrants dying in the Mediterranean Sea (Razum and Bozorgmehr 2015). This can be seen as the consequence of fading solidarity (Bozorgmehr and Wahedi 2017) between central and coastal European countries, and between European citizens and desperate people seeking a better life in safer and economically wealthier countries. The policy responses of ceasing the EU-led life-saving search and rescue-operations, and criminalising the rescue-operations led by non-governmental organisations, dramatically show how different policy sectors such as migration policies and border management, internal affairs, and health and humanitarian policies may conflict.

This is an extreme example of how the political economy affects the distribution (or withdrawal) of health-relevant resources in the context of forced migration. Still, resource allocation in the health system itself is also considerably shaped by normative and socio-political considerations which touch ground in legal policies, or formal and informal practice. Today, nation-states adapt normative stances regulating the breadth of health services granted to forced migrants, whether their entitlements are equal or different from those of the resident population. Furthermore, inequalities in entitlements are created within the heterogeneous group of displaced populations based on residence status or country of origin. While international law regards inequalities based on residence status, ethnicity or country of origin as violation of the human right to health (CESCR 2000), such discriminatory practices are reality in many countries (IOM 2016).

The degree to which any entitlement is translated into realised access to health care depends additionally on the way health services are organised, whether or not the required services are in place, and if they are adequate, sufficient in numbers, and of good quality. Failure of health systems to provide equitable health services may cause inefficiencies, e.g. through over-supply of resources, mismatch between need and services provided, or late diagnosis and treatment due to poor access or restricted entitlements, causing higher costs than early detection or prevention of disease.

Health assessments and screening measures play an important role in early detection and prevention of disease among forced migrant populations. However, these measures are often implemented in differing ways between and within countries. From a health policy and systems perspective, measures implemented for assessment and screening should be evidence-based, cost-effective, consider individual risk profiles (based, e.g., on age, sex, pre-existing illness, country of origin, route of migration, etc.), address issues of relevance to individuals and public health alike, ensure linkage to needed care, and respect ethical as well human right aspects. Furthermore, they should be practicable, feasible, and scalable to address population dynamics when and where needed. All relevant health and socio-demographic data, including population denominators, should be routinely collected and evaluated in regular intervals by the health information system to ensure that planning, care provision, and quality assurance is based on sound data and scientific evidence. However, this is currently far from being reality in many countries, even in those with strong health systems (Bozorgmehr et al. 2018, 2019). Health data in the context of forced migration are often scarce, of poor quality, and fragmented. The question is thus how data availability and integration can be improved, and how data can be better used in dynamic or protracted situations to proactively plan health services, detect health risks, and promote health among displaced populations.

The reality is that assessment and screening policies are often a blend of measures rooting in clinical or public health and socio-political or security considerations. A health policy and systems perspective can investigate policies for forced migrants to examine the overt or covert agendas and motivations to help answer "security of what, for whom, and at which price?"

Health financing systems are an essential component of every health system. Although financial considerations play a major role for equitable health systems, very few studies consider the economics of migration or financial aspects in the context of health research. The role of a health financing system is to raise funds for health services, ensure financial protection of the population, and provide pooling of risks and funds. Health financing systems in the context of forced migration are, however, often fragmented, haphazard, and set up in parallel to those of national health systems. This bears several challenges with respect to administrative and technical efficiency, equity in financing, and purchasing of needed services. The lack of quality assurance in many settings and contexts in which health care is provided to forced migrants, e.g. reception centres, can lead to lack of value for money, resource waste, or missed opportunities to translate invested resources into better health for the displaced population.

A health system must respond to, and uphold its functions under, multiple challenges in the context of forced migration. This applies to dynamic numbers, transient populations, complex health risk profiles, varying expectations of health services, multiple languages and cultures, complex legal regulations intersecting with health and migration policies, humanitarian emergencies, and difficult care settings in protracted camps or gated reception centres. The extent to which a health system is prepared for and responds to such challenges can be regarded as its resilience. We understand resilience of a health system as its absorptive, adaptive, and transformative capacities (Blanchet et al. 2017). A resilient health system would respond to rising numbers of forced migrants by providing and scaling up services when and where they are needed; by adapting its structures and services to reach out to new populations or address new health needs; and by implementing system-level policies to improve its performance. A resilience lens can help to analyse strengths and weakness in health system responses to forced migration (Razum and Bozorgmehr 2017). It can moreover identify areas and building blocks which require policy reform to increase system performance.

Health Policy and Systems Responses: The Specific Contribution of the Book Chapters

All chapters in this book make a specific contribution to one or more system building blocks, and to the "software" of health systems and policy. In the second chapter, Sara Barragán Montes delineates the contemporary political economy in which health policy and system responses to forced migration in the context of forced migration are embedded. She examines how the political and economic structures which distribute power and resources have shaped policies on forced migration in European countries, including issues of policy space but also the normative and legal architecture surrounding forced migration. By focusing on the institutional architecture and governance of forced migration and health issues, lessons are drawn for the fiscal and economic sectors of European societies, including the health sector.

As financing of health systems and services is crucial, a total of three chapters have been devoted to this topic. Paul Spiegel and colleagues address the need for developing and implementing innovative humanitarian financing mechanisms for refugee health in a context in which humanitarian crises are becoming more common and increasingly protracted. As the current mechanism for funding emergencies related to forced migration are unsustainable, the authors introduce and discuss various approaches and financing tools which could be used to integrate health of forced migrants into country health systems to the benefit of displaced persons and host populations alike, avoiding parallel service provision for forced migrants.

Neha Singh and colleagues analyse health care financing arrangements and service provision for 1.5 million displaced Syrian refugees in Lebanon with a focus on women, children, and adolescents. The challenges of mobilising sufficient funds to sustain an equitable and needs-based provision of services are highlighted, including those related to integration of refugees in the host society.

Louise Biddle and colleagues further add to the financing discussion by outlining three scenarios towards responsive financing systems for the health of asylum seekers in Europe. They analyse shortcomings of the current financing system, which is restricted to national boundaries, and discuss—based on existing financial mechanisms—potential financing schemes which would increase solidarity among member states of the European Union.

Karl Blanchet and colleagues introduce and discuss the concept of health system resilience based on systems thinking and complexity theory. They highlight the utility and relevance of the concept in the context of forced migration, improving our understanding of the capacities of the health system to adapt and transform itself towards the challenge of providing effective and high-quality health care to displaced and mobile populations. On a very practical level, the authors demonstrate how the concept can be utilised for health systems strengthening in the context of forced migration by highlighting key areas for development and improvement.

The resilience of a health system closely relates to two important concepts of global health—health security and universal health coverage—which shape both policy and practice in the field of forced migration. Maike Voss and colleagues scrutinise essential and fundamental tensions between the two concepts, which are embedded in different normative boundaries, but also identify synergies that may be used to maximise the health gain for the population of forced migrants and resident populations alike. A shift towards a mutual base on the right to health, and a broader understanding of what constitutes security, may facilitate such synergies and lead to more rational, effective, and efficient interventions to address health of displaced populations.

To this end, appropriate assessment of health needs is required to identify individuals with particular health needs and vulnerabilities. Dominik Zenner and colleagues provide an overview of the current evidence and practice of health assessments among forced migrants. They review current practices and policy frameworks, including both assessments conducted prior to and after migration. Using country examples, the authors discuss ethical and practical questions regarding linkage to care and health care access, and highlight the significant research gaps which remain with regard to the (cost-)effectiveness of current practice.

Health information systems are an essential, but often neglected, component of health systems. Medical care, health care planning, and public health monitoring relies on information on the health-related history of migrants and refugees. However, due to the nature of displacement, information on test results, vaccinations, diagnoses, health status and medications are often not available, resulting in fragmentation, discontinuity of care, and the lack of reliable and timely data for health care provision and planning. Valentina Chiesa and colleagues review the evidence on health records for migrants and refugees, presenting evidence on records implemented specifically to address the needs and requirements of a mobile population. Comparing different types of records, they discuss strengthening health information systems through improved recording and sharing of data, as well as associated challenges related to ethics and data protection.

Beyond quality and efficiency, health system responsiveness is a key measure to be considered during the assessment of health system functioning and performance. This outcome, which gives an indication of patient experiences in the healthcare encounter, is a key factor influencing health system accessibility and continuity of care. Daniela Fuhr and colleagues provide a conceptual framework to guide the assessment of health system responsiveness to the mental health needs of refugees. They apply rapid appraisal methodology to assess responsiveness among Syrian refugees in the Netherlands, and find several obstacles to achieving responsive mental health care provision, including a lack of language interpreters and culturally appropriate mental health services.

At a national level, policies concerned with the health of migrants intersect with other national priorities, including security, housing, labour and education policies. A concern is that migration itself is increasingly securitised, and forced migrants are framed and partially perceived as a threat to societies and social stability. Border control and management, restrictive entry and residence policies, as well as strong encampment and expulsion policies are often the results of securitisation of migration. Using the United Kingdom as an example, Philipa Mladovsky highlights the impacts and consequences of prioritising security aspects over health. She highlights the mechanisms by which mental health of forced migrants is created and exacerbated by social and migration policies which prioritise security concerns, with questionable benefits to society both in terms of health and security.

The fundamental question remains why health systems responses in the area of forced migration often fail to embrace the human right to health more visibly or effectively. Yudit Namer and colleagues show that the broader societal and health system response which can be observed in many European and North American countries is rooted in discrimination and infrahumanising discourses which delegitimise the automatic right to health for forced migrants. The authors highlight and discuss the role of socio-psychological and biopolitical aspects of discrimination, which result in health system responses that may create hostile environments through surveillance and securitised screening practices. They conclude that an updated ethics of care is needed for better inclusion of (forced) migrants in health care systems.

Health systems intersect with other systems of global reach, such as those dealing with trade, development or labour issues. Hence, it is important to understand the interrelations between global health governance (i.e. dedicated health organisations such as the World Health Organization) and governance in global organisations outside the health sector with relevance for health in the area of forced migration. These interrelations become important in light of the Sustainable Development Goals, which reach out beyond the health sector. In the final chapter of this volume, Alexandra Kaasch analyses the status quo of current governance systems with respect to forced migration and discusses global social governance and its effects on health for people experiencing forced migration. After contextualising the right to social protection and the right to health as part of international legal frameworks, she analyses why the right to health for forced migrants is not yet a global reality, and proposes a strengthening of regional governance efforts to further develop the right to health agenda.

Conclusion

This chapter has outlined the need for a health policy and systems perspective on forced migration, and introduced key concepts related to health policy and health systems. By focusing on the building blocks of a health system, the book aims to make a bold and analytical contribution to the field. Additionally, the authors of the different chapters scrutinise important parts of the "software" of health systems, which currently determines and largely affects policy and systems responses to forced migration, including the political economy, concepts of security and universality with different norms and values, as well as outright rejection and discrimination of forced migrants in health systems. We shed light on a wide range of policies and practices related to health screening, recording and sharing of health information, provision of migrant-sensitive health services, and financial health protection, and the ways these practices may affect system performance related to equity, efficiency, quality, and responsiveness.

Despite our attempts to be as comprehensive and analytical as possible, some blind spots remain. First, the building block of human resources remains largely unaddressed. The mobilisation, training, and strategic placement of a strong health workforce are crucial for fostering the resilience and responsiveness of the health system. Further evidence and knowledge on the development of a qualified health workforce to respond to the challenges of forced migration are needed, including system-level strategies or local good practice with potentials for scale-up. Second, given the dynamic and fluid nature of forced migration, even more emphasis could be placed on the prospects of cross-border governance in selected health areas, and on potential strategies to enhance cross-border health governance in the future. Third, more learning and exchange is required on how to influence policy in the context of forced migration, especially in areas where policy-making and evidence-informed recommendations diverge. To further push the agenda on effective, efficient, and high-quality health systems in the context of forced migration, we need two elements: firstly, examples and best practices from regions where evidence-informed recommendations effectively influenced the policy-making process; and secondly, better engagement with decision-makers and policy actors.

Our aspiration is that the evidence, ideas, and discussions presented in this volume will inspire researchers, practitioners, policy-makers, and students to consider the system perspective of forced migrants' health. We hope that many will join us in making health systems work for those that need them most, including populations who have been forcibly displaced from their homes.

References

Abubakar, I., Aldridge, R. W., Devakumar, D., Orcutt, M., Burns, R., Barreto, M. L., et al. (2018). The UCL-Lancet commission on migration and health: The health of a world on the move. *The Lancet, 392*, 2606–2654.

Biswas, D., Toebes, B., Hjern, A., Ascher, H., & Norredam, M. (2012). Access to health care for undocumented migrants from a human rights perspective: A comparative study of Denmark, Sweden, and The Netherlands. *Health and Human Rights, 14*, 49–60.

Blanchet, K., Nam, S. L., Ramalingam, B., & Pozo-Martin, F. (2017). Governance and capacity to manage resilience of health systems: Towards a new conceptual framework. *International Journal of Health Policy and Management, 6*, 431.

Bozorgmehr, K., & Jahn, R. (2019). Adverse health effects of restrictive migration policies: Building the evidence base to change practice. *The Lancet Global Health, 7*, e386–e387.

Bozorgmehr, K., & Wahedi, K. (2017). Reframing solidarity in Europe: Frontex, frontiers, and the fallacy of refugee quota. *The Lancet Public Health, 2*, e10–e11.

Bozorgmehr, K., Stock, C., Joggerst, B., & Razum, O. (2018). Tuberculosis screening in asylum seekers in Germany: a need for better data. *Lancet Public Health, 3*(8), Pe359-e361. https://doi.org/10.1016/s2468-2667(18)30132-4

Bozorgmehr, K., Biddle, L., Rohleder, S., Puthoopparambil, S., & Jahn, R. (2019). What is the evidence on availability and integration of refugee and migrant health data in health information systems in the WHO European Region? Health Evidence Network (HEN) Synthesis Report (Vol. 66). Copenhagen: WHO Regional Office for Europe.

Buse, K., Mays, N., & Walt, G. (2005). *Making health policy*. Milton Keynes: Open University Press.

CESCR. (2000). Substantive Issues Arising in the Implementation of the International Covenant on Economic, Social and Cultural Rights: General Comment No. 14 (2000) – The right to the highest attainable standard of health (article 12 of the International Covenant on Economic, Social and Cultural Rights). UN Economic and Social Council.

de Savigny, D., & Adam, T. (2009). *Systems thinking for health systems strengthening*. Geneva: World Health Organization.

European Commission. (2013). Directive 2013/33/EU of the European Parliament and of the Council of 26 June 2013 laying down standards for the reception of applicants for international protection. *Official Journal of the European Union, L180*, 96–116.

Gilson, L. (2013). Introduction to health policy and systems research. In L. Gilson (Ed.), *Health policy and system research: A methodology reader: The abridged version*. Geneva: World Health Organization.

Gilson, L., Hanson, K., Sheikh, K., Agyepong, I. A., Ssengooba, F., & Bennett, S. (2011). Building the field of health policy and systems research: Social science matters. *PLoS Medicine, 8*, e1001079.

IOM. (2004). *International migration law: Glossary on migration*. Geneva: International Organization for Migration (IOM).

IOM. (2016). *Summary report on the MIPEX health strand & country reports*. Brussels: International Organization for Migration (IOM), Regional Office Brussels, Migration Health Division.

IOM. (2019). *International migration law: Glossary on migration*. Geneva: International Organization for Migration.

Lazaridis, G., & Wadia, K. (2015). *The securitisation of migration in the EU: Debates since 9/11*. Berlin: Springer.

Mulvey, G., & Davidson, N. (2019). Between the crises: Migration politics and the three periods of neoliberalism. *Capital & Class, 43*, 271–292.

Norredam, M., Mygind, A., & Krasnik, A. (2006). Access to health care for asylum seekers in the European Union—A comparative study of country policies. *European Journal of Public Health, 16*, 286–290.

Razum, O., & Bozorgmehr, K. (2015). Disgrace at EU's external borders. *International Journal of Public Health, 60*, 515–516.

Razum, O., & Bozorgmehr, K. (2017). Refugee migration to Germany: Did the health system show resilience? *European Journal of Public Health, 27*. https://doi.org/10.1093/eurpub/ckx187.589

Rechel, B., Mladovsky, P., Ingleby, D., Mackenbach, J. P., & McKee, M. (2013). Migration and health in an increasingly diverse Europe. *Lancet, 381*, 1235–1245.

Sheikh, K., Gilson, L., Agyepong, I. A., Hanson, K., Ssengooba, F., & Bennett, S. (2011). Building the field of health policy and systems research: Framing the questions. *PLoS Medicine, 8*, e1001073.

Stahl, R. M. (2019). Ruling the interregnum: Politics and ideology in nonhegemonic times. *Politics and Society, 47*(3) 1–28.

Stubbe Østergaard, L., Norredam, M., Mock-Munoz de Luna, C., Blair, M., Goldfeld, S., & Hjern, A. (2017). Restricted health care entitlements for child migrants in Europe and Australia. *European Journal of Public Health, 27*, 869–873.

Sweileh, W. (2017). Bibliometric analysis of medicine – related publications on refugees, asylum-seekers, and internally displaced people: 2000 – 2015. *BMC International Health and Human Rights, 17*, 7.

Sweileh, W., Wickramage, K., Pottie, K., Hui, C., Roberts, B., Sawalha, A., et al. (2018). Bibliometric analysis of global migration health research in peer-reviewed literature (2000–2016). *BMC Public Health, 18*, 777.

UNHCR. (2016). *The 10-point plan in action—Glossary*. Geneva: United Nations High Commissioner For Refugees.

UNHCR. (2019). *Global trends: Forced displacement in 2018*. Geneva: United Nations High Commissioner for Refugees.

Walt, G., & Gilson, L. (1994). Reforming the health sector in developing countries: The central role of policy analysis. *Health Policy and Planning, 9*, 353–370.

WHO. (2007). *Everybody's business: Strengthening health systems to improve health outcomes: WHO's framework for action*. Geneva: World Health Organization.

WHO. (2009). In D. Savigny & T. Adam (Eds.), *Systems thinking for health systems strengthening*. Geneva: World Health Organization.

Zimmerman, C., Kiss, L., & Hossain, M. (2011). Migration and health: A framework for 21st century policy-making. *PLoS Medicine, 8*, e1001034.

Chapter 2
The Political Economy of Health and Forced Migration in Europe

Sara Barragán Montes

Abbreviations

AU	African Union
DG SANTE	Directorate General for Health and Food Safety
EC	European Commission
EU	European Union
GDP	Gross Domestic Product
GBV	gender-based violence
HiaP	Health in All Policies
HIC	high-income country
IDPs	internally displaced people
IOM	International Organization for Migration
LMIC	low- and middle-income country
MdM	Medecins du Monde (Doctors of the World)
MIPEX	Migrant Policy Integration Index
MSF	Medecins Sans Frontieres (Doctors Without Borders)
ODA	official development assistance
OECD	Organization of Economic Cooperation and Development
PICUM	Platform for International Cooperation on Undocumented Migrants
WHA	World Health Assembly
WHO	World Health Organization
UN	United Nations
UNHCR	United Nations High Commissioner for Refugees

S. B. Montes (✉)
Global Health Policy, Independent Consultant, Madrid, Spain

© Springer Nature Switzerland AG 2020
K. Bozorgmehr et al. (eds.), *Health Policy and Systems Responses to Forced Migration*, https://doi.org/10.1007/978-3-030-33812-1_2

Introduction

The increase of forced migration to countries of the European Union (EU) in 2015–2016 has positioned migration policy at the centre of the political debate, and challenged the capacity of national governments and EU institutions to put forward joint and comprehensive migration policies. Unprecedented international efforts to strengthen migration governance, including within the health sector, have faced the active opposition of various national governments. Where these have been passed, their non-legally binding nature limits enforceability. Nonetheless, the economic and fiscal impact of migration on European countries is estimated to be largely positive. Within the health sector, higher costs are associated with restrictions in access to primary health care and preventive programmes. This chapter uses a political economy approach to examine how politico-economic structures determine the uneven distribution of health inequities across migrant groups. Furthermore, it analyses the socio-political, economic and fiscal impact of forced migration to European countries, and how this influences decision-making, including in the health sector.

Section "Introduction" introduces the concept of political economy and its main contemporary applications. Additionally, it provides an overview of the movements of forcibly displaced people across EU countries in 2015–2016. Section "Institutional Context: The Governance of Forced Migration and Health" describes the institutional architecture that governs forced migration in general, and the health of forcibly displaced people in particular, elucidating how it impacts differently the health and well-being of various categories of migrants. Section "Socio-Political Impact of Forced Migration and Implications for Health Policy" examines the political and social effects derived from an increase of forced migration to European countries in recent years. Finally, Section "Economic and Fiscal Impact of Forced Migration, and Implications for Health Policy" analyses its potential impact on the European economic and fiscal fabric, including the health sector. The key messages of the chapter are summarised in Box 2.1.

What is Political Economy?

There is no universally agreed definition of political economy. Since its conception in the eighteenth century, this term has prompted enduring and rather unsettled intellectual debates about the relationship between power, on the one hand, and the production and distribution of wealth, on the other. There are two prevailing and sometimes overlapping contemporary applications of the term political economy: as a field of study in itself, and as a set of methodological approaches applied to various disciplines (Wittman and Weingast 2008).

Political economy as a field of study operates in the interplay between what we know today as political science and economics. Early conceptions in this area include the seminal works of Adam Smith or Karl Marx. Smith highly influenced neoclassical economists primarily concerned with the efficient allocation of limited

> **Box 2.1 Key Messages**
>
> - Migrant health is structurally determined. Policies and institutions that operate at international, national and sub-national levels, both within and outside of the health sector, determine the differential exposure to health risks and assets for the various categories of migrants throughout the journey.
> - The increase of forced migration to EU countries in 2015–2016 has challenged the capacity of national governments and EU institutions to put forward joint and comprehensive migration policies, despite unprecedented efforts. Where international health policy frameworks have been agreed, these are not legally binding and their implementation is subject to national legislation.
> - The rise of forced migration to the EU has positioned migration management at the centre of the political debate. While overall attitudes towards migration remained stable during the peak years, it triggered pre-existing latent anti-migrant sentiments that prioritise national security.
> - The economic and fiscal impact of migration on wealthy countries is largely positive. Nonetheless, it is subject to the formal inclusion of displaced individuals into the workforce. In the health sector, barriers to access primary health care services for forced migrants have led to an overuse of emergency services, resulting in higher costs.

resources. Marx largely informed a social perspective of economics focused on explaining the unequal distribution of power and resources among interest groups.

Modern critical thinking labelled as postmodernism or poststructuralism has further developed the discipline of political economy by downplaying the importance of material and structural relations. These schools of thought apply discursive analyses to explain the asymmetrical distribution of power and representation, and the exercise of control and domination, through the role of ideas and narratives (Calkivik 2017). These approaches have been largely used to examine political economy through the lenses of culture, gender or ethnicity.

Power is a central concept in the field of political economy. Its highly contested nature has led to diverging theories about its conception, manifestation and distribution. For example, pluralist scholars such as Robert Dahl focus on the study of *overt* power in democracies, and argue that the exercise of decision-making in these contexts is highly fragmented (Dahl 1958). Critics of this view argue that the real form of power is *covert* and lies within the capacity to define the intellectual boundaries of what is acceptable to enter the political debate in the first place (Schattschneider 1960). Furthermore, Steven Lukes proposes an additional subtle form of power, the *three-dimensional view*, which refers to the ability of systems to influence the dominant values, preferences and behaviours through the unconscious, but socially and culturally rooted, action and inaction of the individuals, groups and institutions that conform them (Lukes 2005).

Lastly, the twentieth century witnessed the expansion of political economy as a set of methodological approaches used in the study of political and economic phenomena, particularly in Western democracies. These approaches aim to understand the emergence of political or economic outcomes through the study of the behaviours of relevant actors. Two main approaches can be distinguished: the economic approach (also known as public choice or rational choice theory), which is concerned with the study of individual rationality; and the sociological approach, which focuses on the role of social and historical factors in the study of institutional behaviour (Wittman and Weingast 2008).

Sizing the Issue: Forced Migration in Europe

The volume of forced displacement has experienced a dramatic rise worldwide, reaching 68.5 million people in 2017. Refugees are the second largest group among all involuntarily displaced, surpassed only by internally displaced people (IDPs). The overwhelming majority of forced migrants live in low- and middle-income countries (LMICs) outside of Europe (UNHCR 2018a).

Despite the relatively small role that Europe plays in hosting people who are involuntarily displaced compared to other regions, it has experienced an increase in the number of forced migrants arriving in the last decade, particularly during the years 2015–2016. EU countries have previously received high numbers of asylum seekers, such as in the early 1990s as a result of the war of Yugoslavia. Nonetheless, 2015 was the first year when the total number of new applications in the EU exceeded one million. This threshold was also surpassed in 2016. Applications were received mostly from people arriving from conflict-affected countries, such as Syria, Afghanistan and Iraq (Eurostat 2016, 2018). However, applications dropped significantly to about 700,000 in 2017, following the entry into force of several measures to counter migration in the EU and neighbouring countries (Eurostat 2018).

The overall number of accepted applications in the EU has also varied throughout these years. Protection status was granted to over 710,000 people in 2016, more than double compared to the previous year (Eurostat 2017a). However, accepted applications decreased by almost 25% in 2017, when around 560,000 persons were granted protection (Eurostat 2018).

The distribution of first-time applicants across the EU has been uneven during the peak years (Table 2.1). Countries have been unequally exposed to migratory pressures depending on their geographical location, as well as the degree of openness of their migration policies. These differences have had profound implications at both national and European levels. They have positioned migration management at the heart of the political debate, playing a key role in national elections across the EU, and have challenged the capacity of national governments and EU institutions to put forward joint and comprehensive migration policies.

The shifts observed in the distribution of first-time applicants across EU countries during these years, as reflected in Table 2.1, are the result of multiple factors.

Table 2.1 First-time asylum applicants in EU countries in 2015 and 2016 (Eurostat 2017a)

	Number of first-time applicants		
	2015	2016	Change (in %)
EU	1,257,030	1,204,280	−4
Belgium	38,990	14,250	−63
Bulgaria	20,165	18,990	−6
Czech Republic	1235	1200	−3
Denmark	20,825	6055	−71
Germany	441,800	722,265	+63
Estonia	225	150	−34
Ireland	3270	2235	−32
Greece	11,370	49,875	+339
Spain	14,600	15,570	+7
France	70,570	75,990	+8
Croatia	140	2150	+1413
Italy	83,245	121,185	+46
Cyprus	2105	2840	+35
Latvia	330	345	+5
Lithuania	275	410	51
Luxembourg	2360	2065	−13
Hungary	174,435	28,215	−84
Malta	1695	1735	+2
Netherlands	43,035	19,285	−55
Austria	85,505	39,860	−53
Poland	10,255	9780	−5
Portugal	870	710	−18
Romania	1225	1855	+51
Slovenia	260	1265	+389
Slovakia	270	100	−63
Finland	32,150	5275	−84
Sweden	156,110	22,330	−86
United Kingdom	39,720	38,290	−4

Number of first-time applicants is rounded to the nearest 5. Calculations are based on exact data

These include unilateral decisions to close borders in countries located across migratory routes; consequent changes in these routes altering the number of arrivals in neighbouring countries; and variations in the volume of quotas accepted by EU members that were not located across the main routes (Geddes 2018).

Similarly, large variations exist across EU countries with regards to the final decisions taken by immigration authorities on the provision of legal protection to asylum seekers. Germany recorded the highest number of positive applications by far both in 2016 (445,210) and 2017 (325,000). These accounted for over 60% of all applications granted in the EU in both years. Other countries that recorded high numbers of accepted final decisions were Sweden (69,350), Italy (35,450), France (35,170), Austria (31,750) and the Netherlands (21,825) in 2016; and France

(40,600), Italy (35,100), Austria (34,000) and Sweden (31,200) in 2017 (Eurostat 2017a, 2018).

Asylum statistics provide a useful official estimation of the impact of forced migration to EU countries during these years. However, it is important to note that asylum seekers do not account for all forcibly displaced people. Individuals may try to avoid requesting legal protection in transit countries with the aim to do so in their preferred destination. This phenomenon led to significant secondary movements of asylum seekers within the EU during these years (Beirens 2018). Many others may simply not apply for asylum and become clandestine, thus going unnoticed in official statistics and posing further difficulties to obtain an accurate estimation of the overall displaced population in Europe. Comparing the official number of asylum applications with the estimated number of arrivals across the Mediterranean Sea in southern European countries may give an idea of the magnitude of this issue. For example, immigration authorities in Greece recorded 11,370 first-time applications for asylum in 2015 (Eurostat 2017b). However, the estimated number of arrivals to Greece by sea in that year alone was 856,723 (UNHCR 2018b).

Institutional Context: The Governance of Forced Migration and Health

The term forced migration is often used to refer to individuals who have been involuntarily displaced, such as refugees or asylum seekers. Different categories of forcibly displaced people are governed distinctively by specific legal frameworks and institutional arrangements at international, national and sub-national levels. As a result, they may enjoy varying degrees of entitlements to public services including healthcare, and be subject to different conditions throughout the journey, which determine their exposure to health risks and assets. Nonetheless, it is important to note that these classifications are a deliberate simplification of the complex reality of involuntary displacement (UNHCR 2010; IOM 2011).

Forced Migration as a Structural Determinant of Health

Health is socially determined. The distribution of health inequities across populations responds to a social gradient: in aggregate terms, the lower the socio-economic status of an individual is, the poorer his or her health status will be (Solar and Irwin 2010). As a result, differences in the social positioning of individuals lead to unfair and avoidable differences in human development and health outcomes (Sen 2002). Additionally, studies of intersectionality have elucidated other factors that influence the distribution of health inequalities beyond socio-economic considerations, such as culture, gender or ethnicity (Gkiouleka et al. 2018).

Differences in the social status of individuals are not arbitrary. Social hierarchies are shaped by the broader socio-political, economic and institutional macro-level structures around which societies organise themselves, and which define and are defined by their political economy (Solar and Irwin 2010). These upstream structural factors produce unequal social positionings—and, by extension, health inequities—through the production and reproduction of imbalances in the allocation of power and resources (Navarro et al. 2006; Mackenbach 2009). Hence, health is not only socially but also structurally determined.

Migration acts as a structural determinant of health in itself. Whether migration has a positive or a negative impact on the health and well-being of those who migrate depends to a large extent on the broader socio-economic, political and institutional architecture that governs population mobility. For example, national legal frameworks provide unequal levels of access to healthcare for different types of forced migrants such as refugees, asylum seekers or undocumented migrants. Immigration policies such as detention and deportation may also have a significantly adverse impact on health outcomes (Sargent and Larchanché 2011; Zimmerman et al. 2011; Castañeda et al. 2015; Gkiouleka et al. 2018). These structural determinants influence health outcomes throughout the different stages of migration such as predeparture, travel, destination, interception and return (Zimmerman et al. 2011).

Furthermore, migration as a structural determinant of health is also socially determined. There is no such thing as one migration journey. The conditions which forcibly displaced people are exposed to when they migrate vary according to the different characteristics of each individual, such as their socio-economic status, gender, sexuality, nationality or ethnicity (Castañeda et al. 2015, Gkiouleka et al. 2018). For instance, an economic migrant from a well-off background will find it easier to migrate, and will not be exposed to the same health-harming circumstances as a refugee who is fleeing from a life-threatening situation; nor will the latter live the same experiences if she or he belongs to a sexual minority. The different environments to which these individuals are exposed to will not only determine their exposure to health risks, but also their capability to optimise their health assets (WHO 2017).

Governing Forced Migration

The politico-economic institutions that govern population mobility affect the health of forced migrants both directly, by defining the level of access to health services, and indirectly, by shaping the conditions which migrants face throughout the journey. A historical approach to the establishment of the current global system of governance of forced migration helps to understand how and why these institutions affect the health of individuals differently.

Although earlier attempts were pursued by the League of Nations in the 1920s, the current international regime of refugee protection was conceived in the aftermath of the Second World War. Its creation under the auspices of the United Nations

(UN) was closely linked to the European geopolitical context of the time, which determined its initial purpose and scope. As reflected in the 1951 Convention Relating to the Status of Refugees (hereinafter referred to as the 1951 Convention), its initial purpose was to manage the flows of political refugees between the Eastern and Western blocks (Barnett 2002; UNHCR 2011).

Nevertheless, the legal definition of refugee was further expanded in 1967 with the entering into force of the Protocol Relating to the Status of Refugees (hereinafter referred to as the 1967 Protocol). This new treaty removed the temporal and geopolitical limitations that anchored the regime of refugee protection to the context of the Cold War, and recognised other causes of forced human displacement that had arisen as a result of the processes of decolonisation. These changes led to a gradual shift of refugee flows from an East-West to a South-North focus, which resulted in a relative decrease in the number of accepted applications. For example, Western European countries accepted only 16% of all applications received in 1996, in comparison with 42% in 1983 (Barnett 2002).

The universal and legally binding definition of 'refugee' included in the 1951 Convention and the 1967 Protocol reflects the state-centric nature of the regime of refugee protection. Firstly, being outside the country of nationality or residence is stated as a precondition for the capacity to apply for legal protection. Secondly, human rights and refugee law provide for the right of an individual to claim legal protection, but they do not include an equivalent obligation for the state to grant it. While states have a responsibility to provide temporary protection throughout the process of asylum determination, the ultimate decision to recognise refugee status lies with national governments given the provisions enacted by the principle of sovereignty (Barnett 2002; Phoung 2005).

The creation of the EU led to the establishment of further international legal instruments to seek common approaches among its Member States for the regulation of human mobility in general, and forced migration in particular. These were refined through several agreements, such as the Schengen Agreement of 1985 and the Dublin Convention of 1990. These agreements were established amid past peaks of asylum seekers arriving to Europe as a result of the disintegration of the former Soviet Union and Yugoslavia, respectively, and were driven primarily by security concerns (Hatton and Williamson 2004; Guiraudon 2017; Geddes 2018).

The Dublin Convention dealt particularly with asylum policy, and specified that the responsibility for the determination of asylum in the EU lies within the first EU country to which the asylum seeker arrives, with the exception of cases of family reunification. The Dublin Convention, however, did not introduce any new provisions for the responsibility to grant legal protection, as the final decision falls under the sovereignty of each Member State (Hatton and Williamson 2004; Geddes 2007). As mentioned in the previous section, secondary movements of asylum applicants in 2015–2016 have challenged EU asylum policy, and questioned the effectiveness of the Dublin Convention.

The increase of forced migration since 2015 has also led to the adoption of new institutional agreements by the EU, both in its 'internal' and 'external' dimensions of migration governance. Internally, some national governments headed by Germany and EU institutions called for political responsibility to relocate asylum seekers through a system of quotas. This move attempted to overcome criticisms of the Dublin System by EU countries of first arrival. However, such efforts encountered both the active opposition to 'secondary movements' from some EU countries, particularly the Visegrad Group (Czech Republic, Hungary, Poland and Slovakia), and the passive inaction of others (Geddes 2018). In September 2015, EU Interior Ministers approved a 2-year scheme to relocate 160,000 asylum seekers from Greece and Italy, of which only around 20,000 were relocated, and an additional 27,800 pledged by Member States within the agreed timeframe (UNHCR 2017).

Externally, the EU has promoted institutional agreements with neighbouring countries that have resulted in a rapid decrease in the volume of arrivals. Several supranational institutions, both within the EU and the UN, such as the United Nations High Commissioner for Refugees (UNHCR) and the International Organization for Migration (IOM), have had an increasingly prominent role as operational partners in the management of migration in Europe amid the implementation of these inter-country deals (Geddes 2018).

The first of these deals was the EU-Turkey Statement of 2016, which led to a sharp reduction of arrivals to Greece, from 176,000 in 2016 down to 35,000 in 2017. This agreement caused shifts in the migratory routes to Europe and resulted in Italy becoming the major point of arrivals immediately after (Geddes 2018).

Additional agreements reached in 2017 between the EU and the Libyan government, and between the EU, the African Union (AU) and the UN led to the strengthening of maritime surveillance and border controls by Libyan authorities; the increase of returns from Libya to countries of origin; and the consequent sharp reduction of arrivals to Italy (EC 2017, 2018a). Over 23,000 new arrivals through the Mediterranean Sea were registered in Italy in 2018, in comparison with almost 120,000 in the previous year (UNHCR 2018b).

While these agreements have reduced the flow of immigration to Europe, they have been strongly criticised for failing to secure safe and adequate spaces and putting the health of those being returned to transit countries at risk, particularly vulnerable people such as pregnant women, breastfeeding mothers, victims of gender-based violence (GBV) and children (Women's Refugee Commission 2016; Amnesty International 2017).

The increase of involuntary displacement to Europe in 2015 also contributed to substantial multilateral efforts to design a common programme for improving the governance of human mobility worldwide. The New York Declaration for Refugees and Migrants was adopted at the UN General Assembly in 2016, setting the course for the development and endorsement in 2018 of a Global Compact on Refugees, and a Global Compact for Safe, Orderly and Regular Migration (thereinafter referred to as Global Compact on Migration). These instruments recognise that the management of migration is subject to the principle of national sovereignty; but acknowledge that international cooperation in this matter is in the interest of all, and that a comprehensive cross-sectoral approach to migration is required to address its multiple demographic, environmental, economic, social and political factors and drivers. Both global compacts are not legally binding and build on existing international law and standards. However, they have encountered the opposition of various governments at a time when migration has occupied the centre of the political debate. The USA and Hungary were the only countries who voted against both global compacts (SDG Knowledge Hub 2018); while the Czech Republic, Israel and Poland voted against the adoption of the Global Compact on Migration (UN 2018).

Governing the Health of Forced Migrants

The management of both the health of forced migrants and the public health aspects derived from forced migration is subject to a complex system of multi-level and multisectoral governance. Politico-economic institutions, both governmental and non-governmental, which operate at international, national and sub-national levels, determine access to health care for and shape health outcomes across different migrant groups (see also Chap. 13 "Global Social Governance and Health Protection for Forced Migrants").

The 2015–2016 peak of forced migration in Europe has led to the proliferation of multiple initiatives in the area of migration and health, which focus on diverse aspects. These include, among others, the provision of technical assistance and policy advice; the development of public health policies and system-wide reforms; the collection and analysis of health data or the performance of outreach and advocacy activities. These initiatives have originated from multiple actors, who hold diverse mandates, operate at different levels, and have various institutional capacities. Table 2.2 provides examples of different types of actors classified according to the level of governance in which they operate. In spite of their many differences, there are multiple examples of cross-financing and joint initiatives among them (Kentikelenis and Shriwise 2016).

Entitlements to health care services are usually regulated by national governments. Disparities persist across European countries regarding the level of access to healthcare provided on the basis of legal status. In a secondary analysis of data gathered by the Migrant Policy Integration Index (MIPEX), Italy scored highest among all EU countries with regards to the inclusiveness of its health system for both documented and undocumented migrants (Abubakar et al. 2018). Differences in entitlements across countries within the EU are strongly correlated with variations of the gross domestic product (GDP); however, other factors have also been found to help in explaining these variations. For example, countries that accessed the EU before 2004 have more inclusive health systems, irrespective of their GDP (Ingleby et al. 2018).

Even in countries where the same access to health care is provided for refugees, asylum seekers and regular migrants as for native citizens, these groups are not exempt from barriers. In tax-based health systems, coverage may be subject to the length of stay in the country; while in insurance-based systems, it is often tied to employment status. Other barriers to access healthcare are informal (see also

Table 2.2 Classification of types of actors involved in migration and health issues in Europe (Source: author's own)

Level of governance	Type of actor	Examples
International and regional	Intergovernmental	United Nations (UN) agencies such as the World Health Organization (WHO), the United Nations High Commissioner for Refugees (UNHCR) and the International Organization for Migration (IOM); regional organisations such as European Union (EU) institutions
	Non-governmental	Not-for-profit organisations such as Doctors Without Borders (MSF), Doctors of the World (MdM) and the Platform for International Cooperation on Undocumented Migrants (PICUM); philanthropic organisations; and for-profit or corporate actors
National	Governmental	Health Directorates and National Institutes of Public Health (Ministries of Health), Migration Directorates (Ministries of Internal Affairs, Labour or Social Affairs), national armed forces (Ministries of Defence) and public academic institutions
	Non-governmental	National Red Cross and Red Crescent Societies, not-for-profit organisations, philanthropic organisations and corporate actors
Sub-national	Governmental	Regional and local departments for health, labour, social affairs or housing
	Non-governmental	Local civil society groups, migrant and diaspora groups

Chap. 12 "Health Systems Responsiveness to the Mental Health Needs of Forcibly Displaced Persons"). For example, 14 out of 38 European countries analysed in 2015 did not have in place policies to provide medical interpretation services, and only half had developed guidelines for the provision of culturally competent and diversity-sensitive care (Ingleby et al. 2018).

Furthermore, in most European countries undocumented migrants do not have full access to health care services. Health workers in some EU countries are required to report undocumented migrants who access heathcare to immigration authorities, while in others, they are prohibited from providing care to this population group in the first place, and may face economic sanctions if they do so (Ingleby et al. 2018).

National governments in the EU also have the sole responsibility for the organisation and delivery of their health services. According to the EU legal principle of subsidiarity, exemptions apply only in areas of common concern to EU Member States, and which individual countries are unable to satisfactorily address nationally, such as in public health matters (European Parliament 2018). National government authorities thus hold the ultimate responsibility in the administration, financing, organisation, and delivery of health care services and health promotion activities for forced migrants.

How these functions are organised within national borders largely depends on national specificities, such as the degree of decentralisation of health systems, or the distribution of responsibilities and resources across governmental sectors. For example, health services in detention or reception centres often fall under the competence of ministries other than health, such as interior or education (WHO 2016a). In this regard, the lack of multisectoral collaboration on migration and health has been widely acknowledged as a key challenge in addressing conflicting objectives across policy sectors. Cross-sectoral engagement to overcome these conflicts is often limited to issues of national health security (Khan et al. 2016). See also Chap. 8 "Security over health: the effect of security policies on migrant mental health in the United Kingdom".

Sustained collaboration across sectors such as health, immigration enforcement, labour, trade, housing or international aid and development cooperation is necessary in order to address competing interests and tackle the underlying determinants of health of forced migrants beyond health security (Peiro and Benedict 2010; Zimmerman et al. 2011; WHO 2016b; Abubakar et al. 2018). Yet, only 20% of the 38 European countries analysed by MIPEX in 2015 were found to have ever applied a 'Health in All Policies' (HiAP) approach to migrant health policies (Ingleby et al. 2018).

In the last years, sub-national actors have emerged as central players in the area of migration and health in Europe. As camps are increasingly used as temporary means of last resort only, urban areas host the vast majority of forcibly displaced people, estimated at around 60 and 80% of all refugees and IDPs, respectively, in the world (UNHCR 2016).

Whereas the entitlement to health care is commonly subject to national legislation, local actors play an extensive role as providers of health services including prevention and promotion programmes. For example, in the city of Barcelona, forcibly displaced people including undocumented migrants whose request for asylum has been rejected have equal access as citizens to all local services. Nonetheless, local authorities set up in 2018 an ad-hoc municipal office to improve access to healthcare, legal and language services to vulnerable populations such as displaced families, children and victims of human trafficking (IRC 2018).

Local actors may face barriers for the provision of healthcare to migrants, even when these are legally entitled. Switzerland implemented the Migrant-Friendly Hospitals-project from 2003 to 2007 as part of its strategy to improve integration policy for regular migrants and asylum seekers. However, hospitals had to assume the costs of the programme, thus reducing their incentive to provide responsive healthcare through, for example, interpretation services (Abubakar et al. 2018).

The political relevance of sub-national actors as advocates in the area of migration and health has also increased during the last years. Multiple transnational networks of sub-national actors have emerged in European countries and beyond, which provide an international platform for local voices. Many of these have been created under the auspices of international organisations, such as the UN Urban Agenda, the WHO Healthy Cities Network and the WHO Regions for Health Network, or philanthropic organisations, such as the 100 Resilient Cities established by the Rockefeller Foundation.

At supranational level, the rise of forced displacement in Europe has also caused the increasing involvement of international and regional organisations. EU institutions complement national legislation, both through *hard* power means, such as setting standards through EU Directives, and *soft* power means, such as promoting inter-country cooperation and exchange of good practices. After the increase of arrivals in 2015–2016, a greater role on migration has been observed across all Directorate Generals of the EC (Geddes 2018), including the Directorate General for Health and Food Safety (DG SANTE) (PICUM and IRCT 2017).

Similarly, *soft* power initiatives have been commonly used by international organisations to promote inter-country approaches on migration and health; one example being the development and adoption of the 2016 Strategy and action plan for refugee and migrant health in the WHO European Region, and its accompanying resolution. Through their endorsement in September 2016, the 53 Member States of the WHO European Region committed to an ambitious agenda for the protection and promotion of the health of these mobile groups. Other examples of similar instruments where the right to health for forced migrants is enshrined include the 2008 World Health Assembly (WHA) Resolution 61.17 on the Health of Migrants, and the 2017 WHA Resolution 70.15 on Promoting the Health of Refugees and Migrants.

However, in addition to these documents not being legally binding, they specify that the actions agreed should be implemented in accordance with national legislation, and in line with national priorities (WHO 2016b). Therefore, whether these commitments translate into action in countries will depend to a large extent on the successes of health diplomacy (Zimmerman et al. 2011).

Socio-Political Impact of Forced Migration and Implications for Health Policy

Large-scale migration, both actual and perceived, has important political implications, as it may prompt shifts in both priorities by policy-makers and changes in public perceptions, and impact on the results of political elections, as the 2015–2016 increase of forced migration in Europe has shown. Evidence suggests that public opinion towards migration can be influenced by both objective data, as well as subjective values and emotions at social and individual level (Dempster and Hargrave 2017; Geddes 2018).

Assessing the political and social effects derived from forced migration is not an easy task. Firstly, the diversity of contextual, social and individual factors that play a role in shaping social and political values hinders the estimation and isolation of variables. Secondly, self-reported data collected through surveys may not always capture the complexity of such socio-political phenomena. Nevertheless, most research on public perceptions relies on quantitative analysis of opinion polls, including those conducted by the EC.

In order to assess the public opinion of EU citizens with regards to the integration of migrants in the aftermath of the peak of arrivals in 2015–2016, the EC conducted in October 2017 the Special Eurobarometer 469. Results from this survey show that respondents in all EU Member States substantially overestimated the number of non-EU immigrants living in their countries, with the exception of

Croatia and Estonia. The estimated figure was at least twice the actual number of immigrants in 19 EU countries, reaching over eight times the actual number in Romania, Bulgaria and Poland, and almost 14 times the actual figure in Slovakia (EC 2018b).

Immigration has played a central role in national elections across the EU in 2017–2018. Countries such as France, Germany, Italy and Sweden have experienced the re-entry or rise of far-right political parties that have an open opposition against immigration. These changes in the EU political landscape have been associated with an increase of anti-immigration public sentiment (see also Chap. 11 "Discrimination as a Health Systems Response to Forced Migration"). However, some scholars have argued that the increasing support for these political parties can be explained through the high levels of issue salience (Dennison and Geddes 2017; Geddes 2018).

In line with this hypothesis, results from the Standard Eurobarometer 89 conducted in March 2018 showed that immigration was considered the most important issue at European level in 21 EU countries, a considerable increase in comparison with 14 in the previous year (EC 2018c). However, despite the growing relevance of immigration and the general overestimation of the migrant population, data from the Special Eurobarometer 469 conducted in 2017 shows that 42% of all EU respondents considered the overall impact of migration to be positive; 30%, negative; and 23%, neutral (EC 2018b). Additionally, most respondents in all EU countries, except for Hungary, agreed with the statement that providing immigrants with the same rights as citizens, particularly in access to healthcare, education and social protection, would increase their prospects for a successful integration (EC 2018b).

Furthermore, results from the European Social Survey conducted in 2014 and 2016 show that, out of the 14 EU countries scrutinised, support for immigration either remained stable or even increased during this period, when the highest numbers of arrivals to Europe were recorded, except in Austria and Poland.

If opinion polls show that attitudes towards immigration have remained relatively stable despite the increase of human displacement to the EU in 2015–2016, how can the rise of anti-migration political parties across many EU countries be explained? Scholars have suggested that the failure of the EU to provide a coherent and orderly institutional response, coupled with widespread media scaremongering, may have triggered pre-existing latent attitudes that have materialised in a shift of some of the conservative vote towards political options that prioritise national security (Geddes 2018). Therefore, the increase of forced migration in 2015–2016 would not have caused a rise of anti-migrant sentiments per se, but rather an awakening of latent beliefs confined to part of the conservative electorate (Geddes 2018).

Aside from political beliefs, the Special Eurobarometer 469 on the integration of migrants by socio-economic status shows that the younger the respondent, the longer he/she has remained in education, the fewer the financial difficulties he/she has experienced, and the more urbanised his/her environment is, the more likely he/she is to agree on the positive effects of immigration (EC 2018b).

There is no consensus among scholars regarding the extent of the impact of economic and fiscal considerations on the public attitudes of resident communities towards migrants. Some studies suggest that economic concerns are central to the rise of xenophobic sentiments (Facchini and Mayda 2009). However, regardless the impact of economic determination, most social scientists and economists agree that attitudes towards migration have a social component that goes beyond economic considerations. For this reason, they argue that factors such as ideology and political beliefs may explain better the differences in public support for migration (Dustmann and Preston 2007).

Identity politics is also considered to play a central role in the maintenance of the politico-economic status quo (Lukes 2005). Charles Tilly described identity as a valued end that helps maintaining the compliance of subordinate groups with, and their lack of active opposition against, politico-economic structures, even when these produce unequal social and power relations (Tilly 1991), which result in inequities in socio-economic and health status.

Negative perceptions about the health of migrants may also have direct effects on cross-border policies (see also Chap. 7 "Health Security in the Context of Forced Migration"). Various non-EU countries impose travel restrictions on health grounds, such as being HIV-positive, suffering from a contagious or infectious disease, having a drug dependency, being mentally ill, or being pregnant (Abubakar et al. 2018). Moreover, as noted previously, in European countries where undocumented migrants are not entitled to health care services, health workers may be obliged to report them to immigration authorities, or even be prohibited from providing them with care. Organisational failures may have exacerbated these negative perceptions. For example, the lack of coordination among institutional actors and across countries contributed to the failure to provide comprehensive services for the prevention and control of infectious diseases among refugees and migrants in European countries (Bozorgmehr et al. 2017). This may have fuelled ill-founded public fears and political scaremongering over the spread of infectious diseases in Europe from large-scale migration.

Economic and Fiscal Impact of Forced Migration, and Implications for Health Policy

Migrants accounted for 70% of the growth of the European labour market from 2002 to 2012. Most analyses on the economic and fiscal impact of migration in the EU focus on labour migrants. Immigration flows in the past 50 years to countries of the Organization for Economic Cooperation and Development (OECD) have not been found to have a major fiscal effect, positive or negative, in most economies in countries of destination. Nevertheless, international migrants, and particularly labour migrants, often contribute more to the financing of public services and infrastructure through taxes than they receive in individual benefits (OECD 2014). An IMF study released in 2016 concluded that a 1% increase in the adult migrant population of advanced economies raises their GPD per capita by 2% (Jaumotte et al. 2016).

However, there is a lack of quantitative analyses on the economic and fiscal effects of forced migration in particular. Some attempts have been made by the EC to foresee the potential impact of the increase in forced migration in 2015–2016. These quantitative studies provide an estimation of the direct economic costs and benefits of forced migration in Europe, accounting for all effects such as the costs of integration, the benefits resulting from increased consumption and participation in the labour market, or variations in unemployment rates, among others. EC estimates suggest that the recent rise of forced migration to the EU could contribute to a long-term increase of around 0.2–1.4% of the overall GDP above the baseline growth, provided that the displaced community is integrated into the workforce of the country of destination speedily. These estimations include the full repayment of the related integration costs after a period of 9–19 years (Kancs and Lecca 2017).

Integration policies, particularly those designed to facilitate the formal inclusion of displaced individuals into the workforce, appear to be one of the most important factors for forced migrants to have a positive economic and fiscal impact in hosting communities (OECD 2014; Dadush and Niebuhr 2016; Kancs and Lecca 2017). These potential positive effects in the fiscal fabric of the EU are explained through the contribution of forced migrants to tax generation, as well as to the increase of both the level of consumption in the short run, and of services supply in the long run (Kancs and Lecca 2017). Nevertheless, these predictions may vary according to the specificities of EU countries, such as differences in their levels of unemployment (Dadush and Niebuhr 2016). Additionally, forced migrants may play a fundamental role as facilitators of foreign trade and investment with countries of origin, as analyses of trade flows between Turkey and Syria suggest (Çağatay and Menekse 2014; Dadush and Niebuhr 2016). Countries of origin also benefit of international migration through remittances. These were estimated at US$613 billion globally in 2017. In LMICs, they accounted for three times the total amount of official development assistance (ODA) received in that year (World Bank 2018). In addition to the economic and fiscal benefits of integrating forced migrants into the workforce, such measure would have a largely positive impact in the lives of displaced people and their families. Integrating migrants in the labour market should therefore be seen as an investment that generates both economic and social returns (OECD 2014).

The health sector in HICs also benefits from international migration in various ways. For example, migrants contribute significantly to the health workforce as both formal and informal health care providers, and as workers in related services such as residential homes. Moreover, many health workers in high-income countries (HICs) obtain their medical qualifications abroad; in the United Kingdom, 37% of doctors are trained in another country (Abubakar et al. 2018).

Economic costs associated with the delivery of health care to migrants in Europe are often caused by an unnecessary and avoidable overuse of emergency care services. On average, migrants use emergency care more often than native citizens in European countries, and they record longer length of stays. However, the contrary has been found for preventive care such as screening services. These differences are the result of multiple factors including lack of entitlement to access primary health care, free access to emergency care, cultural and language barriers, and lack of knowledge on the health system, among others (Graetz et al. 2017).

Temporary restrictions in granting regular access to refugees and asylum seekers in Germany have been found to cause delays in health care delivery and increase related costs (Bozorgmehr and Razum 2015). Overcoming both formal and informal barriers in access to primary health care for all migrants would therefore prevent the unnecessary use of costly emergency care.

Further research on the cost-effectiveness of health policies and interventions is necessary in order to promote policies and reforms that are evidence-informed. However, it is widely acknowledged that migration and health policies are often not driven by evidence, and are subject to political and ideological considerations (Abubakar et al. 2018; Wickramage and Annunziata 2018). Emphasis should also be placed upon how to better address this dichotomy between politics and science.

Various sociologists have warned of the increasing emphasis towards economic and fiscal considerations within narratives of legal protection, which are leading to a further neoliberal economisation of migration governance. The prevalence of market rules in this area may override the protection responsibilities of the state, diluting political values of equality and solidarity and contributing to a commodification of the concept of citizenship (Ong 2006; Mavelli 2018).

Conclusion

Using a political economy approach is essential to the understanding of how political and economic structures and processes determine the uneven exposure to health risks and assets and shape the access to resources for the various categories of migrants, thus shaping the distribution of health inequities. The increase of forced migration in Europe in 2015–2016 has prompted unprecedented efforts to design international instruments to govern human displacement, including within the health sector. Nonetheless, these have encountered active opposition from various national governments. Additionally, their non-legally binding nature renders their implementation subject to national and sub-national considerations. As a result, the extent to which European countries provide for comprehensive, responsive and inclusive health care to forced migrants varies widely.

Overall attitudes towards immigration remained relatively stable in EU countries during 2015–2016. Nonetheless, migration policy occupied a central position in political elections, triggering pre-existing latent anti-migrant sentiments that prioritise national security. While the economic and fiscal impact of migration on wealthy countries is largely positive, access to employment remains the most important variable. Within the health sector, failures to overcome formal and informal barriers to access primary health care services and prevention programmes have led to an overuse of emergency services, resulting in higher costs. While further evidence on the cost-effectiveness of health interventions for forced migrants is needed, health policies are not always informed by evidence, even when this is available. Political and ideological considerations play a central role, and its impact should by further explored through interdisciplinary research.

References

Abubakar, I., Aldridge, R. W., Devakumar, D., Orcutt, M., Burns, R., Barreto, M. L., et al. (2018). The UCL-Lancet commission on migration and health: The health of a world on the move. *The Lancet, 392*, 2606–2654.

Amnesty International. (2017). *Libya's dark web of collusion: Abuses against Europe-bound refugees and migrants.* London: Amnesty International.

Barnett, L. (2002). Global governance and the evolution of the international refugee regime. *International Journal of Refugee Law, 14*(2), 238–262.

Beirens, H. (2018). *Cracked foundation, uncertain future: Structural weaknesses in the Common European Asylum System.* Brussels: Migration Policy Institute.

Bozorgmehr, K., & Razum, O. (2015). Effect of restricting access to health care on health expenditures among asylum-seekers and refugees: A Quasi-Experimental Study in Germany, 1994–2013. *PLoS One, 10*(7), e0131483.

Bozorgmehr, K., Samuilova, M., Petrova-Benedict, R., Girardi, E., Piselli, P., & Kentikelenis, A. (2017). Infectious disease health services for refugees and asylum seekers during a time of crisis: A scoping study of six European Union countries. *Health Policy, 123*, 882–887.

Çağatay, S., & Menekse, B. (2014). *The impact of Syria's refugees on Southern Turkey.* Washington, DC: The Washington Institute for Near East Policy.

Calkivik, A. (2017). Poststructuralism/Postmodernism. International Studies Association. Retrieved 13 June 2018 from http://internationalstudies.oxfordre.com/view/10.1093/acrefore/9780190846626.001.0001/acrefore-9780190846626-e-102?print=pdf.

Castañeda, H., Holmes, S. M., Madrigal, D. S., Young, M. E. D., Beyeler, N., & Quesada, J. (2015). Immigration as a social determinant of health. *Annual Review of Public Health, 36*, 375–392.

Dadush, U., & Niebuhr, M. (2016). *The economic impact of forced migration.* Rabat: OCP Policy Center.

Dahl, R. (1958). *A critique of the ruling elite model.* Yale: American Political Science Association.

Dempster, H., & Hargrave, K. (2017). *Understanding public attitudes towards refugees and migrants.* London: Overseas Development Institute.

Dennison, J., & Geddes, A. (2017). *Are Europeans turning against asylum seekers and refugees?* Florence: European University Institute.

Dustmann, C., & Preston, I. P. (2007). Racial and economic factors in attitudes to immigration. *The BE Journal of Economic Analysis & Policy, 7*(1). https://doi.org/10.2202/1935-1682.1655

EC. (2017). *EU Trust Fund for Africa adopts €46 million programme to support integrated migration and border management in Libya.* Brussels: European Commission.

EC. (2018a). *European Agenda on Migration: Continuous efforts needed to sustain progress.* Brussels: European Commission.

EC. (2018b). Special Eurobarometer 469. Report: *Integration of immigrants in the European Union.* Retrieved July 2, 2018, from https://ec.europa.eu/commfrontoffice/publicopinion/index.cfm/Survey/getSurveyDetail/instruments/SPECIAL/surveyKy/2169

EC. (2018c). Standard Eurobarometer 89. *First results: Public opinion in the European Union.* Retrieved July 2, 2018, from https://ec.europa.eu/commfrontoffice/publicopinion/index.cfm/Survey/getSurveyDetail/instruments/STANDARD/surveyKy/2180

European Parliament. (2018). *The principle of subsidiarity.* Retrieved September 15, 2018, from http://www.europarl.europa.eu/ftu/pdf/en/FTU_1.2.2.pdf

Eurostat. (2016). *Record number of over 1.2 million first time asylum seekers registered in 2015.* Retrieved July 2, 2018, from https://ec.europa.eu/eurostat/documents/2995521/7203832/3-04032016-AP-EN.pdf/790eba01-381c-4163-bcd2-a54959b99ed6

Eurostat. (2017a). *EU member states granted protection to more than 700,000 asylum seekers in 2016.* Retrieved July 2018, from http://www.europeanmigrationlaw.eu/documents/Eurostat-AsylumDecisions-2016.pdf

Eurostat. (2017b). *1.2 million first time asylum seekers registered in 2016.* Retrieved July 2, 2018, https://ec.europa.eu/eurostat/documents/2995521/7921609/3-16032017-BP-EN.pdf/e5fa98bb-5d9d-4297-9168-d07c67d1c9e1

Eurostat. (2018). *EU member states granted protection to more than half a million asylum seekers in 2017*. Retrieved July 2, 2018, https://ec.europa.eu/eurostat/documents/2995521/8817675/3-19042018-AP-EN.pdf/748e8fae-2cfb-4e75-a388-f06f6ce8ff58

Facchini, G., & Mayda, A. M. (2009). Does the welfare state affect individual attitudes toward immigrants? Evidence across countries. *Journal of Population Economics, 30*(1), 265–306.

Geddes, A. (2007). *Immigration and European Integration: Beyond Fortress Europe?* Manchester: Manchester University Press.

Geddes, A. (2018). The politics of European Union Migration Governance. *Journal of Common Market Studies., 56*, 120–130.

Gkiouleka, A., Huijts, T., Beckfield, J., & Bambra, C. (2018). Understanding the micro and macro politics of health: Inequalities, intersectionality & institutions—A research agenda. *Social Science & Medicine, 200*, 92–98.

Graetz, V., Rechel, B., Groot, W., Norredam, M., & Pavlova, M. (2017). Utilization of health care services by migrants in Europe—a systematic literature review. *British Medical Bulletin, 121*, 5–18.

Guiraudon, V. (2017). The 2015 Refugee Crisis Was Not a Turning Point: Explaining Policy Inertia in EU Border Control. *European Political Science, 17*(1), 151–160.

Hatton, T. J., & Williamson, J. G. (2004). *Refugees, asylum seekers and policy in Europe*. Bonn: Institute for the Study of Labor.

Ingleby, D., Petrova-Benedict, R., Huddleston, T., & Sanchez, E. (2018). The MIPEX Health strand: A longitudinal, mixed-method survey of policies on migrant health in 38 countries. *European Journal of Public Health, 29*, 458–462.

IOM. (2011). *Glossary on migration*. Geneva: International Organization for Migration.

IRC. (2018). *How cities are building inclusive communities*. New York: International Rescue Committee.

Jaumotte, F., Koloskova, K., & Saxena, M. S. C. (2016). *Impact of migration on income levels in advance economies*. Washington, DC: International Monetary Fund.

Kancs, A., & Lecca, P. (2017). *Long-term social, economic and fiscal effects of immigration into the EU: The role of the integration policy*. Luxembourg: Publications Office of the European Union.

Kentikelenis, A., & Shriwise, A. (2016). International organizations and migrant health in Europe. *Public Health Review, 37*, 19.

Khan, M. S., Osei-Kofi, A., Omar, A., Kirkbride, H., Kessel, A., & Abbara, A. (2016). Pathogens, prejudice, and politics: The role of the global health community in the European refugee crisis. *The Lancet, 16*, e173–e177.

Lukes, S. (2005). *Power: A radical view*. New York: Palgrave Macmillan.

Mackenbach, J. P. (2009). Politics is nothing but medicine at a larger scale: Reflections on public health's biggest idea. *Journal of Epidemiology and Community Health, 63*, 181–184.

Mavelli, L. (2018). Citizenship for sale and the neoliberal political economy of belonging. *International Studies Quarterly, 0*, 1–12.

Navarro, V., Muntaner, C., Borrell, C., Benach, J., Quiroga, Á., & Rodríguez-Sanz, M. (2006). Politics and health outcomes. *The Lancet, 368*, 1033–1037.

OECD. (2014). *Is migration good for the economy?* Retrieved from December 22, 2018, https://www.oecd.org/migration/OECD%20Migration%20Policy%20Debates%20Numero%202.pdf

Ong, A. (2006). Mutations in citizenship. *Theory, Culture & Society, 2*(3), 499–505.

Peiro, M. J., & Benedict, R. (2010). Migrant health policy: The Portuguese and Spanish EU presidencies. *Eurohealth, 16*(1), 1.

Phoung, C. (2005). *Identifying state's responsibilities towards refugees and asylum seekers*. Geneva: EASIL Research Forum on International Law.

PICUM and IRCT. (2017). *Framing document thematic network on "Migration and Health" November 2017*. Retrieved from September 17, 2018, http://picum.org/wp-content/uploads/2017/11/EUHealthPolicyPlatform_Framing-Document_Nov2017.pdf

Sargent, C., & Larchanché, S. (2011). Transnational migration and global health: The production and management of risk, illness, and access to care. *Annual Review of Anthropology, 40*, 345–361.

Schattschneider, E. E. (1960). *The semi-sovereign people: A realist's view of democracy in America*. New York: Holt, Rhinehart & Winston.

SDG Knowledge Hub. (2018). *UNGA votes to adopt global compact on refugees*. Retrieved from December21,2018,https://sdg.iisd.org/news/unga-votes-to-adopt-global-compact-on-refugees/

Sen, A. (2002). Why health equity? *Health Economics, 11*, 659–666.

Solar, O., & Irwin, A. (2010). *A conceptual framework for action on the social determinants of health. Social Determinants of Health Discussion Paper 2 (Policy and Practice)*. Geneva: World Health Organization.

Tilly, C. (1991). Domination, resistance, compliance … discourse. *Sociological Forum, 6*(3), 593–602.

UN. (2018). *General assembly endorses first-ever global compact on migration, urging cooperation among member states in protecting migrants*. Retrieved from December 21, 2018, https://www.un.org/press/en/2018/ga12113.doc.htm

UNHCR. (2010). *Convention and protocol relating to the status of refugees*. Geneva: United Nations High Commissioner for Refugees.

UNHCR. (2011). *The 1951 convention relating to the status of refugees and its 1967 protocol*. Geneva: United Nations Hugh Commissioner for Refugees.

UNHCR. (2016). *The power of cities*. Retrieved from September 15, 2018, http://www.unhcr.org/innovation/the-power-of-cities/

UNHCR. (2017). *UNHCR calls for the EU relocation scheme to continue*. Retrieved from July 2, 2018, http://www.unhcr.org/news/press/2017/9/59ca64354/unhcr-calls-eu-relocation-scheme-continue.html

UNHCR. (2018a). *Global trends forced displacement in 2017*. Geneva: United Nations High Commissioner for Refugees.

UNHCR. (2018b). *Operational portal refugee situations: Mediterranean situation*. Retrieved from July 2, 2018, https://data2.unhcr.org/en/situations/mediterranean

WHO. (2016a). *Health 2020: Multisectoral action for the health of migrants*. Copenhagen: World Health Organization.

WHO. (2016b). *Strategy and action plan on refugee and migrant health in the WHO European Region*. Copenhagen: World Health Organization.

WHO. (2017). *Beyond the barriers: Framing evidence on health system strengthening to improve the health of migrants experiencing poverty and social exclusion*. Geneva: World Health Organization.

Wickramage, K., & Annunziata, G. (2018). Advancing health in migration governance, and migration in health governance. *The Lancet, 392*, 2528–2530.

Wittman, D. A., & Weingast, B. R. (2008). The reach of political economy. In D. A. Wittman & B. R. Weingast (Eds.), *The Oxford handbook of political economy*. Oxford: Oxford University Press.

Women's Refugee Commission. (2016). *EU-Turkey agreement failing refugee women and girls*. Retrieved from September 15, 2018, https://www.womensrefugeecommission.org/images/zdocs/EU-Turkey-Refugee-Agreement-Failing.pdf

World Bank. (2018). *Migration and remittances: Recent developments and outlook*. Retrieved from December 22, 2018, https://openknowledge.worldbank.org/handle/10986/29777

Zimmerman, C., Kiss, L., & Hossain, M. (2011). Migration and health: A framework for 21st century policy-making. *PLoS Medicine, 8*(5), e1001034.

Chapter 3
Innovative Humanitarian Health Financing for Refugees

Paul Spiegel, Rebecca Chanis, Thea Scognamiglio, and Antonio Trujillo

List of Abbreviations

CCRIF   Caribbean Catastrophe Risk Insurance Facility
CCT   Conditional cash transfer
CERF   Central Emergency Response Fund
FTS   Financial Tracking Service
INGO   International nongovernmental organization
LIC   Low-income country
LMIC   Low- and middle-income country
MIC   Middle-income country
NGO   Nongovernmental organisation
ODA   Overseas development assistance
OECD   Organisation for Economic Co-operation and Development
P4S   Pay for success
PEF   Pandemic Emergency Financing Facility
UCT   Unconditional cash transfer
UHC   Universal healthcare coverage
UNHCR   United Nations High Commissioner for Refugees
WHO   World Health Organization

Introduction

In 2017, there were 68.5 million forcibly displaced persons and 23.2 million refugees worldwide (Urquhart and Tuchel 2018). Whether refugees live in camps or are integrated into host populations, and whether they are settled in low-income or middle-income countries, governments often struggle to meet the health needs of

P. Spiegel (✉) · R. Chanis · T. Scognamiglio · A. Trujillo
Johns Hopkins Center for Humanitarian Health and Johns Hopkins Bloomberg
School of Public Health, Baltimore, MD, USA
e-mail: pbspiegel@jhu.edu

© Springer Nature Switzerland AG 2020
K. Bozorgmehr et al. (eds.), *Health Policy and Systems Responses to Forced Migration*, https://doi.org/10.1007/978-3-030-33812-1_3

these populations. Host countries' existing health systems are often weak, and the added burden of providing for refugees can make them even more fragile.

An important and relatively new goal of humanitarian health assistance is to have a healthcare system for refugees that is integrated into a functioning national system; if implemented correctly, this integration will be beneficial to the refugees and the host populations. Providing sustainable healthcare to refugees (as well as other displaced populations) requires facilitating their access to existing health systems, improving the capacity and quality of such services to ease the strain on host countries, and addressing the financing of these services. Health financing refers to (1) raising monetary resources; (2) the flow of money into the system; and (3) the allocation of monetary resources by public or private means. Innovative financing mechanisms are defined as non-traditional applications of overseas development assistance (ODA), joint public–private mechanisms, and flows that fundraise by tapping new resources or that deliver new financial solutions to humanitarian and/or development problems on the ground (World Health Organization 2009).

This chapter concerns itself primarily with refugees in low- and middle-income countries (LMICs), but many of its conclusions may be applicable to other displaced populations and high-income countries. Refugee contexts and their various attributes can be categorised in numerous ways (Table 3.1). For this chapter, we created the following framework:

How and what type of refugee healthcare is established in a host country depends upon some of the factors listed above. For example, types of services and their quality may differ between the acute emergency phase, where this is often limited capacity and security, compared with the protracted phase, where there is more stability. Parallel health systems are often established in camp settings compared with out-of-camp settings, where refugee healthcare is often integrated within existing national systems. Types of services and ability to refer may differ between urban and rural settings as well as low-income countries and middle-income countries. Although it is difficult to clearly define functioning and non-functioning national or district health systems, district or regional health services have differing abilities to integrate refugees while providing sufficient access and quality of services, and so may require parallel services for refugees. Given the variety of contextual factors, humanitarian health financing is diverse and adaptive. As a result, each financing

Table 3.1 Refugee contexts (Spiegel et al. 2018)

Phase	Location	Host income level	District health system
Preparedness (pre-emergency) Acute emergency Protracted Durable solutions Voluntary repatriation Local integration Resettlement	Camp, out of camp Urban, rural	Low-income country (LIC) Middle-income country (MIC)	Functioning Semi-functioning Non-functioning

tool must be evaluated by governments, international organisations, and stakeholders as appropriate for a certain displaced population in a specific country before implementation.

The objective of this chapter is to explore different innovative humanitarian financing mechanisms for refugee health care, emphasising the need for integrating refugees into host country health systems. It focuses on varied sources of funding and a broad range of financial instruments that can provide health services to refugees in an integrated and sustainable manner. The contents of this chapter were modified from the report to the World Bank Group on this topic as well as the published paper (Spiegel et al. 2017).

Challenges in Traditional Humanitarian Funding

Refugees, like all other persons in the world, have a right to equitable, high quality healthcare. But the humanitarian health response is currently overstretched and underfunded, and cannot meet the current demands of multiple and increasingly protracted humanitarian emergencies (Bennet 2016). International humanitarian assistance funding has grown, rising from $18.4 billion in 2013 to $27.3 billion in 2017. But, as overall humanitarian funding increased, the requested needs and contributions to UN-coordinated appeals also increased. As a result, in 2017 there was a humanitarian assistance funding shortfall of 40% or $10.3 billion, the largest amount to date (Urquhart and Tuchel 2018). Moreover, between 2016 and 2017, contributions from EU institutions and governments stagnated while contributions from private donors grew. Thus, as public contributions stagnate and shortfalls increase, need for new, additional financing continues to rise.

Although not sufficiently researched, most revenue for refugee health financing comes from three sources post-emergency: (1) the host government's social spending; (2) Western government donations; and (3) refugees' out-of-pocket expenses (Spiegel 2017). Most government donations are managed by UN agencies, international and national nongovernmental organisations (NGOs), and faith-based organisations. But, due to limited international funding, host governments often end up paying significant amount of money from their own budgets to provide health care for refugees, particularly out-of-camp refugees. For example, in Jordan, the burden of Syrian refugees on the health care system and the amount of money the Jordanian government was providing for services to refugees was extremely high (JOD 34 million). Ultimately, the Jordanian government changed its policy and stopped providing free health care to Syrian refugees at the end of 2014 (Malkawi 2014).

Once international and host country financing is depleted, it is left to refugees to pay for their care on their own. Various health access and utilisation surveys show that refugees pay out-of-pocket expenses for their health care, particularly refugees living outside of camps. A rather extreme example is in Jordan, where the non-Syrian refugees pay expensive non-Jordanian health care rates as opposed to the Syrian refugees. According to a survey conducted in December 2016, 44% of non-Syrian refugee households spent almost half of their monthly income in the past month on healthcare. (United Nations High Commissioner for Refugees 2016).

While the burden for financing their healthcare falls on refugees if governments and international actors cannot pay, they face additional barriers to earning an income. In many countries, refugees are not officially allowed to work, so they get their money from unofficial work, borrowing, and remittances. A "remittance agency" refers to money transfer agencies or other financial service providers. Anti-money laundering laws often require proof of identity to remit money. In certain settings, refugees may not have sufficient documentation, or the identification provided (e.g. from the host government or an international agency) may not be recognised by the remittance agency. In some circumstances, remittances may be transferred via telecommunication technology instead of a remittance agency. But some refugees do not have access to mobile telephones, although this situation is rapidly changing. All of the above limits refugees' ability to pay for their healthcare if the international and government cannot.

This enormous financing gap and burden not only perpetuates health disparities between refugees and their host populations, but also creates global disparities among refugees: a few high-priority emergencies consume the majority of humanitarian financing, meaning small but serious emergencies are under-resourced. In 2016, the top ten recipients accounted for 60% of all humanitarian funding, with Syria receiving the most ($2.6 billion) (Urquhart and Tuchel 2018). The top three recipients of humanitarian assistance financing in 2018, Syria, Yemen, and South Sudan, alone received one-third (36.9%) of all humanitarian funding (Financial Tracking Service 2018), a substantial increase from 2012 (Urquhart 2018). As a result, many emergencies have been chronically and increasingly underfunded for years.

In addition to having scarce resources, humanitarian health financing donors do not provide multi-year funding to allow for predictable and sustainable programming. The vast majority (86%) of all humanitarian aid goes to countries facing medium- and long-term crises (Urquhart and Tuchel 2018). Multi-annual humanitarian planning and financing would greatly benefit humanitarian responses in these countries, by allowing actors to think in the long-term as well.

Moreover, there is no large-scale assessment of the costs, effectiveness, or efficiency of different refugee healthcare delivery models (Fig. 3.1). At present, financing parallel service delivery for refugees is the norm—but is not sustainable. However, integrating humanitarian healthcare delivery into domestic healthcare could impact the quality and cost of health services provided to the host country population, as short-term supply is fixed but demand increases rapidly with the inclusion of refugees. If done poorly, integrating services could overburden medical personnel, deplete healthcare resources, or create long waiting lists for care. The relative economic and social costs of providing integrated service delivery versus parallel services are unknown and need to be researched.

Finally, the type and channel of funding available for humanitarian relief is often suboptimal. Humanitarian financing is overwhelmingly for post-emergency response and rarely goes directly to the host governments or local NGOs providing

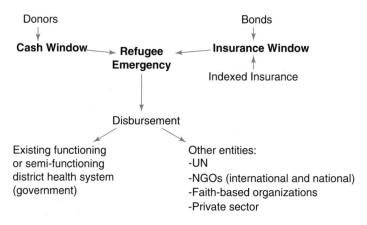

Fig. 3.1 Refugee health financing model (modified from PEF)

services to refugees. Instead, multilateral organisations received 49% of all humanitarian relief financing in 2016. An additional 20% went to NGOs, but only 5.3% went to the public sector and 0.4% to national and local NGOs (Urquhart and Tuchel 2018). Moreover, the majority of humanitarian financing is earmarked. Moving from earmarked to unearmarked humanitarian relief financing would result in quicker responses, better accountability, lower administrative costs, and less reporting (Lattimer 2016). However, unearmarked humanitarian relief funding given to UN agencies actually decreased between 2013 and 2017, from 22% to 18% (Urquhart and Tuchel 2018).

In short, traditional funding for humanitarian emergencies is insufficient and unsustainable. New approaches to financial planning, new sources of funding, and new ways of resource allocation, are essential if the needs of persons affected by humanitarian emergencies are to be met.

Financing Integrated Health Care for Refugees

Host governments must accept that refugees will likely be on their soil for many years and integrate refugees into existing health services. If planned and implemented well, then integration should improve health services for host country nationals and refugees alike by combining national and international financing for a single health service delivery system (see also Chap. 5 "Health Financing for Asylum Seekers in Europe: Three Scenarios Towards Responsive Financing Systems"). Doing so requires multi-year funding from donors addressing humanitarian emergencies, collaboration with national and international actors, and a nuanced toolkit of innovative financing mechanisms.

If a health system cannot integrate services for refugees, even with support from international organisations, only then alternatives should occur, such as providing parallel services. This may be due to national health systems at the regional or district level not being functional or able to address the emergency needs of refugees. Entities providing parallel services include the UN, international nongovernmental organizations (INGOs), faith-based organisations, and in some rare circumstances the private sector (e.g. mostly privatised health systems, such as Lebanon). Private sector participants would have to earn a profit to cover operational costs, making adverse selection a problem, and should be avoided if possible. Since refugees should eventually be integrated into the national health system, incentives and agreements should be put into place to ensure that once the situation is more stable, refugees will move from these "parallel" systems to national systems. Most likely, doing so will also require capacity building the latter.

At present, many refugee camps throughout the world continue to provide parallel health services to refugees. Some are located in remote areas, while others are near more populated locales. The United Nations High Commissioner for Refugees (UNHCR) continues to provide funding for those parallel health services, primarily to NGOs. For the most part, refugees have limited or no livelihoods in these camps (World Bank 2017), and thus health services remain free of charge. They rely on predominantly post-emergency donations for revenue. In long-term protracted refugee camps, compared to host country nationals refugee morality rates are generally lower and maternal-child health outcomes are generally better (Hynes 2002, Spiegel 2002). Consequently, in many of these camps, between 5% and 20% of patients are nationals themselves (Spiegel 2017).

In the past, missions have been undertaken in various African countries to turn these camps into "villages". The objective is to integrate services for refugees into national health and educational systems, which in turn should improve those services for nationals. There is the possibility that the quality of services for refugees would fall as the parallel services provided by NGOs and funded by UNHCR are stopped. However, the principle is to provide a comparable level of care to refugees and host country nationals (Urquhart and Tuchel 2018, United Nations High Commissioner for Refugees, 2014).

There are many complex considerations for providing refugee services in general, let alone moving from parallel to integrated services in these long-term refugee camps. Refugee demand for health services is also shaped by a myriad of incentives: costs, preferences, knowledge, various social determinants, and culture. Refugees are unwilling to purchase health services if they are too costly, if they are socialised to believe it is unimportant, or if they lack knowledge about the services available to them.

If social and political complications are surmounted, experience suggests that in some settings an initial injection of funds is necessary; although there is insufficient documentation as to the cost of undertaking such a process. This would generally not be undertaken in isolation, but rather in conjunction with education and the development plans for that region of the country. Existing health systems, whether functional or semi-functional, will likely need increased capacity and support from the UN and INGOs. When possible, disbursed funds should go to national, regional, or district level offices that manage national health systems and are responsible for integrating refugees.

Other policies support the integrating of health services for refugees as well. Allowing refugees to work will provide them with a means to cover their costs. Subsidies for vulnerable refugees should match those for nationals. If health insurance is mandatory for nationals, incorporating refugees in the insurance scheme can increase the risk pool sufficiently to support their inclusion. If national health systems cannot provide health insurance to both nationals and refugees, then external financial assistance and expertise may help some national systems improve sufficiently to provide health insurance for their citizens and refugees. Numerous countries in Africa have included universal health care into their national frameworks, but progress towards implementation is challenging. As more countries in Africa transition to UHC, the more feasible it will be for refugees to integrate into such systems.

A unique example of a combination or parallel and integrated service delivery purchasing occurred in Lebanon, due to its highly privatised health care system (see also Chap. 4 "Health Financing for Refugees in Lebanon"). A third-party auditor was contracted by UNHCR to control costs incurred by UNHCR for secondary health care in Lebanon, while ensuring an appropriate level and quality of care was provided. This was the first time UNHCR has undertaken such a process due to the unique circumstances of Lebanon. However, such a system may be considered in the future in countries that have a highly privatised health care system (Box 3.1).

A wide variety of financing instruments are available to encourage integrating refugees into host county health systems.

Box 3.1 Third-Party Auditor for Healthcare Delivery in Lebanon to Syrian Refugees

The health care system in Lebanon is complex and highly privatised. As part of the 2013 partnership agreements with UNHCR, partners were tasked to assist refugees with access to secondary health care by providing the following sets of activities: (1) validating entitlements, getting pre-treatment approval, conducting peer reviews, and auditing hospital bills; (2) paying hospitals for hospitalisation/treatment services based on the audited bills; and (3) ensuring hospitals bills for refugees would not exceed the Ministry of Public Health flat rates.

As a result of various challenges, including the complex hospital care system in Lebanon and the limited capacity of UNHCR Lebanon partners to provide secondary health care to refugees, a competitive bidding process was undertaken by UNHCR and a third-party auditor was selected. This company was a private for-profit company.

This company was used by many Lebanese to control their health care costs. In effect, it acted as an HMO to control costs incurred by UNHCR for secondary health care in Lebanon, while ensuring an appropriate level and quality of care was provided.

Innovative Humanitarian Health Financing

Financing tools for humanitarian healthcare have two components: risk and timing. Risk is defined as the potential for or probability of a loss, while timing refers to when the risky outcome occurs. Risk-retention tools hold host countries responsible for risk, which allows host countries to spend at their discretion (and within their budgets) during emergencies. Risk-transfer tools allow host countries to transfer risk to another entity, so host countries no longer shoulder the costs of emergencies. In general, risk-retention instruments are more appropriate for recurrent losses and risk-transfer instruments are preferable for occasional, larger losses (Clarke and Dercon 2016). Both types of tools vary in their timing, some relying on pre-emergency planning while others only include post-emergency response (Clarke and Dercon 2016).

There are a variety of financing instruments available for preparing and responding to humanitarian emergencies, which combine different features of timing and risk (Clarke and Dercon 2016). Below are several examples (Table 3.2).

Table 3.2 Financing instruments according to risk and time (Spiegel et al 2018)

	Dependent upon planning	Not dependent upon planning
Risk retention (refugee host countries are responsible for risk)	• *Domestic contingency funds or budget allocations*: money for emergency relief set aside prior to event • *Taxes* and *subsidies* to alter incentives for providing funding • *Line of contingent credit*: a loan disbursed under certain circumstances	• Budget *reallocation* • *Tax* increases • Post-emergency *credit* • User *fees* • *Taxes* and *subsidies* to alter incentives for providing funding • *Tariffs* or *subsidies* to reduce prices of goods during emergencies
Risk transfer (refugee host countries transfer risk to another entity)	• *Traditional insurance or reinsurance*: contract where insured pays insurer a premium, and insurer agrees to pay for pre-specified and post-verified losses • *Indexed insurance*: insurance contract where insurer makes payments based on certain external, measurable parameters or index (e.g. Sovereign Risk Insurance Pools, Pandemic Emergency Financing Facility) • *Capital market instruments*: financial instruments that can be bought or sold on capital markets, and investors shoulder risk (e.g. catastrophe bonds and swaps, Pandemic Emergency Financing Facility) • *Contingency pooled UN funds* (e.g. Central Emergency Relief Fund and Country-Based Pool Funds)	• *Discretionary post-emergency aid*: includes in-kind and cash transfers • Discretionary post-emergency aid is the most common instrument for aid delivery in humanitarian emergencies and is provided primarily by Western governments

Deciding which tool to use when is the responsibility of governments and international actors. Each instrument should be assessed according to context, so that it considers available financing and sustainability, appropriate responsibilities for implementers, the needs and priorities of beneficiaries, and quickness of response.

Improving financing for humanitarian emergencies requires a paradigm shift: moving from post-emergency financing to pre-emergency planning. An innovative health financing plan would establish funding mechanisms prior to emergencies, setting rules for pay out. It would specify actors and roles, triggers for payment, and allow for flexibility in response according to context (Clarke and Dercon 2016). These rules, responsibilities, and triggers must also mitigate moral hazard, in which countries allow populations to be displaced because they know there will be financing for it. Moreover, the plan must be adaptable to various post-emergency conditions and scalable in LMIC contexts. For example, if a humanitarian financing plan will establish an insurance scheme or specific services, it should define who is covered and for what services, clear inclusion or exclusion for pre-existing conditions, who delivers services and how, and which actors pay for which aspects of coverage. The development of an innovative health financing plan is the first step towards improving humanitarian response funding.

Planned or otherwise, innovative financing mechanisms that create revenue address the immediate challenge of a financing shortfall. Many revenue generation tools exist, but only loans, bonds, solidarity levies, and remittances will briefly be discussed here, as they are the most politically viable tools available.

Many development institutions and banks offer loans to LMICs for improving domestic social services. A loan transfers money from one party to another, with the promise of repayment with interest. Concessional loans have lower interest rates and more flexible repayment terms than market loans, and are often the kind made by development institutions to governments. Concessional loans are not in widespread use for financing refugee healthcare, as they require repayment from host governments. If a host government took a loan for providing refugee health services, it must use its tax revenue to pay the loan back. Doing so is often politically untenable, since LMICs would have to justify to constituents spending scarce resources on non-citizens rather than citizens.

As a result, concessional lending is not politically viable for providing parallel services for refugees. However, if refugees are integrated into existing services, then a loan for refugee healthcare would improve domestic health services in general and benefit host country nationals as well. In 2016, the International Development Association pledged $2 billion for 3-year grants and concessional loans to low-income countries hosting refugees. As the IDA18 progresses, these concessional loans may prove an appropriate vehicle to allow for such a transition from camps to "villages" with integrated services for nationals and refugees, particularly in Africa where many long-term camps exist.

Development institutions, like the World Bank, also use bonds to support developing countries facing large scale disasters. Bonds are a common capital market tool that can be used to finance responses to humanitarian emergencies. A creditor loans money to a public, corporate, or other entity, which issues them a bond. The bond lasts until a pre-set date (maturity date), and once matured then the loaned funds (bond principal) are returned. Interest is usually paid out periodically until maturity. Bonds have either a set or variable interest rate (coupon).

Box 3.2 Example of a Solidarity Levy (Unitaid 2016)

Governments participating in the Unitaid solidarity levy charge a small fee on airline passengers and then donate the proceeds to Unitaid. Currently, ten countries collect air ticket levies for Unitaid: Cameroon, Chile, Congo, France, Guinea, Madagascar, Mali, Mauritius, Niger, and the Republic of Korea (Unitaid 2017b). Since 2006, France has contributed more than €1 billion through the solidarity tax (Unitaid 2013), and overall levy proceeds constitute more than half of Unitaid's budget (Unitaid 2017a)

Catastrophe bonds are special type of bond, in which a public entity, insurance company, or other organisation issues a bond to an investor, with a high coupon rate, usually to reinsure another party. If a catastrophe (currently, most are for natural disasters) occurs, the investor defers or forfeits payment of the interest and/or principal. Instead the money is used to address the catastrophe. If there is no catastrophe, the bonds typically mature within three years, and investors are paid back the principal with interest. Catastrophe bonds are high risk for investors, and as a result can be difficult to find financing for. However, development institutions have successfully implemented them to mitigate natural disasters, and may able to do so with other humanitarian emergencies.

Another common tool is a solidarity levy. A solidarity levy is a government-imposed tax, levied on consumers or tax payers to provide funding towards set projects. The tax can be paid by individuals, business owners, or corporations. The air ticket levy is one such example (Box 3.2) (UNITAID n.d.). While a solidarity levy may be one mechanism to increase revenue for refugee health services, there is much competition. Many international agencies and causes would also like to use this mechanism and that may limit its efficacy.

Finally, remittances are an important and untapped flow of revenue to and from displaced populations. Migrants sent earnings to families and friends living in developing countries at levels above $441 billion in 2015, which was three times the volume of official aid flows (World Bank 2016). Remittances constitute more than 10% of GDP in approximately 25 developing countries (World Bank 2016).

Research on remittances during humanitarian emergencies is scarce, but it is assumed that remittances have a positive impact on the well-being of those receiving them. Remittances may help refugees pay user fees or for medicines, but they should not be relied on as a substitute for health financing. Rather, facilitating remittances can complement other initiatives. It is important to note that, in some cases, refugees may be the ones remitting back home.

Little is known about the flow of and channels for remittances in refugee contexts, but certain actions should be explored to make remittances flow more fluidly and efficiently in such settings. While refugee healthcare should not rely on remittances for funding, international actors could encourage remittances to partially finance refugee healthcare. Agencies could work with partners to reduce or eliminate transfer surcharges specific to refugees; match refugee remittances; ensure that remittance agencies accept certain types of refugee identification; provide mobile phones to refugees; and collaborate with host governments to create appropriate national policies and regulations (Humanitarian Policy Group 2007). All would increase the amount of revenue available for refugee healthcare.

In addition to generating more revenue, there are other pre-emergency financial management practices that will allow humanitarian funding to go father. Pooling revenue allows funds to be held in one place and managed by one entity, and sets rules for how people can access those funds. Pooling does not increase the amount of financing available, but more evenly distributes financing and facilitates pre-emergency planning. Pooled funds can be deployed faster and with greater discretion than post-emergency aid.

Box 3.3 UN Pooled Funds

The United Nations Central Emergency Response Fund sets aside donations and aid money to be immediately available to UN agencies and the International Organization for Migration for emergency responses to humanitarian crises. Between 2010 and 2015, around one-third of the UN's pooled funds for humanitarian relief were from CERF, all of which supported humanitarian relief operations in 45 countries (Lattimer 2016). Roughly half of CERF funding is used for purchasing supplies, with the rest evenly allocated as funding to UN agencies or as partner sub-grants (Urquhart and Tuchel 2018).

Global contingency funds set aside money to cover possible humanitarian emergencies or disease outbreaks, removing the financial burden from host countries. One example is a United Nations pooled fund called the Central Emergency Response Fund (CERF) (see Box 3.3). It is and will remain an important source of funds for the UN and UN-partners at the beginning of an emergency.

Another unique initiative that leverages financing is Pay for Success (P4S). The Pay for Success model is also referred to as "pay for performance", "social impact bonds", and "development impact bonds" among other names. However, the latter terms are confusing because P4S contracts are not truly bonds; they are more like loans.

P4S contracts with investors, governments, bilateral or multilateral donors, and service providers to improve service delivery outcomes. Investors provide financing for a program that is guaranteed by a payer (usually a government). The program has predefined service delivery targets for providers to achieve; in theory, repayment to investors only occurs if the targets are met and the program is successful, so investors assume the risk (Nonprofit Finance Fund 2018). All program outcomes must be verified by an independent agency. As achieving these targets not only improves service delivery but should also reduce costs, the savings generated by the program could be used for repayment, creating sustainability.

As a result, P4S links payments for service delivery to the achievement of impact indicators (not process indicators, which is what is often measured in such settings) (Nonprofit Finance Fund 2018). Depending upon who provides the revenue, P4S could provide much-needed funding from non-traditional donors, particularly the private sector.

There is mixed evidence that P4S improves service delivery quality, and none that it reduces costs. Moreover, P4S requires time to undertake in-depth assessments requiring significant data, set up the financial arrangements, and negotiate among the various partners. Consequently, P4S is not a panacea but rather one potential option for improving refugee healthcare purchasing.

P4S is only appropriate in protracted refugee settings, particularly camps, when addressing specific health interventions, but not broad health systems issues. P4S requires a great deal of preparation, specific data, and measurement of impact indicators that are rarely available at the beginning and early stages of an emergency. Furthermore, during the acute phase of an emergency, one must address the whole health system in a comprehensive manner, which makes it difficult for P4S to be applied to specific interventions. For example, the causal pathways for the ultimate impact indicator of reducing mortality are often not easily attributable to specific interventions, but rather are due to a combination of complex and interdependent factors.

Consequently, P4S should be used for specific interventions that are relatively easy to measure and where evidence already exists of their efficacy and effectiveness. These include increasing vaccination coverage (measured as fewer measles or cholera outbreaks), improved birth outcomes (measured as deliveries with a skilled birth attendant), and reducing deaths due to a malaria (measured as spraying, bed nets, rapid diagnostic tests, following treatment protocols, etc.). These specific interventions all are possible to implement and measure in protracted refugee settings, particularly in refugee camps. Measurement of numerators and denominators

---

Box 3.4 The African Risk Capacity (ARC) (African Risk Capacity n.d.)

The ARC, managed by the African Union, requires participating governments to buy into a risk pool and maintain disaster response plans, thus guaranteeing financing and timely response for catastrophic extreme weather events. The ARC uses a tool called Africa RiskView, which compiles weather, crop, cost, and population data to set thresholds for ARC payment. If the estimated cost of a disaster response crosses a specified threshold, then the participating government will receive funding from the pool. The ARC was founded in 2014 and currently has 33 member states, five of which formed a risk pool in 2017/2018.

> **Box 3.5 The Caribbean Catastrophe Risk Insurance Facility (CCRIF) (Caribbean Catastrophe Risk Insurance Facility 2015)**
>
> Founded in 2007, CCRIF offers insurance coverage to Caribbean governments for natural disasters, combining it with capital market instruments and a parametric index. Initially a public–private partnership supported by the World Bank and other donors, the CCRIF covers 20 countries for earthquakes, hurricanes, and excessive rainfall. Countries purchase insurance annually and are insured for up to $100 million. If an event occurs, payouts disburse within 2 weeks. The CCRIF uses individual portfolios to manage risk while maintaining a single operational structure. In addition to offering insurance, the CCRIF finances itself through the reinsurance market, catastrophe bonds, and catastrophe swaps.

is more easily obtained than in out-of-camp settings, and partners are often international or national NGOs with clear roles and responsibilities. Refugees also have fewer choices regarding services in camps than out of camp. Therefore, P4S has an important but relatively limited role in the delivery of specific health interventions in protracted refugee settings, particularly camps.

Lastly, traditional insurance, indexed insurance, and reinsurance are not new, but are key to financing efficient and effective health services. Insurance schemes can cover regions, nations, communities, or individuals, and many already offer protection from natural disasters or catastrophes (Lattimer 2016). Insurance mutualises risk, so that when a loss occurs its costs are shared among participants. Governments, businesses, communities, or multilateral agencies create insurance schemes to protect populations against humanitarian crises, linking payment to emergencies, pandemics, or natural disasters (Urquhart 2018, Clarke 2016).

Some examples of insurance combine indexed insurance and catastrophe bonds to respond to natural disasters. These include the African Risk Capacity group and the Caribbean Catastrophe Risk Insurance Facility, and are described in Box 3.4 (African Risk Capacity n.d.) and Box 3.5 (Caribbean Catastrophe Risk Insurance Facility 2015).

Following the recent Ebola epidemics in West Africa, the World Bank together with the World Health Organization (WHO) and other partners are establishing a Pandemic Emergency Financing Facility that has specific triggers for specific pandemics. There is an insurance, bond, and cash window (Box 3.6) (World Bank n.d.).

Creating a similar global insurance mechanism for refugee healthcare would greatly increase available financing, as well as facilitate fast and appropriate service provision. One proposition is a "Refugee Health Financing Emergency Facility". Similar to PEF, resources could be mobilised through cash and insurance windows. Fig 3.1 goes here

Box 3.6 Pandemic Emergency Financing Facility (PEF) (World Bank n.d.)

The PEF is an innovative insurance-based mechanism that provides grants to low income countries to respond to uncommon but serious disease outbreaks as a means of averting pandemics. It targets vulnerable countries with an injection of funds to improve their response capacity and timing before an outbreak occurs. It is a joint project between the World Bank and the World Health Organization, as well as other private and public sector actors.

PEF includes an insurance/bond window and a cash window. The insurance window covers a maximum amount of $425 million, through catastrophic (pandemic) bonds and pandemic insurance paid by development organisations. Payment is capped, linked to parametric indices, which consider outbreak size, seriousness, and area, and is trigged by a severe regional outbreak from a specified list of diseases.

The cash window covers $61 million, replenished annually by donations. The cash window provides financing for disease outbreaks that have exhausted the insurance window, are limited to one country, are not included on the specified list of diseases, and require rapid response. These funds are released by approval from PEF's governance, after expert review.

The Refugee Health Financing Emergency Facility would provide funding, from diverse sources using a variety of financing mechanisms, to health systems for refugees during the acute phase of an emergency. The cash window will be UN pooled funds; a mechanism that exists already. Existing rules of disbursement need to be re-examined and decisions more evidence-based and transparent.

The insurance window will consist of bonds financed from the private sector with clear parametric indices. Bonds could be short term, in that they are meant to bridge a gap due to insufficient funds at the beginning of an emergency. Guarantees from donors or UN agencies to repay the bond at specific time could be provided to reduce risk. However, with this mechanism, funds from different sources, likely more traditional ones, would have to be found to eventually pay back the bond holders. Or, bonds could be longer-term with no guarantee of repayment of principle. These bonds may have higher yields than the "short-term" bonds discussed above.

The insurance window will consist of insurance financed from the private sector, donors, and UN agencies (e.g. UNHCR) with clear parametric indices. (UNHCR expends hundreds of millions of dollars each year on health services for refugees. Some of these funds could be "set aside" for health insurance pre-emergency.) Indices considered could include the Fragile States Index produced by the Fund for Peace. It is a critical tool in highlighting not only the normal pressures that all states experience, but also in identifying when those pressures are pushing a state towards the brink of failure. Another potential index would be a certain number of refugees crossing a border. However, it is important to note that academics and actuaries would need to undertake considerable analysis to decide if the risk is measurable and predicable.

In addition to a global insurance mechanism, another option is traditional insurance for refugees. At the country level, insurance companies pool risk by having the insured pay premiums. Should any insured entity suffer a loss, the insurance company will cover them. Insurers also often buy reinsurance from a third party. Reinsurance shares risk (and gain) and reduces loss in the case of an extreme event that the insurer cannot pay for.

A government or organisation looking to insure for humanitarian emergencies needs to determine how much risk it retains and how much it transfers. There are various types of insurance schemes, which can be publicly or privately funded, be managed by public, for-profit or non-profit organisations, and have mandatory or optional participation (Sekhri 2005). In protracted settings, when the health situation is relatively stable, health insurance for refugees should be considered. UNHCR developed a guidance note on health insurance schemes for refugees and other persons of concern to UNHCR that provides strong direction ((United Nations High Commissioner for Refugees, 2012). Providing refugees with voluntary health insurance protects them from catastrophic health expenses, while securing much-needed health services and a card as proof of identity (Box 3.7). However, care would need to be taken to guarantee equity, as the most vulnerable or those with pre-existing conditions could be excluded from the risk pool.

For health insurance for refugees to be feasible and sustainable, however, refugees must earn livelihoods to pay for their premiums and co-share costs. The issue of livelihoods is complex and will not be discussed in detail here. However, they are essential to reduce refugee dependency as well as the amount of donor assistance. The World Bank's 2016 report entitled "Forcibly displaced: toward a development approach that supports refugees, the internally displaced, and their hosts" shows that refugee influxes often benefit the local economy, although who benefits within that community is more nuanced.

There will always be vulnerable populations in all societies that cannot afford to pay for health insurance. Decisions as to who is vulnerable and who will help to pay (fully or partially) for these vulnerable persons will need to be made. Depending upon the number of refugees contributing to the national system, the risk pool may have sufficiently grown to allow for subsidising the insurance premiums and co-payments for these refugees as occurs with nationals. Other sources of revenue could come from UNHCR, which is currently funding hundreds of millions of dollars in health care services via government and NGOs, many of which are parallel services.

The provision of private health insurance for refugees is also a possibility, but it is generally significantly more expensive than national health insurance for refugees. In general, any parallel services for refugees should be comparable to that of the "average" national (United Nations High Commissioner for Refugees 2014). In most countries where refugees are located, it is unlikely that the "average" national can afford private health insurance. Thus, it is unlikely that refugees will be able to afford private health insurance. In summary, health insurance for refugees in protracted settings may be an option for many host countries.

In addition to health insurance, cash transfers may encourage refugees to utilise domestic health services. Unconditional cash transfers (UCTs) give money to individuals or families without making receipt conditional on using specific services or behaviours. Evidence remains scarce, but appropriately timed UCTs (e.g.: immediately before birth) may incentivise families to purchase health services ((United Nations High Commissioner for Refugees, 2015). Conditional cash transfers (CCTs), on the other hand, demonstrably improve health outcomes by tying receipt to certain actions or services. Similar to CCTs, vouchers require participants to redeem their vouchers for specific services. Consequently, they may improve health outcomes while simultaneously strengthening the financial stability of the health marketplace (United Nations High Commissioner for Refugees, 2015). All three must offer an appropriate amount, couple their program with marketing, and target a clearly defined population to be effective. As both CCTs and vouchers are tied to a specific service, they are most appropriate for preventative, primary, and chronic care (United Nations High Commissioner for Refugees, 2015).

Moreover, Islamic social finance is a nascent and underutilised financing opportunity. Traditional Muslim finance instruments, such as the waqf (endowment), zakat (charity), and sukuk (bonds), have rarely been used to raise revenue for refugee health relief (World Humanitarian Summit 2016), despite the fact that Yemen, Syria, and Iraq received the most humanitarian health aid in 2016. Harnessing Islamic social finance for humanitarian relief would open both culturally appropriate and previously ignored capital (World Humanitarian Summit 2016).

Box 3.7 Refugee Health Insurance in the Islamic Republic of Iran

The Islamic Republic of Iran and UNHCR launched the health insurance scheme for Afghan refugees in 2011 through a semi-private insurance company (HISE). HISE was made available to registered refugees on an individual and voluntary basis with the overall goal of improving equity and financial access to in-patient services, with a special focus on vulnerable populations. Launching of HISE also aimed at generating additional opportunities for further improvement of refugees' access to healthcare and creating a positive impact on their health status. Through minimising the financial burden of vulnerable refugees, HISE also aimed at indirectly generating positive impacts on the prevention of gender-based violence, school drop-outs, and other issues. The scheme provided complementary health insurance coverage to 331,003 Afghan refugees, including 214,652 vulnerable persons and 116,351 non-vulnerable refugees. Registered refugees in Iran have the possibility to have work permits and thus livelihoods. This allows some of them to pay for their premiums and co-payments themselves. For those who could not but fit the vulnerability criteria, UNHCR covered their costs.

In 2015, negotiations were concluded with the government to allow refugees access to the national health insurance scheme.

Conclusion

There are innovative health financing instruments that currently exist for development and natural disaster settings that could be adapted to refugee health settings, according to different contexts (see also Chap. 5 "Health Financing for Asylum Seekers in Europe: Three Scenarios Towards Responsive Financing Systems"). Recent developments show that innovative health financing mechanisms are feasible and there is strong interest by donors and the private sector.

Furthermore, primarily due to the Syrian crisis, bilateral and multilateral organisations are re-thinking how humanitarian aid and development assistance are provided. All of this provides a fertile environment to proactively consider how innovative humanitarian health financing can be explored and implemented in refugee settings. Innovative health financing mechanisms will increase access to care, but equally importantly, they will allow host country healthcare providers and health authorities to set up operational contracts that allow them to plan the provision of health services over the long run. In time, doing so will help to control costs without impacting the quality of services.

There remain, however, many unanswered questions that need to be explored. This chapter marks the beginning of discussing innovative financing for refugee healthcare.

Acknowledgments This chapter was developed in part with funds from the World Bank Group.

References

African Risk Capacity. (n.d.). *How the African risk capacity works* [Online]. Retrieved 14 July, 2019, from https://www.africanriskcapacity.org/about/how-arc-works/

Bennet, C., Foley, M., & Pantuliano, S. (2016). *Time to let go: remaking humanitarian action for the modern era*. London: Humanitarian Policy Group.

Caribbean Catastrophe Risk Insurance Facility. (2015). *Understanding CCRIF: A collection of questions and answers* [Online]. Retrieved 14 July, 2019, from https://www.ccrif.org/sites/default/files/publications/Understanding_CCRIF_March_2015.pdf

Clarke, D., & Dercon, S. (2016). *Dull disasters? How planning ahead will make a difference*. New York: Oxford University Press.

Financial Tracking Service. (2018). *Global overview: Total reported funding 2018* [Online]. United Nations Office of the Coordination of Humanitarian Affairs. Retrieved 14 July, 2019, from https://fts.unocha.org/global-funding/overview/2018

Humanitarian Policy Group. (2007). Remittances during crises: Implications for humanitarian response. In K. Savage & P. Harvey (Eds.), *HPG report 25*. London: Humanitarian Policy Group.

Hynes, M., Sheik, M., Wilson, H. G., & Spiegel, P. (2002). Reproductive health indicators and outcomes among refugee and internally displaced persons in postemergency phase camps. *JAMA, 288*, 595–603.

Lattimer, C. (2016). *Global humanitarian assistance report*.

Malkawi, K. (2014). *Gov't had no other choice but to stop providing free healthcare to Syrians–Hiasat* [Online]. Retrieved 14 July, 2019, from http://www.jordantimes.com/news/local/govt-had-no-other-choice-stop-providing-free-healthcare-syrians-%E2%80%94-hiasat

Nonprofit Finance Fund. (2018). *What is pay for success?* [Online]. Retrieved 14 July, 2019, from http://www.payforsuccess.org/learn/basics/

Sekhri, N., & Savedoff, W. (2005). Private health insurance: Implications for developing countries. *Bulletin of the World Health Organization, 83*, 127–134.

Spiegel, P. (2017). *RE: Personal communication.*

Spiegel, P., Chanis, R., & Trujillo, A. (2018). Innovative health financing for refugees. *BMC Medicine, 16*, 90–99.

Spiegel, P., Chanis, R., Trujillo, A., & Doocy, S. (2017). *Innovative humanitarian health financing for refugees.*

Spiegel, P., Sheik, M., Gotway-Crawford, C., & Salama, P. (2002). Health programmes and policies associated with decreased mortality in displaced people in postemergency phase camps: A retrospective study. *The Lancet, 360*, 1927–1934.

Unitaid. (2013). *French levy on airline tickets raises more than one billion euros for world's poor since 2006* [Online]. Unitaid. Retrieved 14 July, 2019, from https://unitaid.org/news-blog/french-levy-on-airline-tickets-raises-more-than-one-billion-euros-for-worlds-poor-since-2006/#en

Unitaid. (2016). *Innovation for global health.* Geneva: Switzerland.

Unitaid. (2017a). *Strategy 2017-2021.* Unitaid.

Unitaid. (2017b). *Unitaid: Accelerating innovation in global health* [Online]. Unitaid. Retrieved 14 July, 2019, from http://unitaid.org/assets/factsheet-about-unitaid-en.pdf

Unitaid. (n.d.). *Innovative financing: The air ticket levy* [Online]. Retrieved 14 July, 2019, from http://www.unitaid.eu/en/how/innovative-financing

United Nations High Commissioner for Refugees. (2014). *Global strategy for public health: A UNHCR strategy 2014-2018.*

United Nations High Commissioner for Refugees. (2016). *Health access and utilization survey: Access to health services in Jordan among refugees from other nationalities.*

Urquhart, A., & Tuchel, L. (2018). *Global humanitarian assistance report.*

World Bank. (2017). *Forcibly displaced: Toward a development approach supporting refugees, the internally displaced, and their hosts.* Washington, DC: World Bank.

World Bank. (n.d.). *Pandemic emergency facility: Frequently asked questions* [Online]. Retrieved 14 July, 2019, from http://www.worldbank.org/en/topic/pandemics/brief/pandemic-emergency-facility-frequently-asked-questions

World Health Organization. (2009). Progress report to taskforce. In Taskforce for Innovative International Financing for Health Systems (Ed.), *Working group 2: Raising and channelling funds.* Geneva: WHO.

World Health Organization. (2016). *UHC in Africa: A framework for action.* Geneva: WHO.

World Humanitarian Summit. (2016). *High-level panel on humanitarian financing report to the secretary-general: Too important to fail - addressing the humanitarian financing gap.*

Chapter 4
Healthcare Financing Arrangements and Service Provision for Syrian Refugees in Lebanon

Neha S. Singh, Antonia Dingle, Alia H. Sabra, Jocelyn DeJong, Catherine Pitt, Ghina R. Mumtaz, Abla M. Sibai, and Sandra Mounier-Jack

List of Abbreviations

3RP	Syrian Regional and Refugee Resilience Plan
ANC	Antenatal care
CRS	Creditor reporting system
D	Donor
DAC	Development Assistance Committee
EU	European Union
GDP	Gross domestic product
IA	Implementing agency
INGO	International Non-governmental Organisation
LCRP	Lebanon crisis response plan
LCC	Lebanese Cash Consortium
LNGO	Local Non-governmental Organisation
MENA	Middle East and North Africa
MoPH	Ministry of Public Health
MoSA	Ministry of Social Affairs
MMU	Mobile medical units
MPCA	Multipurpose cash assistance
MSF	Medecins Sans Frontières
NGO	Non-governmental organisation

N. S. Singh (✉) · A. Dingle · C. Pitt · S. Mounier-Jack
Department of Global Health and Development, London School of Hygiene and Tropical Medicine, London, UK
e-mail: neha.singh@lshtm.ac.uk; antonia.dingle@lshtm.ac.uk; catherine.pitt@lshtm.ac.uk; sandra.mounier-jack@lshtm.ac.uk

A. H. Sabra · J. DeJong · G. R. Mumtaz · A. M. Sibai
Faculty of Health Sciences, American University of Beirut, Beirut, Lebanon
e-mail: jd16@aub.edu.lb; gm15@aub.edu.lb; am00@aub.edu.lb

© Springer Nature Switzerland AG 2020
K. Bozorgmehr et al. (eds.), *Health Policy and Systems Responses to Forced Migration*, https://doi.org/10.1007/978-3-030-33812-1_4

ODA   Official development assistance
OECD   Organisation for Economic Co-operation and Development
PHC   Primary healthcare
PHCC   Primary healthcare centres
PNC   Postnatal care
RMNCH   Reproductive, maternal, newborn and child health
TPA   Third-party administrator
UAE   United Arab Emirates
UK   United Kingdom
UNICEF   United Nations International Children's Emergency Fund
UNFPA   United Nations Population Fund
UNHCR   United Nations High Commissioner for Refugees
UNOCHA   United Nations Office for the Coordination of Humanitarian Affairs
UNRWA   United Nations Relief and Works Agency for Palestine Refugees in
           the Near East
USA   United States of America
WFP   World Food Programme
WHO   World Health Organization

Introduction

The Syrian crisis, which started in 2011, has caused Syrians to flee violence and persecution both internally within its borders and externally as refugees and asylum seekers seek refuge in other countries. As of August 2018, the United Nations estimated that six million refugees had fled Syria, with the majority hosted by the neighbouring countries of Egypt, Lebanon, Jordan and Turkey (UNHCR 2018b).

By September 2018, Lebanon alone hosted an estimated 1.5 million displaced Syrians (UNHCR 2018b). As a result, Lebanon is the country with the highest per capita density of refugees in the world, with one in four people a refugee or displaced person. Refugees in Lebanon include Syrian refugees (UNHCR 2017a; Government of Lebanon and UNHCR 2018), Palestinian refugees recently arrived from Syria, Palestinian refugees already residing in Lebanon as well as Iraqi and other refugees (UNHCR 2018b). This substantial population shift has placed tremendous strain on the country's economy, infrastructure and public services. The World Bank estimates that by the end of 2015, the Syrian crisis had cost the Lebanese economy $18.15 billion due to the economic slowdown, loss in fiscal revenues and additional pressure on public services (World Bank 2017). As the Syrian crisis persists, signs of heightened tensions and host-community fatigue have emerged (Government of Lebanon and UNHCR 2017).

Lebanon's non-encampment policy means that Syrian refugees are widely dispersed throughout the country's urban and rural areas, with the highest concentration in the Beka'a Valley bordering Syria. A 2017 interagency vulnerability assessment of Syrian refugees reported that 73% of Syrians lived in residential buildings or apartments, 17% in improvised shelters such as informal tented settlements and 9% in unofficial urban housing including garages, workshops and farmhouses (UNHCR 2017c). Almost three-quarters of Syrians in Lebanon live below the poverty line proposed for Lebanon by the World Bank in 2013 ($3.84/person/day), without legal residence, and with an average household debt of $798 (Government of Lebanon and UNHCR 2018). Of the 1.5 million refugees, less than two-thirds ($n = 952,962$) were officially registered with the UNHCR in September 2018, and the majority do not have a legal right to work (UNHCR 2018b). Many Syrians in Lebanon are not registered with the United Nations High Commissioner for Refugees (UNHCR), in part because the Lebanese government asked UNHCR in 2015 to stop registering Syrians unless they were newborns of Syrian parents previously registered with UNHCR in Lebanon (Janmyr 2018). The lack of legal status of Syrians in Lebanon contributes to widespread poverty, lack of access to essential services, a risk of statelessness for the refugees' newborn children and barriers which contribute to keeping many Syrian children out of school. Three quarters of those displaced by the Syrian conflict are women and children (UNFPA 2018), while the majority are also under 19 years. In 2018, 57% of displaced Syrians registered with UNHCR as refugees were children (0–18 years), 23% were adolescents (10–19 years) and 17% were youth (20–24 years) (Ministry of Social Affairs Lebanon and UNHCR 2018).

Displaced Syrians in Lebanon are provided access to subsidised care within Lebanon's largely privatised health system, under both UNHCR and the Lebanese government's mandates, irrespective of whether they are formally registered with UNHCR (DeJong 2017). However, Syrian refugees report that access to medical specialists is challenging, with 76% stating that services are unaffordable and 70% that they face barriers in accessing medication (John Hopkins University (JHU), M. D. M., International Medical Corps, Humanitarian Aid and Civil Protection, American University of Beirut and UNHCR 2015). The latter finding is particularly concerning given the predominance of women and children within the Syrian refugee population in Lebanon, as women and children disproportionately account for the morbidity burden in conflict-affected populations (Sami et al. 2014; DeJong et al. 2017). Inadequate or interrupted access to reproductive, maternal, newborn and child health (RMNCH) services can increase the number of people affected by crises, generating a high risk of unintended or unwanted pregnancies, complications related to unsafe abortions, sexual and gender-based violence and an increased incidence of sexually transmitted infections (United Nations 2014; Glasier et al. 2006). These consequences, in turn, limit women's empowerment and their participation in the recovery process, resulting in violations of their human rights, and a reduction in the resources available to alleviate suffering (Singh et al. 2018).

Lebanon has undergone extreme changes in its population structure, its economy and its societal fabric as a result of the unfolding Syrian crisis over the last 7 years. A humanitarian crisis on the scale of the Syrian war has profound effects on the health of those affected by the conflict, as well as on the health system of the countries in which they seek refuge.

This chapter aims to provide a detailed analysis of healthcare financing arrangements and service provision for Syrian refugees in Lebanon, with a focus on women, children and adolescents. Specific objectives are to (1) provide a situational analysis of the Syrian crisis and its impact on the Lebanese health system; (2) analyse health and humanitarian aid to Lebanon from 2002 to 2016; and (3) describe the health sector response to Syrian refugees in Lebanon, including how aid and healthcare is financed, in particular for Syrian refugee women, children and adolescents.

Box 4.1 Methodology

We reviewed existing literature and data on health financing, systems and provision of health services to Syrian refugees in Lebanon and analysed aid to Lebanon.

Data and Literature Search

Eligibility criteria: We included literature and datasets related to health financing in Lebanon, as well as financing arrangements and health services (including RMNCH) for Syrian refugees. We included all primary quantitative and qualitative research studies from peer-reviewed journals as well as grey literature in the public as well as private domains, as well as any reports and datasets with information on health financing and health service provision to Syrian refugees in Lebanon.

Search strategy: We searched for relevant data and published and grey literature in English and Arabic in both public (e.g. international databases, open access governmental and non-governmental websites) and domestic (e.g. Ministry of Public Health, Ministry of Finance) domains from 2011 to 2018. We searched on terms related to the following categories in combination: health financing OR access OR preferences AND general health services OR RMNCAH services AND Syrian refugees and Lebanon. The following databases were searched for published literature: EMBASE, EconLit, MEDLINE and PsychINFO and BASE for grey literature in addition to the online resources – UNICEF, UNHCR, WHO and Lebanon governmental websites. We also screened reference lists for additional relevant literature. Individuals working in governmental (e.g. national statistics office), non-governmental, academic and United Nations (e.g. UNICEF) institutions were asked for data not available online and for additional relevant literature.

Data extraction: We recorded descriptive information on data in an Excel spreadsheet, to provide an overview of what the data contains, who it is owned by, whether the questionnaire is available to the study team, whether it is publicly available and if it is not, then who the point person is. For included literature, we also recorded descriptive information in an Excel spreadsheet, to provide an overview of the author, year, title, type of literature, brief summary and relevant data for the chapter.

Analysing Humanitarian and Health Aid to Lebanon
We analysed aid to Lebanon from 2002 to 2016 using the Creditor Reporting System (CRS), a database compiled by the Organisation for Economic Co-operation and Development, to which donor countries and multilateral institutions report annually (Organisation for Economic Cooperation and Development 2018). We included official development assistance (ODA) and private grants from institutions and calculated annual disbursements to Lebanon in total, for the humanitarian and health sectors, and by purpose and channel within the humanitarian and health sectors. We also analysed aid to Lebanon for the humanitarian sector by donor and examined the largest humanitarian disbursements in greater depth. To determine the key humanitarian and health organisations operating in Lebanon with international funding, we analysed both humanitarian and health aid by channel, i.e. disbursements from multilateral organisations' core budgets (where the multilateral agency was effectively the donor agency) and disbursements channelled through multilaterals by bilateral donors to implement specific activities (where the multilateral was the implementing agency). We made comparisons between humanitarian and health aid received by Lebanon and its neighbours Turkey and Jordan. We downloaded disbursement data from the CRS in July 2018 and reported them in constant 2016 US dollars. Data on refugee populations was obtained from the World Bank, downloaded in September 2018.

Overview of the Lebanese Health System

The health system in Lebanon is a public-private partnership with a number of sources of funding and delivery channels. Despite the fact that the country fosters a very high number of health insurance operators, the majority of the population cannot afford to pay for full coverage (Salti et al. 2010). In principle, the Ministry of Public Health is the funder of last resort, i.e. it is committed to pay if people do not have health insurance. Public healthcare provision is therefore required to cater for expensive long-term treatments. As such, the National Social Security Fund (NSSF), Lebanon's national social insurance system which provides employees with health insurance cover and retirement pensions, has been recording a deficit for several years. Almost 50% of Lebanon's population is financially covered by the NSSF or by other governmental (i.e. civil servants cooperative and military) schemes or private insurance bodies (Salti et al. 2010). These schemes provide financial coverage with variable patient co-payments, and non-adherents are entitled to the coverage of the Ministry of Public Health (MoPH) for secondary and tertiary care at both public and private institutions.

MoPH provides in-kind support to a national network of primary healthcare (PHC) centres (PHCCs) across Lebanon including non-governmental and faith-based organisations (Government of Lebanon and UN 2018). These centres provide consultations with medical specialists at reduced cost, as well as medicines for chronic illness and vaccines funded by the MoPH (Ammar et al. 2016). It is estimated that 68% of the primary healthcare centres in the national network are owned by non-governmental organisations (NGOs) while 80% of hospitals belong to the private sector (Government of Lebanon and UNHCR 2018). The strong presence of the private sector in service delivery has led to an oversupply of hospital beds and technology, and while there is an oversupply of physicians, there is a shortage of nurses (A. H. C. G. Report 2016; Kassak et al. 2006). Moreover, in 2006 the World Health Organization (WHO) estimated that only 8% of the population benefitted from government primary care, revealing a failing primary healthcare system (WHO 2006).

Although recent data on domestic financing for healthcare in Lebanon are unavailable, data from 2006 show that Lebanon spends almost 11.5% of gross domestic product (GDP) on health compared to an average of 5% in the Middle East and North Africa (MENA) region, of which 75% is out-of-pocket expenditure not including insurance cover (Akala and El-Saharty 2006). Three quarters (75%) of public health spending in Lebanon funds hospital-based curative care (Akala and El-Saharty 2006). Moreover, the public sector is the major financing agent for services rendered in the private sector. According to the Ministry of Finance 2006 budget proposal, private sector hospitalisation accounts for 48% of total public health expenditure, which constitutes a significant drain on public sector finance (Salti et al. 2010). In addition, health services in Lebanon are some of the most expensive in the MENA region (Salti et al. 2010; WHO 2006).

Humanitarian and Health Aid to Lebanon

Humanitarian aid comprises a large proportion of total aid to Lebanon. On average, between 2002 and 2016, 25% of all aid to Lebanon flowed to the humanitarian sector, 3% flowed to the health sector and the remaining 72% flowed to other sectors, including education, water, transport, energy, agriculture, construction and general budget support (Fig. 4.3a). Health aid to Lebanon increased from $11 million in 2002 to $44 million in 2016, with funding peaking in 2014 at just over $47 million (Fig. 4.3c). While health aid to Lebanon increased between 2002 and 2016, overall, the proportion of aid for health remained small compared to humanitarian aid and total aid.

In contrast, humanitarian aid averaged $186 million per year, the majority of which supported "material relief assistance and services", which can include health projects as well as provision of shelter, water, sanitation and other non-food relief items (Fig. 4.3b). Humanitarian aid fluctuated considerably over the 15-year period, with three clear peaks coinciding with the first wave of Iraqi refugees entering Lebanon in 2006, the year after the start of the Syrian war, 2012, and then in 2015 with the intensification of the Syrian war coupled with efforts by European donors to keep Syrian refugees in neighbouring territories of Jordan and Lebanon

(Fig. 4.3a). The data presented reflect two distinct but interrelated refugee situations in Lebanon which are important to distinguish – that of the long-term Palestinian refugees spanning the period 2002–2010 and then from 2011/2012 the arrival of Syrian refugees in Lebanon, in addition to Palestinian refugees.

The peaks in humanitarian aid identified in 2012 and 2015, reflecting the Syrian crisis (and to a lesser degree, in 2006 in response to Palestinian refugees in Lebanon), were largely driven by funding from the USA (Fig. 4.3d). US ODA comprised 81% of all humanitarian aid to Lebanon in 2012 (a total of $252 million) and 32% ($191 million) in 2015. European Union (EU) institutions were the second-largest human-itarian donors to Lebanon over the period, contributing $562 million of ODA to the humanitarian sector between 2002 and 2016.

Having disbursed very little humanitarian ODA to Lebanon from 2002 to 2014, in 2015 the UK disbursed $104 million and in 2016 $89 million in humanitarian ODA, making it the second and third largest donor in those respective years. Germany had also contributed relatively little in humanitarian ODA to Lebanon before 2014, when it disbursed $70 million, making it the second largest donor that year after the EU institutions. Germany disbursed $25 million in humanitarian ODA in 2015, followed by $100 million in 2016, making it the largest donor to the humanitarian sector in 2016.

The three implementing agencies in Lebanon with the most aid channelled through them were the United Nations Relief and Works Agency for Palestine Refugees in the Near East (UNRWA) (which only provides services to Palestine refugees), UNHCR and United Nations International Children's Emergency Fund (UNICEF) (Fig. 4.2). However, aid channelled through UNRWA in Lebanon has decreased since 2018 when the USA, the largest single donor to UNRWA, stopped funding the agency.

Although proportionally UNRWA, UNHCR and UNICEF are more dominant within health than the humanitarian sector as classified in the OECD database, the humanitarian sector received a larger proportion of the total available funding between 2002 and 2016 compared to the health sector. Over this period, more than $600 million out of a total $2.8 billion of humanitarian aid was channelled through UNRWA, compared to $230 million out of a total of $390 million of health aid (Fig. 4.1). Within the health sector, these three multilaterals were responsible for allocating the largest amount of funds in 2011 ($29 million) and 2014 ($35 million) (Fig. 4.2).

Since the start of the Syrian crisis in 2011, Lebanon received less humanitarian aid in absolute numbers than its neighbour Jordan, but more than Turkey, both of which also hosted very large numbers of Syrian refugees. However, Turkey received substantially more humanitarian aid per refugee compared to Lebanon and Jordan (Fig. 4.4). Between 2011 and 2016, Turkey received an average of just under $1,685 per refugee per year, while Lebanon received $287 and Jordan an average of $146 per refugee.

At $207 million, Lebanon also received less aid for health from 2011 to 2016 than Turkey ($223 million) and Jordan ($512 million). However, the three countries were comparable in the proportion of aid received for the health sector: 4% in Lebanon, 1% in Turkey and 4% in Jordan.

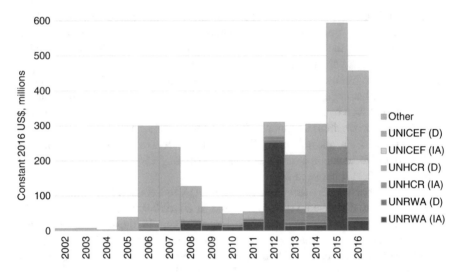

Fig. 4.1 Humanitarian aid to Lebanon by three largest channels. *UNICEF* United Nations International Children's Emergency Fund, *UNHCR* United Nations High Commissioner for Refugees, *UNRWA* United Nations Relief and Works Agency for Palestine Refugees in the Near East, *IA* implementing agency, *D* donor

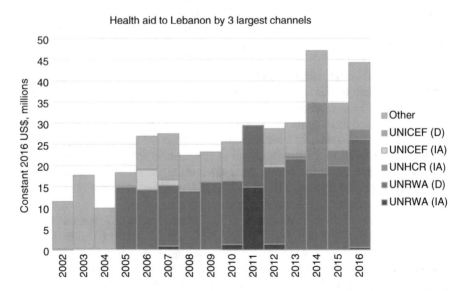

Fig. 4.2 Health aid to Lebanon by three largest channels. *UNICEF* United Nations International Children's Emergency Fund, *UNHCR* United Nations High Commissioner for Refugees, *UNRWA* United Nations Relief and Works Agency for Palestine Refugees in the Near East, *IA* implementing agency, *D* donor

Non-development Assistance Committee Donors

In addition to aid provided by 'traditional' donors—members of the Organisation for Economic Cooperation and Development (OECD) Development Assistance Committee (DAC), e.g. the USA, Germany, the UK—humanitarian aid to the Syrian crisis is also provided by non-DAC donors. Non-DAC donors are any beyond the current 29 DAC members and typically refer to official country donors (i.e., bilateral) as well as private foundations. Some non-DAC donors report their data to the OECD's Creditor Reporting System while others do not. As such, it is challenging to assess the magnitude of aid from non-DAC donors benefiting Syrian refugees in Lebanon.

The UAE is the largest non-DAC donor disbursing aid to Lebanon which reports to the CRS. From 2002 to 2016, UAE disbursed $33.7 million in humanitarian aid (1% of all humanitarian aid) and $12.4 million in health aid (3% of all health aid) to Lebanon. Other non-DAC donors reporting to the CRS include Kuwait, which disbursed 0.1% ($1.9 million) of total humanitarian aid to Lebanon over 2002–2016, and the Organisation of the Petroleum Exporting Companies (OPEC) Fund for International Development, which disbursed 0.3% ($1.1 million) of total health aid to Lebanon between 2002 and 2016. These non-DAC donors are captured within the analysis of aid to Lebanon above (Figs. 4.1, 4.2, 4.3 and 4.4).

Other non-DAC donors understood to be disbursing aid for Syrian refugees in Lebanon include other members of the Gulf Cooperation Council and Iran. In addition, aid to Lebanon is provided by local NGOs, philanthropic organisations, Islamic organisations, civil society organisations and Syrian refugee associations. There is little data available on the scale of contributions from these organisations. Much of their aid goes directly to partners instead of being channelled through the Syrian Regional and Refugee Resilience Plan (3RP). The 3RP, composed of eight sectors including Health, was launched in 2013 for the purpose of improving coordination of the response, with the participation of more than 60 humanitarian implementing partners representing UN agencies, international non-governmental organisations (INGOs) and local NGOs (LNGOs) (3RP 2017).

Limitations

There are limitations inherent in our approach to tracking aid flows for Lebanon. CRS data is widely used when tracking aid for health, as the main publicly available source of data on aid disbursements (Pitt et al. 2018; Grollman et al. 2017). The CRS provides access to data on all main donors of ODA over a long time period. However, there are limitations inherent with using CRS data. Firstly, currently the Bill and Melinda Gates Foundation is the only private foundation that report to the CRS, so the data used do not capture other sources of private grants supporting the health and humanitarian sectors in Lebanon. Secondly, it is challenging to produce

a

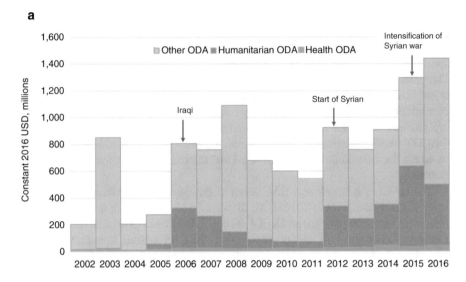

b

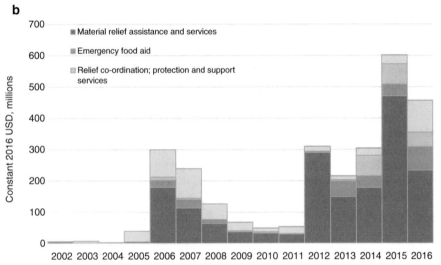

Fig. 4.3 (**a–d**) Aid to Lebanon (USD), 2002–2016. *EU* European Union, *ODA* overseas development assistance, *WFP* World Food Programme

robust estimates of aid flows to a country such as Lebanon, with an integrated refugee population, which uses local education and health services. There is not a clear delineation between aid to the health sector supporting only the Lebanese population and aid to the refugee population. Likewise, aid to the humanitarian sector can actually be supporting health activities for the host population. Finally, to date there is not an accurate picture of the role of nontraditional donors for Lebanon. These

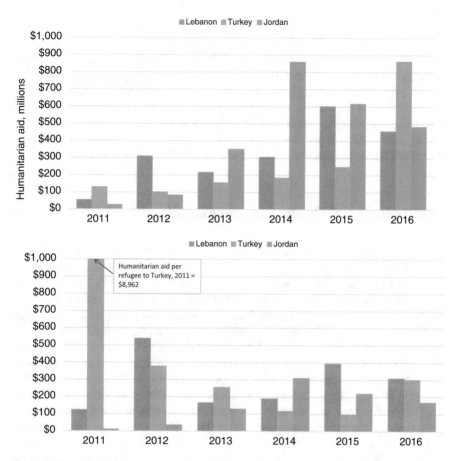

Fig. 4.4 Humanitarian aid to Lebanon in context

may represent a substantial aid envelope for Lebanon, but lack of transparency of data on disbursements from nontraditional donors prevents such insights. Therefore, given the available data, our estimates are the best indication we have of aid flows to the health and humanitarian sectors in Lebanon.

Health Sector Response to the Syrian Crisis

The health sector response in Lebanon involves a total of 24 national, international and governmental implementing agencies and is led by the Lebanon MoPH, WHO and UNHCR. The health sector coordinated response to the refugee crisis targets a population of over 1.5 million people out of a total of 2.4 million population in need (Inter-Agency Coordination Lebanon 2018). The populations targeted by the response plan include not only Syrian refugees but also Palestinian refugees settled in Lebanon or coming from Syria, as well as vulnerable Lebanese host communities. The health sector response lists the following four priority interventions: (1) ensuring access to target populations to a standardised package of basic health service at primary care level, (2) access to life-saving secondary care mainly for the Syrian displaced population, (3) preventing and controlling epidemic outbreaks in high risk areas with the largest number of Syrian displaced population and (4) reinforcing youth health as part of a comprehensive reproductive healthcare and through the school health programme (Ministry of Public Health (MPH) and WU 2015).

Healthcare for all Displaced Syrians in Lebanon

In Lebanon, primary healthcare is available to Lebanese as well as displaced Syrians (i.e. whether registered or unregistered with UNHCR), through a variety of primary healthcare facilities. The Lebanon Crisis Response Plan (LCRP) 2017–2020 set financing arrangements to strengthen and enhance the resilience and capacities of the health system in responding to primary, secondary and tertiary healthcare needs of displaced Syrians, Palestinian refugees from Syria and the most vulnerable in the host communities of Palestinian refugees and Lebanese in Lebanon. According to the LCRP Health sector strategy, subsidised primary healthcare is available to both registered and non-registered Syrian refugees (Ministry of Public Health (MPH) and WU 2015). Primary healthcare includes the following services: vaccination, medication for acute and chronic conditions, non-communicable diseases (NCD) care, sexual and reproductive healthcare, malnutrition screening and management, mental healthcare, dental care, basic laboratory and diagnostics as well as health promotion. Most of these services are provided to Syrian refugees in 111 primary healthcare facilities (including 62 MoPH-PHCCs and 49 dispensaries including 13 Lebanese Ministry of Social Affairs (MoSA) social development centres) (Ministry of Social Affairs Lebanon and UNHCR 2018) for a nominal fee compared to private clinics. Services are delivered with the support of international and local partners to reduce out-of-pocket expenditure, in light of the high economic vulnerability levels of displaced Syrians. Subsidised care is available to a number of vulnerable Lebanese as a way of addressing critical health needs and mitigating potential sources of tension in nearly 75% of the aforementioned facilities. From January to September 2017, approximately 1,058,412 subsidised consultations were provided at the PHC level by LCRP partners, out of which data for Syrian refugees have not been disaggregated, but 17% were consultations for vulnerable Lebanese (Ministry of Social Affairs Lebanon and UNHCR 2018).

In addition to LCRP partners, other organisations, e.g. Médecins Sans Frontières (MSF) Switzerland and MSF-Belgium, provide a number of free PHC services for displaced Syrians, vulnerable Lebanese as well as other population groups. From January to August 2017, MSF-Switzerland and MSF-Belgium provided approximately 225,000 additional consultations, representing an additional 21% of the caseload supported by LCRP partners (Ministry of Social Affairs Lebanon and UNHCR 2018). MSF-Belgium also offers free delivery care for Syrian refugees with very high demand.

In parallel to the provision of PHC services through MoPH PHCCs and dispensaries, specific primary healthcare services are also made available to displaced Syrians through approximately 25 mobile medical units (MMUs), operated by various NGOs, which provide free consultations and medication and often refer patients to PHCCs for services unavailable at MMUs. Though fewer in number than at the onset of the Syrian crisis, MMUs continue to be operational primarily in areas with high distribution of informal settlements and/or in distant rural areas from which PHCs are hard to reach. From January to September 2017, approximately 216,266 free consultations were provided through MMUs by LCRP partners representing an additional 17% of the total consultations supported by LCRP partners (Ministry of Public Health (MPH) and WU 2015). Meanwhile, primary healthcare services are also widely available to displaced Syrians through private doctors' clinics, pharmacies or even hospitals, although these services are much higher in cost, leading to higher out-of-pocket expenditure. Medical services are also available to the displaced population through numerous informal practices run by Syrian doctors or midwives in informal settlements (Syrian Refugees 2014).

Healthcare for Syrian Refugees Registered with UNHCR

To facilitate the process of providing healthcare to registered Syrian refugees, UNHCR contracts a third-party administrator (TPA), including a range of governmental and non-governmental administrators. The TPA is the link between registered Syrian refugees and the facility where they receive healthcare. The TPA contracts a network of public and private hospitals throughout the country where refugees can access care. Inclusion in this network is decided by UNHCR based on proximity to beneficiaries, availability of services and cost-effectiveness. As a general rule, UNHCR does not support care given in hospitals outside of the network.

UNHCR supports provision of referral care to Syrian refugees through a cost-sharing mechanism. The TPA agrees with the contracted hospital on standardised fees following MoPH fixed rates. Since July 2018, for bills between $101 and $2900, UNHCR requires Syrian refugees to pay $100 in addition to 25% of the remaining hospital bill. For bills of $2900 and above, Syrian refugees pay $800 (UNHCR 2018a). The remaining bill is directly paid by UNHCR, conditional on Syrian refugees retaining and submitting the bill for payment. Syrian refugees who are unable to pay their share are not able to receive care.

UNHCR has specified $10,000 as the maximum total cost for a single hospital admission and does not reimburse bills exceeding this amount (UNHCR 2018a). For certain types of care, e.g. neonatal intensive care and burns intensive care, the maximum amount is extended to $15,000. The maximum total amount that UNHCR will provide for one single household during a year is $30,000. As a general rule,

UNCHCR also mandates that governmental hospitals should be prioritised, and if not possible, then the most cost-effective alternative should be sought. Nonurgent cases are often ineligible for UNHCR support. To be declared eligible, a detailed medical report is needed accompanied by appropriate copies of medical investigations performed.

Affordability of Healthcare for Syrian Refugees

Affordability of healthcare has been identified as a major challenge for refugees in accessing healthcare (Ministry of Social Affairs Lebanon and UNHCR 2018). The 2017 vulnerability assessment survey showed that although displaced Syrians can, in theory, access primary healthcare services from a variety of health outlets, their main barrier to accessing services is reported to be cost-related (UNHCR 2017c). The survey found that of those Syrian refugee households that did not receive the required primary healthcare, the main reasons cited were cost of drugs (33%) and consultation fees (33%). Furthermore, out-of-pocket expenditure on health among displaced Syrians comprises 11% of total household expenditure (UNHCR 2017c). The financial cost of covering the healthcare expenses of the displaced Syrian population is reported to exceed by far the resources allocated by both international and national agencies (Ammar et al. 2016).

Meeting the cost of hospital care is challenging for Syrian refugees. Nearly one quarter (24%) of surveyed Syrian refugee households report requiring access to secondary or tertiary healthcare in the previous 6 months, of which one in five did not receive the required care, with 53% of surveyed households cited cost of treatment as the main barrier to accessing care (UNHCR 2017c). There are also reports of hospitals putting in place strategies to recover as much of the Syrian patients' portions of the bills as possible by inflating bills, asking for deposits to be paid prior to admission and retaining corpses/displaced Syrian IDs or UNHCR registration documents until the hospital bill is settled, which raises protection concerns (UNHCR 2017c).

On the supply side, the impact of displaced Syrians on the Lebanese health system remains unparalleled, when examined in proportion to the country's host population (Blanchet et al. 2016; Government of Lebanon and UNHCR 2018). Treating patients who are not able to pay has caused hospitals to accumulate a total debt of $15 million since the onset of the Syrian crisis, according to MoPH records for 2016. This debt has put an enormous stress on the public hospital system and its ability to provide services to Syrian refugees and vulnerable Lebanese (GoL & UN 2018; Ministry of Social Affairs Lebanon and UNHCR 2018). The limited financing of access to secondary care services has resulted in a major gap in service coverage, leading to a heavy financial burden on refugees seeking secondary and tertiary care services. Lebanese hospitals are seeing increased numbers of Syrian patients who are unable to pay their proportion of the bill, as well as Syrian patients whose hospitalisations are not subsidised. Referral of uncovered Syrian patients with complicated morbidities to public hospitals has also become a common practice by private

Box 4.2 *Spotlight:* **Financing Care to Syrian Refugee Women in Lebanon**

Financial constraints limit Syrian refugee women's access to healthcare. Antenatal care (ANC) constitutes an important proportion of medical services provided to Syrian women at primary healthcare level. However, a 2017 UNHCR study found that 73% of women aged 15–49 years and who had been pregnant in the past 2 years reported accessing at least one ANC visit, representing a 3% increase in access compared to 2016 (Government of Lebanon and UNHCR 2017). Among the 27% of pregnant women who did not receive ANC, 47% reported being unable to afford doctors' fees. Moreover, only 28% of women who delivered reported receiving postnatal care (PNC), of which 22% said they could not afford the clinic fees. These findings demonstrate the need to increase uptake of ANC and PNC by displaced Syrian women and address financial barriers.

With regard to family planning, a recent study on the barriers to contraceptive use among Syrian refugees points to cost as the main reported barrier to contraceptive use (UNDP and ARK 2017; Masterson et al. 2014). These findings are echoed by implementing agencies who report a contributing factor as the inconsistent implementation of the official communication of the MoPH related to reproductive health services at MoPH-PHCC level, which both places a ceiling on the cost of reproductive health services and emphasises that family planning commodities are to be distributed free of charge (Government of Lebanon and UNHCR 2018).

Assessing the current health status and healthcare utilisation of Syrian women in Lebanon is challenging due to lack of quality and quantity of timely data. However, a recent study assessing coverage of key evidence-based RMNCH indicators in displaced Syrian women reported that in 2015, out of all referrals for delivery, about one-third (33.7%) of Syrian refugee deliveries in UNHCR-contracted hospitals were Caesarean sections (C-sections) (DeJong et al. 2017). This is also due to the fact that Syrian women are delivering within a Lebanese health system where C-sections rates are high.

Another challenge to Syrian refugee women accessing care is the July 2018 revision to the UNHCR healthcare financing policy stipulating that compared to the earlier policy, only pregnant women who are registered with UNHCR before arriving at the health facility to deliver are eligible to receive financial support from the agency to cover partial delivery expenses (UNHCR 2018c). Pregnant Syrian women who are registered with UNHCR will be required to pay between $150 and 200 for a normal delivery and $225 and 355 for a C-section depending on which hospital they go to, with the understanding that UNHCR will pay the remaining bill if the receipt is retained by the patient. Women who have not already registered with UNHCR will be required to pay the entire hospital bill. Women in need of additional hospital care other than for their delivery are required to pay $100 more than the previous UNHCR policy (UNHCR 2018c).

hospitals, even though care at public hospitals is also not free but only subsidised by UNHCR for registered refugees (A. H. C. G. Report 2016).

Aid Planning and Coordination

UNHCR was given the leading role to coordinate and implement aid to refugees in Lebanon, which is commensurate with it being the second largest channel of health and humanitarian aid in Lebanon after UNRWA, which caters solely to Palestinian refugees. As part of this role, in 2013 UNHCR created a separate coordination platform that it coleads with MoSA representing the Government of Lebanon. The multisectoral 3RP launched in 2013 with more than 60 humanitarian implementing partners aims to also address host community inclusion and create livelihood opportunities via the introduction of new programmes and the enhancement of governmental institutions capacities (3RP 2017). As part of the coordination mechanism, the United Nations Office for the Coordination of Humanitarian Affairs (UNOCHA) monitors gaps and coordination issues among the UN agencies, UNDP coordinates development projects and WFP conducts the annual vulnerability assessment surveys to improve beneficiary targeting.

Funding Levels

Mobilising adequate funding has been a major impediment to the response to the refugee crisis in Lebanon (Fig. 4.5). In 2018, delays in funding were reported to have led to discontinuing financial coverage of pregnant women in Palestine refugees

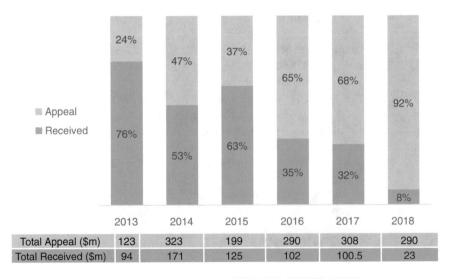

Fig. 4.5 Health sector funding status in Lebanon, 2013–2017 (UNHCR 2018b)

from Syria and resulted in serious shortages of medication for chronic conditions at medical facilities supported by MoPH (Inter-Agency Coordination Lebanon 2018).

Lack of sufficient funding for healthcare in the eighth year of the Syrian crisis poses grave challenges to agencies tasked with delivering services to Syrian refugees. In 2017, the United Nations Children's Fund (UNICEF) appeals to keep basic services functioning for $1.4 billion received less than 25% of its funding requirements, while the UNHCR 3RP appeals seeking $4.63 billion to also only cover essential services received $433 million, i.e. 9% of the request (United Nations Refugees and Migrants (UNRM) 2017; UNHCR 2017b, c). At a donor conference for Syrian refugees hosted in Brussels in 2019, UNHCR appealed for aid citing that the funding gap is leaving Syrian refugees, particularly women and children (over 70% of the refugee population), with substantial cuts in services and a lack of resources to address their growing needs but fell $1 billion short of its target (European Council 2019). In Lebanon, in 2017 UNHCR faced an underfunding of $11.7 million for secondary healthcare needed to reach a minimum of 5000 people per month. Similarly, UNICEF reported it needed $4.7 million to provide child health and nutrition care to 500,000 children under the age of 5 years (3RP 2017).

Evolving Use of Cash-Based Interventions to Deliver Aid to Syrian Refugees

While aid to refugees has traditionally been provided through in-kind contributions, such as shelter and hygiene kits and the direct provision of healthcare services, cash-based interventions have been used increasingly in recent years (see also Chap. 3 "Innovative Humanitarian Health Financing for Refugees"), especially in Lebanon. Cash-based interventions include both unconditional and multipurpose cash transfers, cash transfers with eligibility conditions (including cash for work) and vouchers that can be exchanged for specific items, services or cash. The humanitarian communities in Lebanon, including donors, have been increasingly relying on cash-based interventions—rather than in-kind basic assistance—as a way of delivering assistance to the affected population in Lebanon as part of the Syria response since 2013. For example, food assistance provided by World Food Programme (WFP) has evolved from in-kind support to paper food vouchers and then to electronic cards in 2016 for use in designated shops across Lebanon. As donor appetite for multipurpose cash assistance (MPCA) has grown, cash-based interventions have evolved in Lebanon and have included a wide range of activities across various sectors, including shelter, education, protection, WASH, food security and basic assistance. Considering that Lebanon is a country with well-functioning and elastic markets with a range of goods and services available, cash has been determined to be an appropriate modality to enable every household to prioritise their individual needs. With the Syrian refugee population spread across the country, living in different shelter types and with different needs and priorities, cash offers a flexible solution that enables families to choose for themselves how to address their prioritised needs in a dignified manner.

Despite these advantages, cash has not been deemed by humanitarian actors as a 'silver bullet' and is instead one component of a wider response in which other humanitarian actors have sought to ensure availability and accessibility of quality services such as health, education and water supply for all. Reflecting on the different needs that voucher and cash-based interventions were being used to deliver, six international NGOs delivering assistance in Lebanon opted to form the Lebanese Cash Consortium (LCC) and to develop and roll out a 'multipurpose' cash approach to socio-economically vulnerable Syrian refugee households in Lebanon from 2014. Members of the LCC are Save the Children (Consortium Lead), the International Rescue Committee (Monitoring and Evaluation and Research Lead), ACTED, CARE, Solidarités and World Vision International. This consists of a single transfer that is intended to cover multiple survival needs of a refugee family. After the development of the Survival Minimum Expenditure Basket (SMEB) among cash actors in 2014, an appropriate transfer value was set at $175 per family per month, which has been deemed to be the gap in a family's needs that could not be met through the family's own means or through food assistance, and continues to be provided by WFP. Figure 4.6 provides an overview of programme delivery steps of the LCC's MPCA.

Findings from the most recent vulnerability assessment survey in 2017 (UNHCR 2017c) show that economically vulnerable Syrian refugees continued to receive cash and other types of help including household items, education, subsidised healthcare and shelter assistance. Seventy-one percent of the sampled population reported receiving some form of assistance in the three months prior to the survey. Food assistance delivered by WFP through a common cash card makes up the largest proportion of assistance to Syrian refugees. The level of assistance was maintained at $27 per person per month, and in May 2017, WFP provided food assistance to 692,451 Syrian refugees, which is an increase of over 14,000 refugees compared to June 2016. Compared to food and other assistance, MPCA is delivered to fewer Syrian refugees as it aims to assist the most socio-economically vulnerable households, selected based on predefined criteria, in meeting their basic needs. In May 2017, 29,581 Syrian refugee households were receiving multipurpose cash from UNHCR, and other cash actors were providing multipurpose cash assistance to an additional 17,874 households (UNHCR 2017c). In addition, just over one-third of surveyed Syrian households reported receiving seasonal cash assistance during the winter cycle in 2016–2017 (UNHCR 2017c). The same survey reported 72% of children and youth aged 5–24 currently attending school received some type of school-related support in the 2016–2017 academic year (UNHCR 2017c).

An impact evaluation of the LCC MPCA found that it increased refugees' consumption of living essentials, including food and gas for cooking. Syrian refugees' total monthly expenditures, which include food, water, health, hygiene and other consumables, were on average 21% higher than those of non-beneficiaries (Lebanon Cash Consortium (LCC) 2016). From a social cohesion perspective, LCC beneficiaries felt eight times more secure, as compared to non-beneficiaries. In addition, LCC MPCA appeared to increase by five times Syrian refugees' sense of trust of the community hosting them (Lebanon Cash Consortium (LCC) 2016).

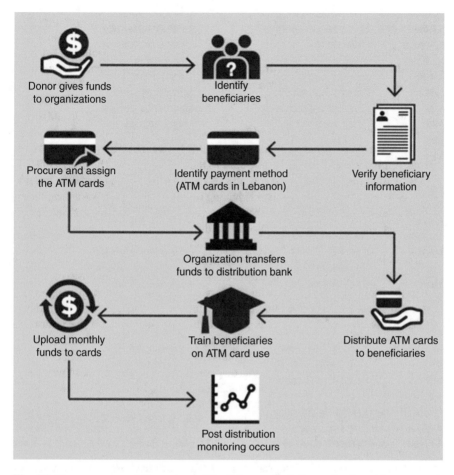

Fig. 4.6 Key programme delivery steps of the Lebanese Cash Consortium's multipurpose cash delivery (International Rescue Committee 2014)

Implications for Research and Practice

Lebanon has the highest per capita density of refugees in the world, with three quarters of this population comprising women and children and the majority under 19 years old. This large refugee population has placed critical strain on the country's economy and public services, including the health system. A complex financing environment exists for displaced Syrians in Lebanon as a result of a high level of health service provision from the private sector, high out-of-pocket expenditure on health services and an increasingly constrained funding landscape (see also Chap. 3 "Innovative Humanitarian Health Financing for Refugees").

We found that aid to humanitarian and health sectors comprised 28% of all aid to Lebanon between 2002 and 2016. In total, $3.2 billion has been disbursed to

Lebanon in both humanitarian and health aid over this period. Clear peaks in humanitarian aid are identifiable in 2012 and 2015, in line with the start (in 2011) and then intensification of the Syrian crisis. These peaks in humanitarian aid were largely driven by disbursements from the USA. Since 2014, Germany and the UK have also become significant donors of aid to Lebanon. Aid to Lebanon has largely been channelled through three organisations—UNRWA, UNHCR and UNICEF. Lebanon has received more total humanitarian aid between 2002 and 2016 than its neighbours Turkey and Jordan, which also host Syrian refugees.

Despite the aid received by Lebanon, the difficulty of mobilising adequate funding has significantly impeded the response to the refugee crisis. The 2017 UNHCR appeal to fund the 3RP received just 9% of the $4.6 billion requested to provide essential services. This funding gap is having a critical impact on Syrian refugees' access to care and well-being in Lebanon, particularly that of women, children and adolescents who comprise the majority of the Syrian refugee population. Cash-based interventions are increasingly being used in Lebanon to deliver both aid and health services to displaced Syrians, in combination with subsidised private sector and free public sector primary health services. A significant gap in coverage is evident in the provision of secondary and tertiary care where subsidies are proportionally much smaller than for primary care, placing the financial burden on refugees requiring this level of care. This is particularly challenging given the protracted nature of the Syrian crisis and that humanitarian agencies have had to reduce their subsidies since July 2018. Displaced Syrians report that costs are the main barrier to accessing health services, and their out-of-pocket expenditure is high. In particular, Syrian women are facing increased financial constraints, for example, as a result of recent policy revisions by UNHCR regarding eligibility for subsidised delivery care for pregnant Syrian women.

Findings from our chapter highlight the challenges of integration for host and refugee populations alike in Lebanon. The country's non-encampment policy is one of few models of deliberate integration of refugees with the host population. It contrasts with Jordan's encampment policy and the UNRWA model for Palestinian refugees. However, it presents similarities with Turkey's refugee policy, which provides its 3.6 million Syrian displaced population (3RP 2019) temporary protection to access services in the national system alongside Turkish nationals, and Uganda's integration policy which offers access to domestic health services to its 1.3 million refugee population, the majority (64.9%) of whom are from South Sudan (UNHCR 2019). Nevertheless, in proportion to its total population, the impact of the Syrian population on the Lebanese health system remains unparalleled (Blanchet et al. 2016; Government of Lebanon and UNHCR 2018). Integrating displaced Syrians with host Lebanese populations has several potential benefits including fostering sustainability without the need to set up parallel systems for health, education, etc. However, integration also raises distinct challenges for refugees and host populations that arise with their mixing, such as barriers to access to secondary care, high out-of-pocket expenditures, variable access to cash-based incentives and basic care needs which are not met for a proportion of refugees and vulnerable Lebanese. Furthermore, these issues pose a threat to Lebanon's integration model, as the immigration of Syrian refugees has had a substantial impact on the country's health system and on low-income Lebanese. For example, overburdening hospitals and health facilities eventually limits care for both the refugee and local population and has led to tensions (APIS Health Consulting Group 2016). Similar challenges are also seen in countries like Turkey where refugees have experienced an increase in out-of-pocket expenditures and challenges in accessing healthcare, while pressure on the health systems has been growing (Samari 2015; Chong 2018; 3RP 2019).

Our literature review and aid analysis highlight several limitations including gaps in data (see also Chap. 9 "The State of the Art and the Evidence on Health Records for Migrants and Refugees: Findings from a Systematic Review"). Firstly, data on domestic financing in Lebanon have not been accessible since 2006, which makes it challenging to understand whether financing arrangements are effective and efficient. Secondly, data on coverage of key interventions for women, children and adolescent refugees are mostly unavailable. These data gaps mean that we have a very incomplete picture of the RMNCH among the whole population of refugees, because of difficulties in sampling given the mobility of refugee populations and the absence of a sampling frame (DeJong 2017, DeJong et al. 2017). Using population as a denominator to calculate coverage of interventions for both host and refugee populations in Lebanon is also challenging because the last census in Lebanon was conducted in 1932, the refugee population is highly mobile and estimates of displaced Syrians in Lebanon are difficult to determine and fluctuate. Thirdly, recent health system data in Lebanon are not available in the public domain, making it difficult to assess health system functionality and to measure the impact of the Syrian crisis on the Lebanese health system. Fourthly, the Syrian refugee and funding situation remains very fluid. To paint a full picture of the situation, this chapter has had to combine data from different years and of different forms. For example, coverage rates of health interventions vary over time according to financing and which health services are funded over time and to what level vary substantially, such as in the case of delivery of care as described earlier.

This chapter also highlights significant gaps in research. To date, there are no comprehensive published studies on the cost-effectiveness of cash-based incentives and their effect on intended outcomes (e.g. health and nutrition) for refugees in Lebanon. Additionally, in terms of estimating coverage rates for RMNCH and other health-related interventions, it is unclear what the comparators for Syrian refugees should be, e.g. Syria pre-conflict or the Lebanese population. This comparator issue is one of the largest conceptual and methodological challenges researchers face when working on refugee populations in all settings (DeJong 2017). Finally, gaps in data and evidence underscore the importance of developing and supporting research capacity in Lebanon, as researchers in such countries are in the best position to collaborate with existing governmental and service providers to maximise the chances of generating relevant research findings that inform positive change in financing as well as provision of health services and programmes (DeJong 2017).

Our findings raise a number of questions for the future of displaced Syrians in Lebanon, as well as their impact on the country's health system and low-income Lebanese populations. The future of financing and delivery of essential services, including RMNCH, for refugees in Lebanon is unclear taking into account increased funding cuts from international donors (e.g. the USA) and grave underfunding of UNHCR. Furthermore, the US announcement of its withdrawal of aid from UNRWA in 2018 will have significant implications for the funding of refugees in Lebanon. The EU and Germany pledged their continued support for UNRWA and are urging other donor countries to do the same (Kitamura et al. 2018), but to date significant funding gaps remain. This systemic underfunding and the strain that the hosting of refugees has placed on Lebanon's health system also have implications for low-income Lebanese populations and their access to essential services.

Our findings echo challenges increasingly being faced by other countries using an integrated health systems model for refugees such as Turkey and Uganda. The recent draft global action 2019–2023 on "Promoting the health of refugees and migrants" endorsed at the World Health Assembly in May 2019 notes that the entitlement of and access to health services by refugees and migrants vary by country and are determined by national law (World Health Organization 2019) (see also Chap. 13 "Global Social Governance and Health Protection for Forced Migrants"). It argues for a mainstreaming of refugee health in country agendas, as well as strengthening capacity of host countries and the provision of evidence-based health services delivery models. With humanitarian crises becoming both more commonplace and increasingly protracted, it is important to understand how an integrated approach to healthcare can be made more effective, efficient and sustainable and how to mitigate for unintended consequences of this model. Innovative models for financing of service delivery are urgently needed to ensure adequate provision of healthcare to refugees outside of the traditional, short-term and camp-based approach and in order to optimise equitable access to healthcare among both host and refugee populations.

References

3RP. (2017). *Regional Refugee & Resilience Plan 2017-2018 - 2017 annual report.* Retrieved 10 September, 2018, from https://reliefweb.int/report/syrian-arab-republic/3rp-regional-refugee-and-resilience-plan-2017-2018-response-syria-0

3RP. (2019). *Turkey: 3RP country chapter - 2019/2020.* Retrieved 14 June, 2019, from https://reliefweb.int/report/turkey/turkey-3rp-country-chapter-20192020-entr

A. H. C. G. Report. (2016). *Syrian Refugees crisis impact on Lebanese Public Hospitals: Financial impact analysis: Generated problems and possible solutions.*

Akala, F. A., & El-Saharty, S. (2006). Public-health challenges in the Middle East and North Africa. *The Lancet, 367*, 961–964.

Ammar, W., Kdouh, O., Hammoud, R., Hamadeh, R., Harb, H., Ammar, Z., et al. (2016). Health system resilience: Lebanon and the Syrian refugee crisis. *Journal of Global Health, 6*, 020704.

APIS Health Consulting Group. (2016). *Syrian Refugees crisis impact on Lebanese Public Hospitals: Financial impact analysis: Generated problems and possible solutions.* Retrieved 9 May, 2019, from https://www.moph.gov.lb/en/Pages/127/9287/syrian-refugees-crisis-impact-on-lebanese-public-hospitals-financial-impact-analysis-apis-report

Blanchet, K., Fouad, F. M., & Pherali, T. (2016). Syrian refugees in Lebanon: The search for universal health coverage. *Conflict and Health, 10*, 12.

Chong, C. (2018). *Temporary protection: Its impact on healthcare for Syrian refugees in Turkey.* Oxford: Oxford University Press.

Dejong, J. (2017). Challenges to understanding the reproductive health needs of women forcibly displaced by the Syrian conflict. *The Journal of Family Planning and Reproductive Health Care, 43*, 103–104.

Dejong, J., Ghattas, H., Bashour, H., Mourtada, R., Akik, C., & Reese-Masterson, A. (2017). Reproductive, maternal, neonatal and child health in conflict: A case study on Syria using Countdown indicators. *BMJ Global Health, 2*, e000302.

European Council. (2019). *Supporting the future of Syria and the region - Brussels III conference, 1214/03/2019.* Retrieved 9 May 2019.

Glasier, A., Gulmezoglu, A. M., Schmid, G. P., Moreno, C. G., & Van Look, P. F. (2006). Sexual and reproductive health: A matter of life and death. *Lancet, 368*, 1595–1607.

Government of Lebanon & UN. (2018). *Lebanon crisis response plan 2017-2020* [Online]. Retrieved 20 September, 2018, from https://data2.unhcr.org/en/documents/download/63238

Government of Lebanon & UNHCR. (2017). *Lebanon crisis response plan (LCRP) 2017-2020.* Retrieved 8 July, 2018, from http://www.un.org.lb/lcrp2017-2020

Government of Lebanon & UNHCR. (2018). *Lebanon crisis response plan 2017-2020 (2018 update).* Retrieved 5 January, 2019, from https://reliefweb.int/report/lebanon/lebanon-crisis-response-plan-2017-2020-2018-update

Grollman, C., Arregoces, L., Martinez-Alvarez, M., Pitt, C., Mills, A., & Borghi, J. (2017). 11 years of tracking aid to reproductive, maternal, newborn, and child health: estimates and analysis for 2003-13 from the Countdown to 2015. *The Lancet Global Health, 5*, e104–e114.

Inter-Agency Coordination Lebanon. (2018). *Health dashboard Jan-April 2018.*

International Rescue Committee. (2014). *Emergency economies: The impact of cash assistance in Lebanon.*

Janmyr, M. (2018). UNHCR and the Syrian refugee response: negotiating status and registration in Lebanon. *The International Journal of Human Rights, 22*, 393–419.

John Hopkins University (JHU), M. D. M., International Medical Corps, Humanitarian Aid and Civil Protection, American University of Beirut and UNHCR. (2015). *Syrian refugee and affected host population health access survey in Lebanon.*

Kassak, K. M., Ghomrawi, H. M., Osseiran, A. M., & Kobeissi, H. (2006). The providers of health services in Lebanon: A survey of physicians. *Human Resources for Health, 4*, 4.

Kitamura, A., Jimba, M., Mccahey, J., Paolucci, G., Shah, S., Hababeh, M., et al. (2018). Health and dignity of Palestine refugees at stake: A need for international response to sustain crucial life services at UNRWA. *The Lancet, 392*, 2736–2744.

Lebanon Cash Consortium (LCC). (2016). *Impact evaluation of the multipurpose cash assistance programme.* Retrieved 10 September, 2018, from https://resourcecentre.savethechildren.net/library/impact-evaluation-multipurpose-cash-assistance-programme

Masterson, A. R., Usta, J., Gupta, J., & Ettinger, A. S. (2014). Assessment of reproductive health and violence against women among displaced Syrians in Lebanon. *BMC Women's Health, 14*, 25.

Ministry of Public Health (MPH) & WU. (2015). *Health: LCRP sector response plan.*

Ministry of Social Affairs Lebanon & UNHCR. (2018). *Lebanon crisis 2017-2020 (2018 update) response plan.* Retrieved from http://www.LCRP.gov.lb

Organisation for Economic Cooperation and Development. (2018). Paris, France. Retrieved 5 July, 2018, from https://stats.oecd.org/Index.aspx?DataSetCode=crs1

Pitt, C., Grollman, C., Martinez-Alvarez, M., Arregoces, L., & Borghi, J. (2018). Tracking aid for global health goals: a systematic comparison of four approaches applied to reproductive, maternal, newborn, and child health. *The Lancet Global Health, 6*, e859–e874.

Salti, N., Chaaban, J., & Raad, F. (2010). Health equity in Lebanon: A microeconomic analysis. *International Journal for Equity in Health, 9*, 11.

Samari, G. (2015). Syrian Refugee Women's Health needs in Lebanon, Turkey and Jordan and recommendations for improved practice. *World Medical & Health Policy, 9*(2), 255–274.

Sami, S., Williams, H. A., Krause, S., Onyango, M. A., Burton, A., & Tomczyk, B. (2014). Responding to the Syrian crisis: The needs of women and girls. *Lancet, 383*, 1179–1181.

Singh, N. S., Smith, J., Aryasinghe, S., Khosla, R., Say, L., & Blanchet, K. (2018). Evaluating the effectiveness of sexual and reproductive health services during humanitarian crises: A systematic review. *PLoS One, 13*, e0199300.

Syrian Refugees. (2014). Syrian health crisis in Lebanon. *Lancet, 383*, 1862.

UNDP & ARK. (2017). *Regular perception surveys on social tensions throughout Lebanon: Wave I*. Retrieved 10 December 2018.

UNFPA. (2018). *Regional situation report on Syria crisis, Issue No. 72, July–August 2018*. Geneva: UNFPA.

UNHCR. (2017a). *Global trends, forced displacement in 2017*. Retrieved 8 September, 2018, from http://www.unhcr.org/5b27be547.pdf

UNHCR. (2017b). *UNHCR warns funding cuts threaten aid to Syrian refugees, hosts*. Retrieved 9 September, 2018, from https://www.unhcr.org/uk/news/latest/2017/4/58e347288/unhcr-warns-funding-cuts-threaten-aid-syrian-refugees-hosts.html

UNHCR. (2017c). *Vulnerability assessment of Syrian Refugees in Lebanon 2017*. Retrieved 12 December, 2018, from https://reliefweb.int/report/lebanon/vasyr-2017-vulnerability-assessment-syrian-refugees-lebanon

UNHCR. (2018a). *Guidelines for referral health care in Lebanon: Standard operating procedures*. Retrieved https://data2.unhcr.org/es/documents/download/64586

UNHCR. (2018b). *Lebanon - Syria Regional Refugee response*. Retrieved 9 October, 2018, from https://data2.unhcr.org/en/situations/syria/location/71

UNHCR. (2018c). *Q&A on UNHCR emergency healthcare new coverage and on support for birth deliveries for refugees in Lebanon*. Retrieved https://www.refugees-lebanon.org/uploads/poster/poster_152993684592.pdf

UNHCR. (2019). *Uganda comprehensive refugee response portal*. Retrieved 14 June, 2019, from https://data2.unhcr.org/en/country/uga

United Nations. (2014). *Report of the secretary-general on women and peace and security*. Retrieved http://www.un.org/ga/search/view_doc.asp?symbol=S/2014/693

United Nations Refugees and Migrants (UNRM). (2017). *UNICEF-backed projects for millions of children in Syria on verge of being 'cut off'*. Retrieved 10 September, 2018, from https://refugeesmigrants.un.org/unicef-backed-projects-millions-children-syria-verge-being-cut

WHO. (2006). *Health action in crises: Lebanon*. Retrieved http://www.who.int/hac/crises/Lebanon_Aug06.pdf

World Bank. (2017). *The toll of war: The economic and social consequences of the conflict in Syria*. Washington DC: World Bank.

World Health Organization. (2019). *Promoting the health of refugees and migrants: Draft action plan, 2019–2023* [Online]. Retrieved from http://apps.who.int/gb/ebwha/pdf_files/WHA72/A72_25-en.pdf

Chapter 5
Health Financing for Asylum Seekers in Europe: Three Scenarios Towards Responsive Financing Systems

Louise Biddle, Philipa Mladovsky, and Kayvan Bozorgmehr

List of Abbreviations

EU   European Union
UHC   Universal Health Coverage
WHO   World Health Organization
UCL   University College London

Introduction

Europe has a long history of forced migration: both giving cause for flight and providing refuge for asylum seekers and refugees in numerous times of conflict in the past century. Since 2015, however, the issue has garnered sustained attention as the numbers of individuals seeking asylum within Europe have increased substantially. 3.7 million first-time applications for asylum have been registered in the 28 member states of the European Union (EU) since 2015, with Greece, Italy, and Spain repre-

L. Biddle (✉)
Department of General Practice and Health Services Research,
University Hospital Heidelberg, Heidelberg, Germany
e-mail: louise.biddle@med.uni-heidelberg.de

P. Mladovsky
Department of International Development, London School of Economics and Political
Science, London, UK
e-mail: p.mladovsky@lse.ac.uk

K. Bozorgmehr
Department of General Practice and Health Services Research, University Hospital
Heidelberg, Heidelberg, Germany

Department of Population Medicine and Health Services Research, School of Public Health,
Bielefeld University, Bielefeld, Germany
e-mail: kayvan.bozorgmehr@uni-bielefeld.de

© Springer Nature Switzerland AG 2020
K. Bozorgmehr et al. (eds.), *Health Policy and Systems Responses to Forced Migration*, https://doi.org/10.1007/978-3-030-33812-1_5

senting the most common entry points and Germany, France, and Greece being the most popular destination countries (Eurostat 2019). The EU is united by the principle of economic solidarity. Yet in the provision of funds for securing the health of asylum seekers, the burden still falls disproportionately on a few countries with already stretched financial systems.

This chapter will explore the possibilities for increased financial solidarity through the use of various financial mechanisms in the EU. We will start by looking at existing financial distribution mechanisms at a European level and current health financing models for asylum seekers in the EU. We will then present three scenarios for a more responsive financing system and discuss these in light of dominant political discourses of security, austerity, and eligibility.

Although the number of asylum seekers is dwarfed by the size of the refugee population in Middle Eastern countries such as Jordan, Lebanon, and Turkey, the political consequences of the recent population movements in Europe have made the issue a particularly salient one. This saliency is partly due to the uneven distribution of asylum seekers throughout Europe. As many asylum seekers from the Middle East and North Africa arrive on boat via the Mediterranean, coastal countries have become some of the largest hosts of asylum seekers within Europe. The Dublin agreement, which came into force in July 2013, upholds that asylum seekers must apply for asylum in the country within which they were first registered. Under its temporary relocation scheme starting in 2015, the European Commission has relocated several asylum seekers to countries such as the Czech Republic, Hungary, Poland, and Slovakia to alleviate some of the burden on arrival countries (European Parliament 2019). However, by March 2018, only 33,846 asylum seekers had been relocated, representing less than 1% of the total number of first-time applicants in the EU in the same period (European Parliament 2019). A comprehensive redistribution quota or a complete repeal of the Dublin agreement has fallen out of favour in the current political climate, as these ideas are superseded by issues of tightening control of the EU's external borders (Niemann and Zaun 2018).

The issue is further complicated by its timing: when the numbers of asylum seekers started increasing in 2013, many European countries were still reeling from the effects of the 2008/2009 financial crisis. Under the conditions of austerity, substantial cuts to social protection and public services were made in many affected countries, including education, social support, and public facilities but also health provision (Vasilopoulou et al. 2014; Legido-Quigley et al. 2013a; Thomson et al. 2015). It has been well documented that during this time, several affected countries became politically polarised, with the rise of new populist, right-wing movements rejecting internationalism and calling for increased restrictions to the free movement of people and goods within Europe (Inglehart and Norris 2016). This is in line with a long tradition of political analysis which has linked social inequality and populist movements (Golder 2016).

Thus, the same coastal countries that are the main countries of arrival for asylum seekers (Spain, Italy, and Greece) instituted severe financial austerity measures in order to comply with bailout demands (Kentikelenis et al. 2014). This had substantial effects on access to healthcare, as several countries decreased healthcare coverage and/or instituted (higher) user fees as part of the austerity package (Kentikelenis et al. 2014; Legido-Quigley et al. 2013a), as can be seen in the example of Spain (Box 5.1). This affected both migrants and the resident population. The potential costs of migrants to the national healthcare system have frequently been used in populist rhetoric as a reason for restricting entitlements and have led to a tightening of restrictions, for example, in Germany since the early 1990s (Pross 1998). The economic argument, and the lack of the European community to systematically address financing issues, has therefore added fuel to populist debates and acted to further drive divisions between those perceived as "deserving" and "not deserving" healthcare entitlements (also see Chap. 11 "Discrimination as a Health Systems Response to Forced Migration").

Box 5.1 Restrictions to Healthcare Under Austerity in Spain

The Spanish health system has a tradition of being very liberal and accessible. The right to equal access to healthcare for all with an "established" residence in the country, irrespective of citizenship, is anchored in the General Health Law of 1986 and has been reinforced in a number of reforms throughout the 2000s (Legido-Quigley et al. 2018). These migrant-friendly reforms established Spain as one of the few countries in the world with universal health coverage.

In 2012, however, the Royal Decree Law 1192/2012 undertook drastic changes to the Spanish healthcare system, replacing the National Health Service with a social health insurance system (Legido-Quigley et al. 2013b). The Spanish government stated at the time that public spending cuts, which also affected other sectors, were necessary to curtail spending in the aftermath of the financial crisis (Legido-Quigley et al. 2013b). These reforms expressly excluded undocumented migrants from comprehensive care, granting access only to emergency, maternity, and paediatric services. It has been estimated that some 500,000 undocumented migrants in Spain lost their health insurance as a result (Legido-Quigley et al. 2013a). In addition, increased co-payments for services and medications as well as the increased privatisation of medical services placed additional burdens on migrants and citizens alike. Although asylum seekers were still formally entitled to the same benefits as nationals, the introduction of the social health insurance system introduced additional bureaucratic hurdles to accessing care. The national non-profit organisation Accem reports that some asylum seekers were denied access because healthcare providers were not familiar with the new rules and regulations (European Council on Refugees and Exiles (ECRE) 2019).

Mounting pressure on the Spanish government led to a partial repeal of the 2012 Royal Decree in 2018, and undocumented migrants' right to universal healthcare has been reinstated (European Council on Refugees and Exiles (ECRE) 2019). However, the future of the Spanish health system is unclear as the political situation remains contested.

In principle, all member states of the European Union subscribe to the principles of Universal Health Coverage (UHC), which ensures that "all people and communities can use the […] health services they need, […] while also ensuring these services do not expose the user to financial hardship" (World Health Organization 2019). However, both the austerity cuts introduced after the economic crisis and the increased numbers of asylum seekers entering Europe have demonstrated that UHC is not always an achievable or desirable objective for national governments. The Refugee Convention (1951) and the International Covenant on Economic, Social and Cultural Rights (1966) state that all individuals should have access to required healthcare services regardless of legal status (UN Committee on Economic Social and Cultural Rights (CESCR) 2000). However, in European law, this principle (equal treatment as nationals) has been translated for recognised refugees only (da Costa 2006), often leaving individuals seeking asylum and undocumented migrants with lower levels of entitlements to healthcare (Fig. 5.1).

Out of the 28 EU member states, 13 provide the same coverage to asylum seekers as to nationals, and 14 other member states have some restrictions in place, while one member state provides only emergency care (Abubakar et al. 2018). Even in those countries in which full coverage is granted, some countries require means testing ($n = 3$), require co-payments ($n = 3$), or are linked to residence in state

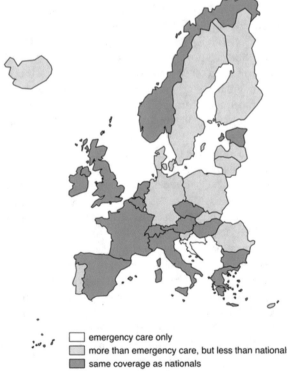

Fig. 5.1 Healthcare entitlements for asylum seekers across the European Union. Source: own illustration of data provided by Abubakar et al. (2018)

☐ emergency care only
☐ more than emergency care, but less than nationals
■ same coverage as nationals

accommodation ($n = 5$) (Abubakar et al. 2018). While these figures apply to individuals formally applying for asylum, the coverage for undocumented migrants is often much worse, as was in the case of Spain (Box 5.1). But even if access is granted legally, a number of financial, bureaucratic, knowledge, and language barriers may prevent access to health services being realised for asylum seekers and refugees (Bradby et al. 2015). In order to increase access for asylum seekers to essential health services, a responsive health financing system would incentivise the removal of barriers and the provision of appropriate care for this population.

Existing Health Financing Mechanisms

To put potential financing mechanisms into context, it is worth exploring first what a "good" health financing system looks like. As defined by the World Health Organization (WHO), health financing systems have three primary functions (revenue collection, pooling, and purchasing) and three primary goals under UHC (utilisation relative to need, quality, and universal financial protection) (Kutzin 2013). In order to meet these goals, Kutzin (2013) defines three key intermediate objectives for universal health coverage (Fig. 5.2), which can be considered as principles of good practice for any health financing system. Firstly, the financing system must ensure equity in resource distribution, which includes both equity in revenue collection (i.e., progressivity of the financing system) and providing incentives for equity in access. Secondly, the financing system must promote technical, bureaucratic, and allocative efficiency (Cylus et al. 2017). In the purchasing of health services, the financing system will be efficient by obtaining value for money for the invested resources (including quantity and quality of services), for example, through health technology assessments or adequate provider payment mechanisms. However, the financing system can also demonstrate efficiency in pooling by using insurance

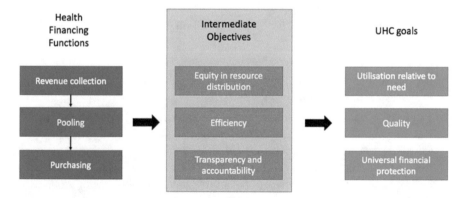

Fig. 5.2 Intermediate objectives of health financing systems. Source: own illustration, adapted from Kutzin (2013)

schemes with large risk pools, thus lowering the risk of the group, leading to lower contributions and a more efficient investment for each individual. Finally, transparency and accountability of the system should be encouraged both by helping individuals understand their rights and entitlements and increasing the accountability of health financing institutions.

Current Health Financing for Refugees: Brief Overview of EU Country Policies

Very few studies to date have examined the financing arrangements for health provision for asylum seekers and refugees across the European region. However, existing studies have shown a high degree of fragmentation of financing sources in arrival, transit, and receiving countries (Bozorgmehr et al. 2018a).

A scoping study of six European member states finds that they can be divided into those who include asylum seekers in existing social health insurance or general taxation schemes and those who have specific ring-fenced budgets held by the ministry of health or the ministry of the interior. Some governments additionally rely on short-term funding from humanitarian agencies or non-governmental organisations (Bozorgmehr et al. 2018a). This pattern is likely to be extended across the European region, with governments using multiple funding mechanisms so help support the additional costs of newly arriving asylum seekers.

It is difficult to say, without further information, whether the current financing mechanisms adhere to the principles of "good" financing systems outlined above. However, the case of Germany (Box 5.2) shows how decentralised financing mechanisms, which are not integrated into existing health financing structures, can lead to problems with equity in resource distribution, efficiency, and transparency. Financial mechanisms operating independently for the group of asylum seekers are likely to suffer from problems related to small financial pools, lack of integration into national payment structures, and revenue collection in already stretched health and social care budgets for those countries operating under conditions of austerity.

Box 5.2 Fragmentation of the Health Financing Landscape for Asylum Seekers and Refugees in Germany

The German healthcare system is a statutory social health insurance system with an opt-out option to private health insurance, characterised by strong fragmentation and decentralisation. In the 1990s, the Asylum Seekers' Benefits Act established a financing system for asylum seekers parallel to the healthcare system of the general population. The financing of health services is strongly linked to the asylum process with shared responsibilities between authorities at different levels of administration. During their stay at one or more state-level reception centres, the state-level authorities cover the costs of health screening and health assessments as well as individual medical care. Dispersal between and within the 16 federal states at the level of reception centres is common, leading to different authorities in charge to cover costs. Once asylum seekers reach their designated state, they are dispersed to one of the 412 districts, cities, and communities which in most cases are the designated authority to cover incurring healthcare costs.

Services provided at the population level in the context of hygiene and prevention and control of notifiable infectious diseases are financed by local public health offices. Further cost bearers, such as social health insurance, play a role depending on residence status, duration of residence, and employment status (Bozorgmehr et al. 2018b). A mixed-method evaluation of the health system response in 2015 (Bozorgmehr et al. 2016) showed that in some cases, there were indications of authorities in charge deliberately delaying delivery of needed health services, such as vaccination of the arriving population and health assessments, with the rationale that individuals would soon be dispersed to other states or districts who would then be in charge of covering costs.

Evaluations of notifiable diseases among asylum seekers (2002–2014) show that incident infections were mainly due to vaccine-preventable conditions, providing evidence of insufficient implementation of vaccination programs (Kuhne and Gilsdorf 2016). While it is hard to determine at the national level the extent to which the financing system contributed to the weak vaccination coverage, it can be argued that it incentivised a "watch and wait" behaviour which was beneficial to the local budget as long as there was no outbreak. Similar situations are observed in the health assessments: when asylum seekers are assigned to another state before undergoing their health assessment, assessments may not be performed in the first federal state as costs would burden the local budget. As such, the lack of timely health assessment (Bozorgmehr et al. 2016) and the lack of concrete regulations in state-level policies regarding the timing of the health assessment (Wahedi et al. 2017) may be a result of a financial disincentive to provide timely care.

Within the schematic laid out in the chapter by Spiegel and colleagues (see Chap. 3 "Innovative Humanitarian Health Financing for Refugees"; Table 3.2), shifting the health financing debate from the national to the supranational level would have several benefits. Akin to shifting from a *risk retention* to a *risk transfer* model, we can consider shifting the financing debate to a European level, that is, transferring financial risk from the host countries to another entity (viz. the EU). In doing so, the size of the financial pool could be substantially increased, thus alleviating the financial burden on those countries receiving the largest number of migrants. This in turn could provide incentives to increase access to appropriate care for this population, as well as instating clear and transparent processes by which revenue is collected and funds are distributed among member states. A larger risk pool also means that crisis planning can be carried out with greater accuracy, allowing for innovative *ex ante* financing mechanisms, rather than relying entirely on *ex post* instruments.

Relevant European Health Financing Mechanisms

Several mechanisms currently exist at the European level to redistribute funds for refugees, asylum seekers, and migrants. These include four funds set up by the European Commission, as well as the European Health Insurance Card scheme. However, these mechanisms currently do not address the specific requirements of redistributing funds for the protection of asylum seekers' right to health.

The Asylum, Migration and Integration Fund has been instituted specifically to support member states accepting a large number of migrants, including asylum seekers, with regard to their asylum process, integration, and potential resettlement. The fund was set up in 2014 and runs for 7 years, replacing several funds which had previously been in place under the "Solidarity and Management of Migration Flows" programme. Initially, €3.137 billion were dedicated to the fund, which was increased to €6.894 billion in light of the increased number of asylum seekers during 2015 and 2016 (Directorate-General for Migration and Home Affairs (European Commission) 2018). All EU member states can apply for the fund by proposing specific project plans in line with stated objectives of the fund, one of which was to strengthen a common European asylum system. Member states are required to contribute 10% of the specified project budget, the remaining 90% being contributed by the fund. The fund specifies several regulation measures for national programmes, including audits, reports, and a midterm review to assess implementation and adjust budgeted funds if necessary (Directorate-General for Migration and Home Affairs (European Commission) 2018).

Two further project-based funds which have supported health and employment initiatives, the Health Programme and European Social Fund, have recently been joined with several other small funds under the new programme European Social Fund Plus. This is intended to strengthen the EU's response to crisis, strengthen health systems, support EU legislation on public health and implementation of best practices (European Commission 2018). Beneficiaries of this programme include national health authorities, public and private bodies, international organisations, and non-governmental organisations, which need to propose projects in line with the fund's objectives.

While these funds address some of the key social and structural determinants of health, none of them cover the financing of frontline healthcare services for the asylum-seeking population. This means that national governments are required to finance service provision, with no method for redistribution at a European level. Given the lack of European solidarity in this matter, national governments have no financial incentive to provide equitable entitlements to asylum seekers or provide high-quality services for this population. Furthermore, the efficiency of the pro-grammes is hampered by the long timescales of the project grants, which usually cover 6 to 7 years and have a lengthy application process. This reflects their aim of supporting long-term structural development. However, it means they are not respon-sive to the short-term changes in the numbers of or the composition of individuals in need of care which affects frontline service provision. A sustainable health financing mechanism for service provision requires balancing long-term financial support with responsive, transparent adjustments to the funding schedule on a shorter timescale. With regard to the more general health system improvement grants, the project-based funds represent an opportunity to shift towards migrant-friendly health sys-tems by specifically addressing issues of crucial importance to refugee health, such as migrant-sensitive health monitoring, staffing, and service provision.

One of the funds that has previously supported the establishment of frontline health services is the emergency support provided by the European Civil Protection and Humanitarian Aid Operations (Civil protection and Humanitarian Aid Operations (European Commission) 2018). This emergency support was adopted in 2016 in the wake of sharply rising refugee numbers and has since supported the establishment of essential services. In Greece, the EU dedicated 643 million euro to support emergency support operation, including housing, healthcare, and hygiene infrastructure. This fund is a typical *ex post* financing mechanism, providing funds after the catastrophe has hit. It has been sharply criticised for failing to alleviate the situation for asylum seekers in Greece and suffering from issues of misallocated funds, lack of planning, and corruption (Leape 2018). Thus, while the distribution of funds through the EU has the potential to offer more transparency, this is not a given. Indeed, it may be particularly difficult to achieve in *ex post* humanitarian aid, where the crisis situation results in untransparent procedures and a lack of regula-tory oversight (Maxwell et al. 2012).

Finally, only one *ex ante* European health financing scheme does not rely on project-based funding. However, it does not cover asylum seekers and refugees. The European Health Insurance Scheme ensures that citizens of EU member states can access public healthcare in any EU member state for temporary visits. Through the European Health Insurance Card, individuals are able to receive the same service package abroad as they would have been provided in their home country, if avail-able. The costs can be claimed either by the member state in which treatment occurs or by the individual. In 2015, 91% of paid claims were issued by member states, demonstrating a high degree of integration of the reimbursement mechanism into existing financial systems (Directorate-General for Employment Social Affairs and Inclusion (European Commission) 2016). This scheme benefits from efficiency in process: funds go directly to frontline service providers rather than passing through the multiple hands of national and regional governments. Furthermore, it promotes equity in treatment as providers can claim the same costs for foreigners from within the EU as they can for nationals, especially when the process is well integrated and reimbursement is timely. Significant effort has gone into making the system trans-parent, by educating both patients and service providers about the rights and entitle-ments of EU citizens in a different member state (Directorate-General for Employment Social Affairs and Inclusion (European Commission) 2016).

In summary, the current funding mechanisms in the European region may offer support to tackle the social and structural determinants of ill health for migrants, but they only offer solutions to support frontline health services in emergency situations. The burden of financing currently lies on national governments, who have largely instituted parallel financing schemes or in some cases have restricted access to services out of fear for the financial burden. There are no Europe-wide financing mechanisms which offer a long-term solution to the problem to an uneven health burden on member states which is responsive to future changes in the number and composition of asylum seekers. Yet the number of asylum seekers and migrants to the European Union is not expected to cease.

In the following section, we explore what a responsive health financing system for asylum seekers, guided by the principles of "good" health financing systems, may look like at a European level. In doing so, we make two key assumptions: first, that there is political will for the principles of UHC and for European solidarity on the issue of forced migration. Although the political climate on the issue between member states is strained, there is reason to believe that the benefits of a European financing scheme would encourage member states bearing the financial burden for asylum seekers' healthcare to build alliances and lobby for change. Second, we assume that sufficient funding is available, or can be raised additionally, for the European budget to support either subsidies or full provision of healthcare by member states. The previous chapter by Spiegel and colleagues (see Chap. 3 "Innovative Humanitarian Health Financing for Refugees") has shown that several financing mechanisms are available which could raise additional funds. Furthermore, the current evidence suggests that funds in refugee health are often used inefficiently, and substantial additional funds could be made available by incentivising and increasing access to essential primary healthcare services (Bozorgmehr and Razum 2015) or avoiding securitisation of health issues (Wahedi et al. 2017) (see also Chap. 7 "Health Security in the Context of Forced Migration"). How and whether these assumptions may hold in each of the three presented scenarios will be discussed in more detail later.

Scenarios for Responsive Financing of Healthcare for Asylum Seekers in Europe

We present three scenarios for responsive financing of healthcare for asylum seekers in Europe. In line with the observations made by Spiegel and colleagues (see Chap. 3 "Innovative Humanitarian Health Financing for Refugees"), these require a shift from *ex post* donations to *ex ante* planning to enable the establishment of sustainable and reliable financing structures. Thus, we consider three mechanisms in the bottom left quadrant of Spiegel and colleagues' classification of financing instruments: traditional insurance, indexed insurance, and contingency pooled funds.

Scenario 1: European Health Insurance for Refugees (Traditional Insurance)

In our first scenario, we consider the opportunities of a comprehensive supranational health insurance programme for asylum seekers. Analogous to the EHIC system for citizens of the European Union, asylum seekers would receive a European health insurance card with which they can access healthcare services in all member states of the European Union according to the respective entitlements of the country's general population in line with the right to health requirements (non-differential treatment based on residence status) (UN Committee on Economic Social and Cultural Rights (CESCR) 2000). However, instead of providers claiming to the national governments of the nation states of the migrants, they claim directly to a large, central European healthcare fund. In practice, this represents a subsidy of the EU to national health systems, as the funds directly flow to the settings of service provision.

Such a system has several benefits. It works within the multiplicity of health systems of the EU and requires no special adaptation of the health system for refugees. This means that asylum seekers can be embedded in existing financing mechanisms without the need to set up parallel budgets for healthcare provision for this population. It guarantees financial protection for host countries, alleviating fears around the reception of asylum seekers on the grounds of healthcare costs. It removes the financial incentive to limit entitlements as costs are covered through EU funds. It also provides a flexible framework which accounts for individuals moving across multiple national or regional borders without the need for further shifting of budgets. It thus gives a financial baseline for an equitable health protection for asylum seekers throughout Europe, making it easier for host states to provide actualised equity through the accessibility of the health system, responsiveness of services, and the removal of other barriers to care for this population.

In addition, there are several financial incentives provided by such a system which makes a European healthcare fund attractive. The existence of a standardised financing mechanism allows for harmonisation of routine data collection mechanisms among asylum seekers across countries, which are currently either excluded from such data collection systems or integrated in systems which lack international comparability and interoperability (see also Chap. 9 "The State of the Art and the Evidence on Health Records for Migrants and Refugees: Findings from a Systematic Review"). This may improve optimisation of service delivery and, ideally, translate into more effective care. A major strength would be that it incentivises the—yet poorly implemented—identification of healthcare needs and vulnerabilities in line with the EU directive on the reception of refugees (European Parliament 2013), as EU-level structures pay for the costs of care without burdening the "own" (national or subnational) budget.

However, several important considerations need to be made before implementing such a financing mechanism. First off, there is the question of the timing of the scheme: when are asylum seekers formally covered by the insurance scheme, and when is the financial responsibility for healthcare conferred to member states? Countries have varying legal processes around the asylum process and the question remains whether the scheme should only cover asylum seekers once a formal claim has been made, or once the intent of claiming has been voiced, either in the hosting country or in transit. The length of the asylum process also varies substantially between states, and an insurance scheme may introduce a financial incentive to extend this period if coverage is provided indefinitely during the process. It seems sensible to set such a limit to the insurance fund at 6 months after an asylum claim has been made—the recommended maximum time in which asylum proceedings should be concluded (European Council on Refugees and Exiles (ECRE) 2016)—with a further 6 months as a potential phase-out period where claims are partly covered. To prevent artificially prolonging an individual's asylum application, all newly arriving asylum seekers' healthcare costs should be covered for the period of 6 + 6 months, irrespective of legal status. A European insurance scheme therefore has the potential to act as a *bonus malus* incentive, where member states are encouraged to complete the asylum case within 12 months, before healthcare costs are transferred to national budgets. However, it needs to be ensured that the entitlements conferred by the insurance scheme are subsequently provided by the member states, even if the asylum process is not yet complete, so no gap in healthcare access is created. Similar considerations need to be made with regard to the population group covered (i.e. formal asylum seekers vs. irregular migrants) and the providers that are able to make claims through this scheme, acknowledging that in many countries, healthcare for asylum seekers is provided by a variety of actors, including non-governmental, charity, and for-profit organisations alongside public provision arrangements.

The introduction of such a scheme at the European level has benefits in terms of the sheer size of the insurance pool but also has drawbacks relating to the potential bureaucracy required to make it work. There is a large potential for high transaction costs in making and processing the claims made by the host countries at a European level, which could delay repayments and decrease the efficiency of the scheme. The successful integration of the EHIC scheme in national financing systems has shown, however, that efficient, expedient, and unbureaucratic claims processing is possible (Directorate-General for Employment Social Affairs and Inclusion (European Commission) 2016).

Finally, there is substantial financial risk involved in the first years following the introduction of the scheme. Due to the lack of routine data for asylum seekers currently utilising health services in Europe, estimations of the possible costs of such a scheme would have to be made with large margins for error. This financial risk is wholly conferred to EU budgets under an insurance scheme and thus requires significant political will from member states. However, increasing access to primary health services under the insurance scheme may even reduce the costs of service provisions overall, as costly specialist and emergency care is avoided (Starfield et al. 2005). Furthermore, net receiving countries will benefit substantially as the risk of financial expenditure is shifted from a national to a supranational budget. Based on the improved data collected through the insurance scheme, adjustments can be made over time to the relative and absolute contribution by member states.

Scenario 2: Refugee Health Budget (Indexed Insurance)

A second option for a redistribution of available resources at a European level would be the institution of a refugee health budget. In contrast to an individual insurance scheme, the budget could "top up" member states' health budgets based on the size and composition of their asylum-seeking population. In contrast to other EU funding mechanisms, it would need to provide funds on a more short-term (e.g. yearly) basis if it is to adequately address the rapidly changing number of and composition in the asylum-seeking population in the member states, and funds must go directly to the financing of frontline services.

A specifically allocated budget has the benefit that it is paid for in advance with a predefined budget size. The specified revenue is pooled from member states' contributions and ring-fenced for the use in health services for asylum seekers. It could, therefore, act as a security blanket for member states in terms of their health expenditure while still protecting the EU budget from financial risk. As the fund is capped, it could not cover the entirety of healthcare spending for member states, leaving these partly responsible for the financing of healthcare services. However, funds could act as a buffer in times of increased in-migration, so that sustainable, long-term financing solutions can be found going forward.

However, such a scheme would also require a discussion of some key considerations before it could be implemented. A key question for consideration is how the budget would be allocated. A fair mechanism would be to link this to the distribution of asylum seekers across the European region. To be equitable in terms of health, however, the allocation would also need to consider the composition of the asylum-seeking population in terms of age, sex, socio-economic status, country of origin, etc.—as proxies for a differential distribution of health risk (Bozorgmehr and Wahedi 2017). Such risk equalisation models have been implemented in several national health insurance systems as a means to increase efficiency and equity of systems facing unequal distributions of risk in the insurance pool (Van de Ven 2011). Unfortunately, required information is usually not generally reliable, if available at all. Thus, member states may only be eligible for participation in the advance risk equalisation scheme if migrant-sensitive data collection mechanisms are strengthened; or else they will receive only post hoc funds as a lump sum based on generic data such as the number of asylum seekers and age/sex distribution. This would be a large drawback for member states as they do not have a concrete figure with which to plan service delivery.

Furthermore, a key consideration is how such a fund would be governed. The fund does not, as with a traditional insurance mechanism, ensure that the money is spent for on-the-ground services. Instead, it relies on the existence of specified budgets for healthcare services for asylum seekers and clear plans for service delivery. However, the way in which healthcare for this population is financed differs markedly between member states, so the question becomes how the allocation of funds for asylum seekers' health can be ensured. In scenario1, considerations regarding the timing of the scheme, migrant groups covered, and type of provider reimbursed are explicitly linked to the release of funds. With a refugee health budget, however, these details can only be implicitly specified but essentially remain at the discretion of member states. Such issues require additional governance and legal arrangements to ensure funds are well spent while acknowledging that countries have different institutional arrangements which must be respected.

Finally, because a refugee health budget for health leaves some of the financial risk with member states, the incentive for increasing access to health services is less strong than it would be under an insurance scheme. Working with a refugee health budget therefore requires political negotiations regarding the size of the benefit package, degree of out-of-pocket-payments, and the population covered if the stipulation of equal treatment for asylum seekers and the general population are to be upheld. Given the current political climate in the European Union, the political will for taking on additional financial responsibilities through the provision of additional services for asylum seekers is likely to be weak, despite the potential reprise from an EU refugee health budget. Thus, the financial certainty of such a scheme potentially comes at the cost of less certainty regarding the equitable treatment of persons across Europe.

Scenario 3: Refugee Health Emergency Fund (Contingency Pooled Funds)

Finally, a third option for the redistribution of funds would be the extension of the current EU emergency funds to specifically cover asylum seekers' health. As with the refugee health budget, this fund would consist of a predefined, ring-fenced budget to be allocated to member states in times of health emergencies. In contrast to the health budget, however, it would not be automatically distributed every year or so based on an allocation formula. Instead, the budget is intended to provide support to member states in times of emergency, as laid down in clear, predefined criteria.

It could be argued that such a mechanism provides the least support to member states and thus provides the least incentives to increase access to full healthcare coverage for asylum seekers. However, it leaves member states in the knowledge that there are additional funds to fall back on if unprecedented costs in the health systems arise due to increased numbers of asylum seekers and thus gives more certainty to provide full access or at least preserve current coverage should numbers of asylum applicants rise again.

Using project-based funds would allow for additional contextual factors, including the intersection with other political, economic, social, or environmental challenges, to be taken into account. It does, however, also render the process much more subjective and prone to political influence and may only function on longer financing timescales due to the delayed release of funds through the application process.

In order to alleviate noted issues with the existing emergency fund, the governance and accountability of the refugee health emergency fund would need to be strengthened. This could be achieved by setting clear eligibility criteria, as well as specifying achievable goals which promote the equity and efficiency of healthcare services for asylum seekers in receiving countries. For example, subsequent rounds of funding could be made dependent on the achievement of specified goals and ongoing qualitative and quantitative evaluations of fund expenditures (Maxwell et al. 2012). However, increasing the efficiency and transparency of how funds are spent locally may come at the cost of increased central overheads for the management and processing of grant applications, monitoring and evaluation, and project management support for receiving countries.

Critical Reflections on Practicability and Feasibility of the Scenarios

We have presented three scenarios implementing the proposed financing mechanisms from Spiegel and colleagues in a European context. The proposed schemes have the potential to increase the responsiveness of refugee health financing at a European level to the needs of both member states and the asylum seekers themselves. However, the question remains whether these arrangements are practically possible, politically feasible, and financially realistic. In order to answer these questions, we will begin by reflecting on the three scenarios in terms of their ability to meet the intermediate objectives of financing systems (Fig. 5.2), before discussing their practical and political implications.

Adherence to Principles of "Good" Financing Systems

Each of the three scenarios presented demonstrates different properties with regard to their ability to achieve equity in resource distribution, efficiency, as well as transparency and accountability, ultimately affecting the utilisation relative to need, quality of care, and universal financial protection of the health system (Fig. 5.2).

In terms of equity, all three financing mechanisms demonstrate equity in revenue collection: revenues are taken from the contributions made by member states, with disproportionally larger contributions made by the wealthier economies. In terms of redistribution of funds, all scenarios presented operate on the principle of a redistribution of funds to those countries receiving the largest numbers of asylum seekers, additionally considering the composition of the population. However, while in all three scenarios distribution equity is ensured for the size and composition of the asylum-seeking population, in scenario 1 and 2, this does not factor in the countries' ability, i.e. their resilience (see also Chap. 6 "Understanding the Resilience of

Health Systems"), to cope with the newly arriving asylum seekers. Thus, allocation of funds for Germany or Sweden, for example, would be carried out just the same as in Italy or Greece, even though their resilience in the face of increased asylum seekers may be quite different. In scenario 3, in contrast, these contextual factors could be taken into account.

Furthermore, the presented scenarios differ in the incentives they give for providing equity in access. It could be argued that these incentives are strongest in scenario 1. As all costs incurred in the provision of care for asylum seekers are covered by the EU insurance pool in this scenario, governments would be encouraged financially to increase entitlements for asylum seekers to match those of the resident population. In scenarios 2 and 3, however, potential equity issues need to be explicitly mitigated. In scenario 3, the strength of incentives depends on the grant structure and the quality of auditing and evaluation processes. In scenario 2, the funding mechanism alone provides arguably the least strong incentives for equity in access to care, as funds are distributed based on a redistribution formula irrespective of local arrangements. In these scenarios, and depending on how comprehensive the scheme is, improving access to healthcare for asylum seekers may actually create inequity in favour of asylum seekers in countries where access to healthcare is limited for the resident population (e.g. Greece). If the specified budget for healthcare is small, on the other hand, this may have no impact on equity, despite the best governance efforts. Furthermore, the pitfalls of specifying a "minimum benefit package" must be acknowledged, which may actually be less comprehensive than what was previously provided, and could thus harm equity as well as quality of care. However, a health budget or emergency fund may provide an additional argument to push for increased equity in access in bilateral and multilateral negotiations, especially if these are supported by strong institutions and governance arrangements.

Turning to the efficiency of the financing system, all three scenarios benefit from the additional technical efficiency gains made through risk pooling at a European level. At the same time, this must be balanced with the potential administrative inefficiencies arising as the result of a centralised management of funds. It could be argued that these are least troubling in scenario 2; as long as adequate information on the size and composition of the refugee population are available, distribution could occur with very little additional managerial burden. In scenario 1, administrative efficiency losses could be minimised if reimbursement mechanisms are well integrated in national financing structures and clear processes have been set up to enable healthcare providers to make claims. The initial evaluation of the EHIC has shown that this is possible (Directorate-General for Employment Social Affairs and Inclusion (European Commission) 2016). Arguably the largest bureaucratic investments would need to be made in scenario 3, the health emergency fund, if it is to support the delivery of effective care in a transparent fashion.

Not only the efficiency of central management, but also of the funds reaching frontline services (allocative efficiency) must be considered. While scenario 1 allows for funds to directly reach the providers of frontline services, with the potential to directly improve quality of care on the ground by linking reimbursement to quality standards and clinical guidelines, scenarios 2 and 3 rely on the existence of good national service delivery plans and efficient local financing arrangements and in absence of these entail the risk of misuse or ineffective use of funds. The allocative efficiency of scenario 1 could be harmed, however, if the insurance scheme promotes moral hazard on the supply or the demand side, for example, through supplier-induced demand or unnecessary utilisation among the asylum-seeking populations. Policy options to counter this issue, including co-payments for specific services or a combination of insurance with global budgets, should be explored (Mossialos et al. 2002). Furthermore, current practices which are not supported by available evidence, such as the indiscriminate screening of newly arriving asylum seekers for rare infectious illnesses (Bozorgmehr et al. 2017)—a practice which has arisen out of fear of immigrants as "carriers" of dangerous epidemics—should be discouraged to maintain the efficiency of the financing schemes and avoid driving up costs for all member states.

Finally, in terms of transparency and accountability, all three scenarios have the potential to provide asylum seekers with an increased understanding of their rights and entitlements to healthcare. However, only scenario 1 provides specific incentives to do so, as member states benefit directly if asylum seekers' care is financed through the European insurance scheme rather than by national budgets. This could directly improve the responsiveness, or non-technical quality of care, of healthcare services (also see Chap. 12 "Health Systems Responsiveness to the Mental Health Needs of Forcibly Displaced Persons"). Scenario 1 also maximises the accountability of financing institutions, as all transaction can be tracked and monitored, potentially exposing fraudulent of inefficient spending, as well as large, unexplained spending discrepancies between member states. In the other two scenarios, accurate monitoring and evaluation mechanisms with regular, transparent reporting would be required to increase accountability and could also be used to ensure eligibility of member states to receive funds.

Practical and Political Implications

Reforming financing systems in Europe to support responsive and equitable healthcare services for asylum seekers requires political will. In order to push for change, those countries which could benefit from the proposed financing mechanisms need to form coalitions to support financial reform. During renegotiations of the Dublin agreement, we saw how difficult it can be to make progress regarding European asylum policies, with those countries in disfavour of alternatives to Dublin gaining the upper hand and pushing instead for stronger political support to secure the EU's external borders (Niemann and Zaun 2018). However, even if the arrival of asylum seekers now occurs on a somewhat smaller scale, current numbers are not expected to cease. Therefore, as the UCL-Lancet Commission on Migration and Health has noted, a discussion needs to take place on the future of national health systems given the reality of increased human mobility across geopolitical borders (Abubakar et al. 2018). What do health systems beyond geopolitical borders look like? What regulatory and governance mechanisms need to be instituted to protect the health of mobile populations? In this chapter, we have provided three options to move towards an international health system, outlining some of the key financial considerations at stake.

On a political level, there is some cause to believe that a financing reform would enjoy greater support than renegotiations of the Dublin agreement. A financing reform would benefit politically powerful member states with many asylum seekers, such as Germany and Sweden, just as it would benefit Mediterranean receiving countries. Arguably, scenario 1 is the most radical reform presented here, requiring a lot of upfront political and technical effort. However, it has several advantages such as flexibility across borders and direct investment in frontline services which make it particularly attractive from a sustainability perspective. Once integrated in current national financing systems, the scheme could work very efficiently. However, the idea may encounter political opposition due to the different health systems the scheme would need to cover. Because health systems across the European region have developed quite differently, with different service configurations, technological developments, payment mechanisms, and entitlements, they are likely to incur varying costs which may cause tensions at a European level if the scheme is perceived not as a subsidy for the healthcare of asylum seekers but instead for the relatively more "expensive" health systems themselves. Within countries, these issues are often addressed through the use of Diagnosis-Related Groups (DRGs), which ensure that treatments for specified illnesses have the same costs despite being carried out in different districts or regions. However, extrapolating this mechanism across national boundaries could be substantially more complicated given different pricing regulations, organisational structures, and health service arrangements. Other supranational financing mechanisms, such as the remuneration of UN staff in countries with different costs of living, have circumvented these problems using weighted contributions. A similar scheme may work in this context to alleviate subsidy concerns. Currently, the overall cost of a comprehensive health insurance scheme is unknown, which may be another factor hindering the implementation of scenario 1. Modelling studies to estimate the overall costs of such a scheme based on the demographic of this population and epidemiological data should be performed in the future to facilitate and inform policy discourses regarding the feasibility an implementation of such a scheme. If scenario 1 is not politically possible, scenarios 2 and 3 represent viable alternative options, but with lower potential impacts on health equity and drawbacks on accountability. These two options could also be helpfully used in conjunction, by providing members states with a needs-adjusted fund to support frontline services (scenario 2) as well as providing emergency relief to those countries showing less resilience in the face of rising numbers of asylum seekers (scenario 3). Since these funds are based on existing European financing schemes, they may require less political will to actualise.

Furthermore, it must be noted that responsive financing reforms for the healthcare of asylum seekers cannot act as a panacea for the failings of the Dublin agreement. Even with sufficient financial resources, leaving the fate of refugees in Europe to a few European member states puts these under substantial economic, infrastructural, and political strain. On the other hand, if Dublin was replaced—either with a quota system or one of free choice of asylum claim (Bozorgmehr and Wahedi 2017)—the issue of responsive financing would not be solved. The alternatives to the Dublin agreement do not necessarily ensure that the burden of health would be evenly distributed among member states, and the problem of individuals seeking care in multiple countries would remain. Thus, the same considerations must be made regarding responsive health financing for asylum seekers at a European level.

This chapter has focused on the financing of services for formal asylum seekers. However, a 2008 estimate suggests that between 1.9 and 3.8 million irregular migrants reside in the European Union (Kraler and Rogoz 2011), a figure which is likely to have increased in recent years. Thus, it is worth exploring the impact of the presented scenarios on the equity of service provision for this group of migrants in the future.

Finally, the political and ideological dimension of healthcare restrictions must be acknowledged. Although the rise of populism can be attributed, in part, to concerns of social and economic inequality, addressing solely the financing dimension of the current refugee debate will not reshape populist discourse. Political and ideological conceptions about refugees, their reasons for migration, and their treatment in host countries are powerful determinants of restrictive health policies. For example, in Germany healthcare restrictions have been expressly instituted not because of a lack of funds but to deter additional asylum seekers from entering the country. In fact, myths around free healthcare as a pull factor for migration remain endemic in several European countries (Bozorgmehr and Razum 2016). In several European countries, discourses around the "deservingness" of asylum seekers to receive free healthcare have blossomed, questioning the automatic right to health of anyone stepping onto the soil of the hosting country (Holmes and Castañeda 2016). In Greece, tensions have flared among citizens as they have to make substantial co-payments to services, while asylum seekers are exempt, being classed as a "vulnerable group". Thus, different ideas about who "deserves" to receive free care on a political level shape the entitlements that are granted. While a responsive health system could help to alleviate the financial strain under which these discourses have arisen, nevertheless they have an ideological dimension which needs to be discussed within each member state. If we want to increase the accessibility of health services for asylum seekers and extend Universal Health Coverage to all migrants, responsive financing systems must go hand in hand with citizen engagement and political collaboration across Europe.

Conclusion

An increasingly mobile population has challenged the financing of health services within geopolitical boundaries. Yet the existing financing mechanisms at a European level are currently not fit to provide responsive and equitable care to the asylum seekers, a particularly vulnerable population group. We have presented three options at the level of the European Union to increase economic solidarity and support member states which currently bear largest responsibility for asylum seekers' health. While the three scenarios have different implications in terms of equity, efficiency, and transparency of the financing system, all three represent viable options to incentivise increased access to essential healthcare services at a national level. Financial reform is sorely needed in order to protect the health of newly arriving asylum seekers to the European Union. However, the technical considerations of the financing options must be accompanied by political leadership, evidence-informed discourses, and citizen engagement in order to succeed.

References

Abubakar, I., Aldridge, R. W., Devakumar, D., Orcutt, M., Burns, R., Barreto, M. L., et al. (2018). The UCL–Lancet Commission on Migration and Health: The health of a world on the move. *The Lancet, 392*, 2606–2654.

Bozorgmehr, K., Nöst, S., Thaiss, H. M., & Razum, O. (2016). Health care provisions for asylum-seekers: A nationwide survey of public health authorities in Germany. *Bundesgesundheitsblatt, Gesundheitsforschung, Gesundheitsschutz, 59*, 545–555.

Bozorgmehr, K., & Razum, O. (2015). Effect of restricting access to health care on health expenditures among asylum-seekers and refugees: A quasi-experimental study in Germany, 1994–2013. *PLoS One, 10*, e0131483.

Bozorgmehr, K., & Razum, O. (2016). Refugees in Germany—untenable restrictions to health care. *The Lancet, 388*, 2351–2352.

Bozorgmehr, K., Samuilova, M., Petrova-Benedict, R., Girardi, E., Piselli, P., & Kentikelenis, A. (2018a). Infectious disease health services for refugees and asylum seekers during a time of crisis: A scoping study of six European Union countries. *Health Policy, 123*, 882–887.

Bozorgmehr, K., & Wahedi, K. (2017). Reframing solidarity in Europe: Frontex, frontiers, and the fallacy of refugee quota. *The Lancet Public Health, 2*, e10–e11.

Bozorgmehr, K., Wahedi, K., Noest, S., Szecsenyi, J., & Razum, O. (2017). Infectious disease screening in asylum seekers: Range, coverage and economic evaluation in Germany, 2015. *Eurosurveillance, 22*, 40.

Bozorgmehr, K., Wenner, J., Noest, S., Stock, C., & Razum, O. (2018b). Germany: Financing health services provided to asylum seekers. In *Compendium of health system responses to large-scale migration in the WHO European Region*. Copenhagen: World Health Organization.

Bradby, H., Humphris, R., Newall, D., & Phillimore, J. (2015). *Public health aspects of migrant health: A review of the evidence on health status for refugees and asylum seekers in the European Region*. Copenhagen: World Health Organization.

Civil Protection and Humanitarian Aid Operations (European Commission). (2018). Echo factsheet: Emergency support within the EU. Brussels. Available from: https://ec.europa.eu/echo/files/aid/countries/factsheets/thematic/eu_emergency_support_en.pdf

Cylus, J., Papanicolas, I., & Smith, P. C. (2017). *How to make sense of health system efficiency comparisons?* Copenhagen: World Health Organization Regional Office for Europe.

da Costa, R. (2006). *Rights of refugees in the context of integration: Legal standards and recommendations, UNHCR*.

Directorate-General for Employment Social Affairs and Inclusion (European Commission). (2016). *The European Health Insurance Card - reference year 2015*. Brussels: European Union.

Directorate-General for Migration and Home Affairs (European Commission). (2018). *Interim evaluation of the asylum, migration and integration fund*. Luxembourg: European Union.

European Commission. (2018). Factsheet: EU health budget for the future. Retrieved 12 June, 2019, from https://ec.europa.eu/health/sites/health/files/programme/docs/2021_budget_factsheet_en.pdf.

European Council on Refugees and Exiles (ECRE). (2016). *The length of asylum procedures in Europe*.

European Council on Refugees and Exiles (ECRE). (2019). *Health care - Spain* [Online]. Retrieved 13 June, 2019, from http://asylumineurope.org/reports/country/spain/health-care

European Parliament. (2013). *Directive 2013/33/EU of the European Parliament and of the Council of 26 June 2013 laying down standards for the reception of applicants for international protection*.

European Parliament. (2019). *Legislative train schedule: towards a new policy on migration* [Online]. Retrieved 12 June, 2019, from http://www.europarl.europa.eu/legislative-train/theme-towards-a-new-policy-on-migration/file-1st-emergency-relocation-scheme

Eurostat. (2019). *Asylum statistics* [Online]. Retrieved 12 June, 2019, from https://ec.europa.eu/eurostat/statistics-explained/index.php/Asylum_statistics

Golder, M. (2016). Far right parties in Europe. *Annual Review of Political Science, 19*, 477–497.

Holmes, S. M., & Castañeda, H. (2016). Representing the "European refugee crisis" in Germany and beyond: Deservingness and difference, life and death. *American Ethnologist, 43*, 12–24.

Inglehart, R. F. & Norris, P. (2016). *Trump, Brexit, and the rise of populism: Economic have-nots and cultural backlash*.

Kentikelenis, A., Karanikolos, M., Reeves, A., Mckee, M., & Stuckler, D. (2014). Greece's health crisis: from austerity to denialism. *The Lancet, 383*, 748–753.

Kraler, A., & Rogoz, M. (2011). *Irregular migration in the European Union since the turn of the millennium–development, economic background and discourses*. Clandestino Project, Database on Irregular Migration.

Kuhne, A., & Gilsdorf, A. (2016). Infectious disease outbreaks in centralized homes for asylum seekers in Germany from 2004-2014. *Bundesgesundheitsblatt, Gesundheitsforschung, Gesundheitsschutz, 59*, 570–577.

Kutzin, J. (2013). Health financing for universal coverage and health system performance: Concepts and implications for policy. *Bulletin of the World Health Organization, 91*, 602–611.

Leape, S. (2018). Greece has the means to help refugees on Lesbos – but does it have the will? *The Guardian*.

Legido-Quigley, H., Otero, L., la Parra, D., Alvarez-Dardet, C., Martin-Moreno, J. M., & Mckee, M. (2013a). Will austerity cuts dismantle the Spanish healthcare system? *BMJ, 346*, f2363.

Legido-Quigley, H., Pajin, L., Fanjul, G., Urdaneta, E., & Mckee, M. (2018). Spain shows that a humane response to migrant health is possible in Europe. *The Lancet Public Health, 3*, e358.

Legido-Quigley, H., Urdaneta, E., Gonzalez, A., la Parra, D., Muntaner, C., Alvarez-Dardet, C., et al. (2013b). Erosion of universal health coverage in Spain. *The Lancet, 382*, 1977.

Maxwell, D., Bailey, S., Harvey, P., Walker, P., Sharbatke-Church, C., & Savage, K. (2012). Preventing corruption in humanitarian assistance: perceptions, gaps and challenges. *Disasters, 36*, 140–160.

Mossialos, E., Dixon, A., Figueras, J., & Kutzin, J. (2002). *Funding health care: Options for Europe*. Buckingham: Open University Press.

Niemann, A., & Zaun, N. (2018). EU refugee policies and politics in times of crisis: Theoretical and empirical perspectives. *JCMS: Journal of Common Market Studies, 56*, 3–22.

PROSS, C. (1998). Third class medicine: Health care for refugees in Germany. *Health and Human Rights, 3*, 40–53.

Starfield, B., Shi, L., & Macinko, J. (2005). Contribution of primary care to health systems and health. *The Milbank Quarterly, 83*, 457–502.

Thomson, S., Figueras, J., Evetovits, T., Jowett, M., Mladovsky, P., Maresso, A., et al. (2015). *Economic crisis, health systems and health in Europe: Impact and implications for policy*. Maidenhead: Open University Press.

UN Committee on Economic Social and Cultural Rights (CESCR). (2000). *General comment No. 14: The right to the highest attainable standard of health* (Art. 12 of the Covenant).

van de Ven, W. P. (2011). Risk adjustment and risk equalization: What needs to be done? *Health Economics, Policy, and Law, 6,* 147–156.

Vasilopoulou, S., Halikiopoulou, D., & Exadaktylos, T. (2014). Greece in crisis: Austerity, populism and the politics of blame. *JCMS: Journal of Common Market Studies, 52,* 388–402.

Wahedi, K., Nöst, S., & Bozorgmehr, K. (2017). Health examination of asylum seekers: A nationwide analysis of state policies in Germany: §62 of the asylum law. *Bundesgesundheitsblatt, Gesundheitsforschung, Gesundheitsschutz, 60,* 108–117.

World Health Organization. (2019). *Health financing for universal coverage* [Online]. Retrieved 12 June, 2019, from https://www.who.int/health_financing/universal_coverage_definition/en/

Chapter 6
Understanding the Resilience of Health Systems

Karl Blanchet, Karin Diaconu, and Sophie Witter

List of Abbreviations

HSA   Health System Assessment
UHC   Universal Health Coverage
MIPEX   Migration Integration Policy Index
UNISDR   United Nations System for Disaster Risk Reduction
EU   European Union
UNRWA   United Nations Relief and Works Agency for Palestine Refugees in the Near East
MHPSS   Mental health and psychosocial support

Introduction

Migration and Health Systems

Globally, displacement is now at the highest level ever recorded. The number of people forcibly displaced by the end of 2016 had risen to a staggering 68.5 million (UNHCR 2018a). Violence, poor economic conditions and political instability have been the main drivers for mobility towards Europe in the recent decade, producing new challenges for national health systems in the Middle East and Europe.

The 2008 World Health Assembly on Migration Health (WHO 2008) highlighted four important issues. Two of them concerned the capacity of national health

---
K. Blanchet (✉)
CERAH - Geneva Centre for Education and Research in Humanitarian Action,
A Joint Centre of Université de Genève/The Graduate Institute (IHEID), Geneva, Switzerland
e-mail: Karl.Blanchet@lshtm.ac.uk

K. Diaconu · S. Witter
Queen Margaret University, Musselburgh, UK
e-mail: kdiaconu@qmu.ac.uk; switter@qmu.ac.uk

© Springer Nature Switzerland AG 2020
K. Bozorgmehr et al. (eds.), *Health Policy and Systems Responses to Forced Migration*, https://doi.org/10.1007/978-3-030-33812-1_6

systems to guarantee access to basic health services for migrants. Practical translation of this implies two key components: (1) development of migrant-sensitive health systems that deliver sufficient services in an inclusive and coordinated manner and (2) support for the creation of health-focused alliances throughout the pathway of the migration process.

However, little information is available on how health systems should adapt and transform themselves to ensure that migrants can actually benefit from basic health services in countries they cross or in countries where they seek asylum. There is wider acknowledgment that the political and social integration of migrants—as well as their inclusion in health systems' Universal Health Coverage (UHC) agenda—particularly affects care experiences and eventually health outcomes (Ager and Strang 2008; Giannoni et al. 2016; Ben Farhat et al. 2018).

In many ways, exploring UHC and migration is about investigating how national health systems can maintain their initial functions while accommodating additional groups of populations who have specific needs and perceptions of healthcare. This dynamic adaptive capacity has been described by some as the resilience of health systems (Folke et al. 2002). Reflecting on the resilience of health systems in the context of migration and health is about challenging perspectives that only view migrants through a global health security lens (see also Chap. 7 "Health Security in the Context of Forced Migration"). Building the resilience of health systems is not therefore about migrants, the "others", but about our own health systems, the foundational values they represent and how health systems can adapt to a changing and future environment.

What Is the Relevance of Resilience for Health Systems Today?

Despite its use across a wide range of disciplines and contexts (including psychology, engineering and environmental science), "resilience" has emerged as a key concept in global health systems research only in the 2010s. The term gained substantive popularity from 2014 and 2015 due to the onset of the Ebola outbreak in West Africa (Kieny et al. 2014; Nam and Blanchet 2014) and has recently gained even further traction due to the Syrian crisis and associated regional instability and displacement in the Middle East and Europe.

There is wide consensus that the global community has to help build more resilient health systems. But do we really know what resilience means, and do we all have the same vision of resilience? Does resilience mean different things to different people, or is it simply a new term replacing previous buzzwords such as "health systems strengthening" or sustainability?

Most definitions of health system resilience have their foundations in the field of environmental science where system resilience is the result of interactions between the human sphere and ecosystems and describes a system's ability to be self-organising, learn and adapt. In health systems research, many definitions focus on the absorptive capacity of the system to resist a one-off event and return to a state of equilibrium (ICRC 2004; Albanese et al. 2008; Tadele et al. 2009; Agani et al. 2010; DFID 2011). The capacity of a health system to learn through experiencing shocks is present in health systems literature (Almedom and Tumwine 2008; Levine and Mosel 2014) but does not have the same importance as it has gained in ecology (Walker et al. 2002; Folke et al. 2005).

Managing resilience is viewed as consisting both in building the configurations of the health system and creating a warning system for the internal and external factors that can affect the structure and functions of the health system. Actors, social networks and institutions manage the resilience of health systems. There is broad consensus in the literature on the importance of change and transformation as an integral part of resilience (Thomas et al. 2013). The degree of change that a health system needs to introduce depends on the scale and intensity of the shock (Hyder et al. 2007). Whatever the degree of intensity, resilience will enable absorption and adaptation to the shock or transformation of the health system.

In the context of health systems research, resilience has thus been used in at least three different ways: (1) thinking about the building blocks of health systems and addressing those elements that are missing or strengthening the components that are weaker; (2) focusing on the enabling institutional environment within which health systems operate and pushing for reforms that might enhance their resilience; and (3) focusing on the organic and systemic properties of health systems which liken health systems to ecological systems and focusing on what might be described as "system stewardship".

The concept of resilience of systems, as defined by the authors of the chapter, is grounded in a view that sees the world as a set of dynamic and interactive systems that operate far from equilibrium. With the emergence of system thinking and complexity science, the world is now described as a network of systems interacting with each other and influencing different levels of society (Blanchet and James 2013; Berkes et al. 2003; Ramalingam 2013). Dynamic systems of different sizes interact across multiple scales (Kieny et al. 2014; O'Neill et al. 1989; Wilbanks and Kates 1999) and affect systems' ability to respond to shocks and stressors of diverse nature, frequency and intensity (Janssen et al. 2006).

Resilience is seen as a "boundary term" (Scoones 2007) that is at the crossroad between politics and science (Gieryn 1999). As such, it may have the function of building political consensus and aligning and enabling the coexistence of several different agendas (Wilson 1992). This can go some way to explaining why the term resilience may remain contested and ambiguous: so as to preserve multiple interpretations from a wide range of stakeholders, from politicians and policymakers, scientists, health service managers or community members. However, it remains important for health systems researchers and practitioners to clarify the meaning of the concept and have common guidance as to its use.

The present chapter offers reflections and a new conceptual framework based on system thinking and complexity theories (Plsek and Greenhalgh 2001; de Savigny and Adam 2009). This chapter also offers examples from resilience-focused migration and health challenges and policies in order to illustrate the utility of the conceptual framework. Through this chapter, we will explore the concept of resilience and how this concept has evolved over time. We will also explore how resilience has been translated into indexes and measures. We reflect on how resilience is relevant for European and neighbouring health systems faced by population flows and conflict. Finally, we make recommendations for a new research agenda.

Towards a New Conceptual Framework

Framework

While definitions between fields of study do not necessarily share the same perspective of resilience, there are common elements in theoretical models of system resilience (Castleden et al. 2011). For example, in the field of health sciences, resilience is often defined as the capacity of individuals, communities, systems and institutions to anticipate, withstand and/or judiciously engage with catastrophic events and/or experiences (Almedom and Tumwine 2008). Drawing on the resilience literature (Carpenter et al. 2001; Holling 2001), it is important to both define what resilience is, in specific contexts, and explain how it can be managed in those contexts.

We propose a new conceptual framework adapted from environmental studies (Lebel et al. 2006) to help analyse the various definitions of health systems resilience, and with a firm grounding in complex systems sciences. In this framework, resilience of health systems is characterised by four main dimensions: (1) capacity to collect, integrate and analyse different forms of *knowledge* and information; (2) ability to anticipate and cope with *uncertainties* and surprises; (3) capacity to manage *interdependence*, to engage effectively with and handle multiple- and cross-scale dynamics and feedbacks; and finally (4) capacity to build or develop *legitimate* institutions that are socially accepted and contextually adapted.

Based on frameworks used in ecology, three levels of resilience can be applied to health systems: absorptive capacity, adaptive capacity and transformative capacity. Within health systems thinking, the absorptive capacity relates to the capacity of a health system to continue to deliver the same level (quantity, quality, and equity) of basic healthcare services and protection to populations, especially vulnerable groups (including migrant populations), despite shocks (Adger et al. 2003). Adaptive capacity is the capacity of the health system actors to deliver the same level of healthcare services with fewer resources or a different combination of resources (Walker et al. 2002; Folke et al. 2002; Thomas et al. 2013). Finally, the transformative capacity describes the ability of health system actors to transform the functions and structure of the health system to respond to a changing environment (Olsson et al. 2006; Castleden et al. 2011; Lebel et al. 2005).

Figure 6.1 illustrates the various resilience capacities and the resilience of health systems. The potential value of this framework is that it integrates all of the different approaches to resilience—the building blocks, the systemic properties and the enabling institutional environment—into one single approach for use by researchers, practitioners and policymakers. Each dimension is described here.

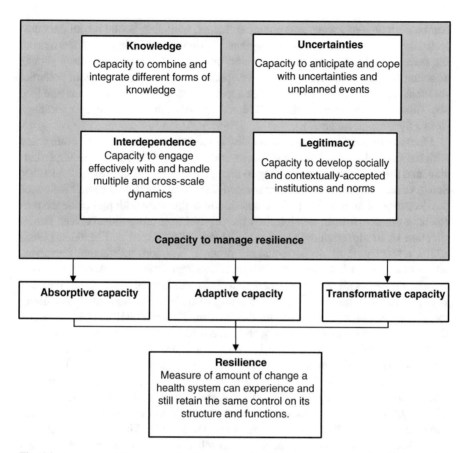

Fig. 6.1 A conceptual framework: the dimensions of resilience management (adapted from Lebel et al. 2006)

Knowledge: Capacity to Combine and Integrate Different Forms of Knowledge

The knowledge that needs to be collected and processed to ensure health system functioning and resilience is wide. For example, health systems planners need to understand current resources available, where gaps in resources exist or where weaknesses in the health system lie. But they also need to understand the current health status of the population and their health priorities. Furthermore, beyond the health system, planners need to be able to monitor risks and threats to individual and population health and the health system, which can sometimes relate to the economic sphere or the political context. In other words, the type of information necessary to make the right decisions to ensure functioning and resilience needs to combine a range of known and potential factors, including public health data collected through, for example, the surveillance system, information about the state of the current health system, the nature and intensity of potential or actual shocks affecting the health system and served population and information about potential solutions and innovations that could be accessible to health systems managers (see also Chap. 9 "Evidence on Health Records for Migrants and Refugees: Findings from a Systematic Review").

Decision-making is a daily task for health service managers who are confronted with the difficulty of anticipating shocks and stresses, which are often unpredictable, and the challenge of responding to disruptive events quickly (Streefland 1995; Senge et al. 2004). Even well documented, evidence-based data cannot influence the decisions of an individual if the decision in conformity with that evidence represents a threat to his/her own interests and survival (e.g. professional career, family situation or life-threatening situation) (Nulden 1996). Ajzen and Madden (1986) added a third type of decision-making process, emotion and factual cognition, which has to do with the impact of action following the decision. According to the authors, managers are very concerned both about whether the action has a chance of working and whether individuals belonging to their social network (particularly those who may bear an influence on the individual's status) will criticise or praise their decision and action. In other words, decision-making processes are complex, combine rational and non-rational behaviours and are influenced by individuals' interests and the opinions of peers who are part of the same social network.

Scholars have found that there is a relationship between the structure of networks, the type of links between actors (i.e. the degree of bonding between actors of the system or bridging links with other systems) and the resilience of social-ecological systems (Burt 2003; Newman and Dale 2005). The capacity to engage with a diversity of actors belonging to various spheres of society has been extensively documented in social network analysis, which highlighted the role of social brokers, i.e. individuals who create links between users and researchers (Borgatti et al. 2009). The brokers in a health system help coordinate actors in times of crises or shocks and build bridges between different groups within the system (Burt 2003; Newman and Dale 2005).

Uncertainties: Capacity to Anticipate and Cope with Uncertainties and Unplanned Events

Resilience can be understood in terms of adaptability of health systems (Carpenter et al. 2001; Walker et al. 2002; Blanchet et al. 2014). Adaptability is the capacity of the actors in a system to respond to stresses and shocks (Westley et al. 2006). Because human actions dominate social-ecological systems, the adaptability of such systems is mainly a function of the actions and decisions taken by individuals, networks and groups managing these systems (Gunderson and Holling 2002; Berkes et al. 2003) and their perception of risks (Slovic 2000). Managing uncertainties and risks relates to the combination of two different organisational and individual capacities: collecting information about the nature and scale of the risk and, from the individual perspective and emotional sphere, about how individuals evaluate these risks (Kasperson et al. 1988). For example, in the case of migration and disease control, anticipating public health outbreaks requires a functional disease surveillance system to inform health service managers on the occurrence of outbreaks and the state of transmission of the disease (Rojek et al. 2018; Moon et al. 2015). Using complex adaptive systems analysis, MacKenzie et al. (2015) showed that the capacity of the health system in Northern Nigeria to adapt to an outbreak required not only a capacity to operate all six building blocks of the health system but also access to flexible resources (e.g. human resources, vehicles, laboratory capacities, drugs and supplies) to respond to unexpected shocks, such as outbreaks. However, the surveillance of contextual factors required to support preparedness goes beyond public health and requires monitoring of external factors that can affect the resilience of health systems: e.g. price of oil, security status in the country, likelihood of natural disasters (Blanchet et al. 2014; Permanand et al. 2016; Rosenkotter et al. 2014). Analysing contextual factors and translating them into health systems terms require the combination of various methodologies and techniques (e.g. systems dynamics, process mapping, social network analysis, scenario technique, cynefin) that all derive from system thinking, recognising the importance of feedback loops and process contexts (de Savigny et al. 2017).

Interdependence: Capacity to Engage Effectively with and Handle Multiple and Wide-Ranging Dynamics

Recognising that health systems are embedded within other complex structures (e.g. political, economic, judiciary, social and ecological systems) alludes to how health systems are affected by factors which may not seem to be directly linked to public health. In the policy context, this was described by Blanchet et al. (2014) who showed that the structure of the physical rehabilitation system in Somaliland was transformed following changes in national security and international donors' strategies. The degree to which health systems are influenced by non-health systems is often all too apparent when health systems are not resilient. For example, the inadequate capacity of fragile health systems underpinned the challenges in responding to the Ebola outbreak, in countries afflicted by decades of conflict, weak economies and entrenched poverty (McPake et al. 2015). Building resilience in the wake of Ebola will need to take all of these factors into account: not treating the crisis solely as a medical emergency but as a profound and long-term failure of economic and social development (Ramalingam 2013).

Legitimacy: Capacity to Develop Socially Accepted and Contextually Adapted Institutions and Norms

Another important component of resilient health systems in the literature relates to the necessity of community trust and ownership. This can be built through an inclusive consultation process engaging communities meaningfully as the users of the health system in the development of policies and management of healthcare services where patients are placed at the centre of the system (Gilson 2005; Wilkinson and Leach 2015). Importantly, person-centred management of health systems needs to happen at every level. Kieny and Dovlo (2015) showed that responding to the Ebola outbreak requires trust and accountability to exist or be built at every level of the health system: from the patient to the community health worker and nurses at the health centre to medical and managerial staff at higher level. This person-centred management is led by accountability and transparency principles.

The Ebola outbreak has demonstrated the importance of building a trusting relationship with populations, to mitigate the situation where communities avoid using health facilities for fear of contamination (UNFPA and Options 2015). The violence against healthcare workers also showed the disconnect between communities and health services (Delamou et al. 2015; Raven et al. 2018). Bloom et al. (2007) further discussed the necessity to build social and health institutions that are recognised as legitimate by communities.

Applications of Health System Resilience

Health Systems Assessment

Linked to the Sustainable Development Goals, there is a shared international commitment to leave no one behind and reduce population risks and vulnerabilities. Building on major global processes, including the 2030 Agenda for Sustainable Development, the World Humanitarian Summit, the New York Declaration and the twin resolutions on Sustaining Peace, new working methods across the humanitarian, development and peace nexus are recognised as imperative.

The UHC2030 working groups on Health Systems Assessment (HSA) and Health Systems in Fragile States have recommended approaches to better assess health systems' performance and inform the health system strengthening interventions to be implemented. These could be applied to any health system and any context. They include:

1. Joint analysis and assessment between all actors (government and civil society, national and external actors), which requires a concerted investment in consistent and sound joint situation and contexts analysis to establish a joint problem statement and shared understanding of priorities based on reliable data as well as the capacities available to address them.

2. Joint planning, which will ensure complementarity of approaches and programmatic activities that will help minimise gaps in the response and increase possibilities of collective efforts towards shared goals.
3. Collective outcomes are at the centre of the commitment to leave no one behind, as it serves to transcend longstanding conventional thinking, silos, mandates and other obstacles.
4. Coordination structures are to be developed that are outcome-based and that bring together emergency and development partners.

A sound analysis of the context, focused on the determinants of the problems, its historical evolution, the constraints posed and the opportunities offered, should be at the basis of any engagement. With regard to the joint analysis for the health system, this should bring together the findings from a health risk analysis, country capacity assessment for preparedness and response as well as HSAs.

Based on the HSA, planning and decisions by national and international actors can be made on an essential package of services, financing, supply management, task allocation among health workforce, etc., in order to ensure, for example, that access to basic health services for migrants is guaranteed. Such HSA is also needed to avoid undermining or fragmenting the national health system (Blanchet et al. 2016). Furthermore, HSAs can also help understand the capacity of essential public health functions and how preparedness functions can be strengthened in such contexts (Rojek et al. 2018).

Taking into account the dynamic characteristics of population displacement, the HSA needs to be done within a relatively short time frame and remain an organic information tool that is regularly updated when there are dramatic changes in the context. The HSA is considered as the first step to guide national, international and local authorities making decisions on allocation of resources and priority setting. As illustrated by country profiles produced by the European Observatory on Health Systems and Policies, the national HSA is structured around the health system foundations and takes into account cross-cutting aspects such as the role of the private sector and civil society, access to health services for minorities. It also includes an analysis and prioritisation of health system bottlenecks that need to be addressed to increase access, coverage, quality and scope of an essential package of quality health services, including the content and implementation modalities of such package of services. With the recent migration in Europe, a full assessment section should be added on displacement and cross-border activities. One way of synthesizing health systems capacities is to use indices.

Use of Resilience Indices

There is a wide range of indicators and indices relating to the governance of countries, their capacity to innovate and change or their capacity of coping with disasters. However, none of them measures the resilience of health systems. There is a need to combine the information gathered by some of the indices to provide information on the general context where health systems operate. Similar exercises could be tested in Europe in order to analyse the capacities of health systems to integrate migrants and asylum seekers into their national health system. Like every index exercise, such initiative will need to be agile and repeated at least every year in order to have any value for decision-makers. Finally, we will need to invest time to create consensus on the indicators that will need to be measured to assess the resilience of health systems and on how such an index could inform local and international planning and action. Kruk et al. (2017), for example, propose a health system-specific resilience index. However, further efforts will need to be invested in order to create consensus on the exact indicators that will need to be measured to assess the resilience of health systems and on how such index could inform local and international planning and action (Ridde et al. 2019).

Measuring resilience through a set of indicators has been widely developed in various ways. They may be called resilience, fragility or readiness indices. Without being exhaustive, we illustrate how these indices are used. In terms of migration in Europe, we suggest to use resilience indices in combination with the Migrant Integration Policy Index (MIPEX). First launched in 2004, the MIPEX is a set of 167 policy indicators that provide a picture on the level of efforts in each EU country on integration of migrants. In terms of resilience index, much can be learned from the humanitarian sector. For example, DARA, an independent think tank, has established an index to measure the quality of the institutional and governance framework in relation to countries' capacity to reduce risk (DARA 2018). Perhaps unsurprisingly, their analysis shows that the bottom six countries (Afghanistan, Chad, Haiti, Somalia, Democratic Republic of Congo and Somalia) are low-income countries that have recently experienced conflict or political crises and despite their very high level of vulnerability to a range of extreme physical events, they have very weak capacity to address the drivers of risk. Similarly, UNISDR has concluded that improving governance is the single most important priority for reducing risk (UNISDR 2015). The Caribbean Catastrophic Risk Insurance Facility (CCRIF) is the world's first regional fund to use parametric insurance to give governments access to low-price earthquake and hurricane catastrophe coverage (CCRIF 2015). With standard insurance approaches, detailed assessments of losses have to be carried out before a payment is made. With parametric insurance, loss is calculated by using a resilience index in which hazard levels—wind, storm surge and waves for hurricane, ground shaking for earthquake—are used as an advance proxy for losses. In the private sector, again, KPMG has developed a Change Readiness Index that is updated every year and classifies countries using indicators grouped looking at the capacities of three different groups of actors: enterprise capability, government capability and civil society capability (KPMG 2018). Somalia, Syria, Chad, Sudan and South Sudan are at the very bottom of the 2017 raking. In the humanitarian sector, the INFORM index identifies countries at risk of humanitarian crisis and disaster. The INFORM index analyses three areas of risk: hazards and exposure, vulnerability and lack of coping capacity (Marin-Ferrer et al. 2017). The index is extensively used by international donors and United Nations agencies.

Migration, Health Systems and Resilience

Recent global events, including the conflicts in Syria and Yemen, have put considerable pressure not only on local and regional health systems but also on countries viewed as potential routes of access and/or promising places of future settlement. Since 2014, more than 1.8 million migrants entered the European continent via Spain, Greece or Italy (Da Rold 2018) with many of them pursuing onward journeys to Germany (Wetzke et al. 2018). Newspaper articles across the European Union report that further inflows of migrants are likely, reinforcing existing worries relating to the health states of those newly arriving and the potential burdens they may place on national systems.

However, despite high political and social importance, research on the effects of migration on EU countries and national health systems responses/adaptations is still in its infancy. Despite this, we note clear synergies between recommendations in this literature and the wider resilience discourses and examples presented in this chapter. Existing literature draws attention to the scale of the shock Western countries experienced during initial waves of migration and settlement between 2012 and 2014 (Wetzke et al. 2018). At this time, national systems were seen as ill-prepared to deal with the complex interacting needs of asylum seekers, including psychological (e.g. being affected by post-traumatic stress disorder), physical (e.g. being a survivor of gender-based violence or of torture) as well as sociolegal needs (e.g. arriving in a country with no legal recourse to legal advice, minimal protection from repatriation) (Rojek et al. 2018; Ben Farhat et al. 2018; Juul Bjertrup et al. 2018).

Available literature highlights how important it was and is for systems to leverage accurate knowledge of target populations, their needs and expectations, as well as secure their engagement in processes of care access and uptake in line with resilience thinking. For example, Wetzke et al. (2018) highlighted the critical role that health services play in the first weeks in refugees settling in new environments. In their study on a 2015 cohort settling in Germany, they noted that health service utilisation was particularly high in first weeks of camp residence (on average 37.1 visits per 100,000 persons); a steady decline was then evident: at 6 weeks of camp inhabitancy, only 9.5 visits occurred per 100,000 persons. Accurate understanding of migrant needs and level of integration—including by age group and taking into account tailoring of services to individual histories and experiences of violence, neglect and medical needs—is critical to meeting migrant health needs. This has been similarly emphasised in the United Kingdom, where Campos-Matos et al. (2016) report Public Health England leading the revision of guidelines for pre-entry health assessment to ensure collaboration with humanitarian agents, migrant specialists and NHS and local authorities (see also Chap. 10 "Assessing the Health of Persons Experiencing Forced Migration: Current Practices for Health Service Organisations").

Similarly, we note calls in the literature for more nuanced and legitimising approaches to migrant service delivery. For example, Grotti et al. (2018) draw attention to the wider discourses on migration—where migrants are viewed as vulnerable populations, often discussed in contexts of limited agency—and how such discourses further reinforce gendered and paternalistic service delivery. While migrant women are vulnerable due to their journey and personal experiences, they are then further constructed as vulnerable by health systems and providers that are meant to address their needs in a new alien environment. Given care services are already overstretched and fragile, this additional labelling may prompt women to seek help informally in their own communities.

Most refugees and migrants are managed within their countries and regions, and there is a growing body of work understanding how these health systems manage the chronic and acute stresses of conflict and population displacement and how this can illuminate strategies to support resilience (Campos-Matos et al. 2016), as illustrated by the following examples on the United Nations Relief and Works Agency for Palestine Refugees in the Near East (UNRWA).

UNRWA is responsible for the delivery of key services such as education and social support for Palestine refugees. As part of its mandate, the organisation offers health services via a network of primary care facilities and ensures access to advanced care via referral. Since 2011, UNRWA health systems in Syria, Lebanon and Jordan have had had to address various challenges due to the Syria conflict.

A collaborative research project between UNRWA, the American University of Beirut and Queen Margaret University, Edinburgh, explored this issue through 97 in-depth interviews, 3 group model building workshops with 46 UNRWA professionals and development of 3 systems dynamics simulation models.

The research indicated that UNRWA health systems have broadly maintained trends in utilisation and delivery of key services by deploying absorptive, adaptive and transformative capacities in their response to the Syria crisis and associated displacement. Key examples of this include:

Absorption: UNRWA reform packages—such as the introduction of an electronic record and queuing system—have assisted clinics in Jordan in managing the increased patient load. Reform packages had successfully been integrated into routine practice by 2012 (peak of the displacement period) and thus assisted health professionals in managing utilisation at their clinics.

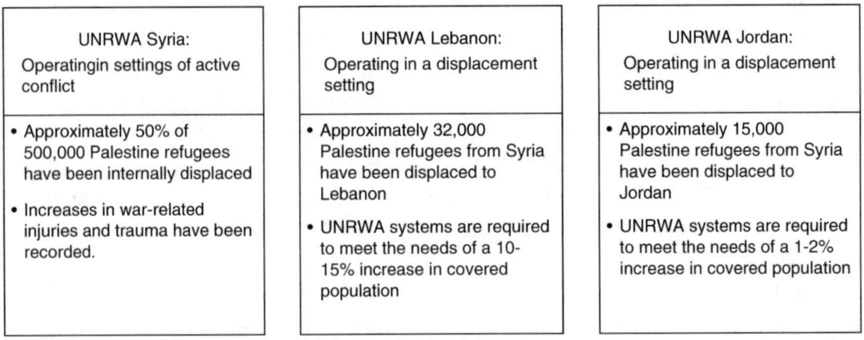

UNRWA Syria: Operatingin settings of active conflict	UNRWA Lebanon: Operating in a displacement setting	UNRWA Jordan: Operating in a displacement setting
• Approximately 50% of 500,000 Palestine refugees have been internally displaced • Increases in war-related injuries and trauma have been recorded.	• Approximately 32,000 Palestine refugees from Syria have been displaced to Lebanon • UNRWA systems are required to meet the needs of a 10-15% increase in covered population	• Approximately 15,000 Palestine refugees from Syria have been displaced to Jordan • UNRWA systems are required to meet the needs of a 1-2% increase in covered population

Fig. 6.2 Challenges encountered by UNRWA health systems in Syria, Lebanon and Jordan

Adaptation: In response to increased and overwhelming utilisation of UNRWA primary care clinics in Lebanon, area and clinic managers were supported by increased devolution of resources, which supported their implementation of innovative solutions. New clinical teams were hired to address the increase in utilisation, and, as needed, new health delivery points were opened in camps experiencing conflict between newly arriving and settled refugees. To address service delivery challenges to the most politically vulnerable Palestine refugees, UNRWA has also engaged in advocacy with national health authorities in order to broker access to much needed secondary care.

Transformation: In Syria, the crisis affected not only communities but also healthcare staff residing in the country. To address the mental health stressors placed on staff, as well as strengthen their wellbeing and in turn staff capacity to respond to the needs of patients, mental health and psychosocial support training was introduced. The training covered both manager- and peer-support mechanisms for enhancing staff wellbeing as well as the introduction of services for patients. Similar trainings have been rolled out in Lebanon and Jordan and are now part of UNRWA's routine service offer.

The empirical case studies from Syria, Lebanon and Jordan suggest that adopting a complex and dynamic systems lens is critical in identifying and exploring resilience (Alameddine et al. 2018). We identified distinct resilience capacities (absorption, adaptation and transformation) and wider organisation and systems elements sustaining them (see Fig. 6.3). Notably, we highlight that both system hardware (e.g. availability of resources) and software (e.g. a culture of learning)

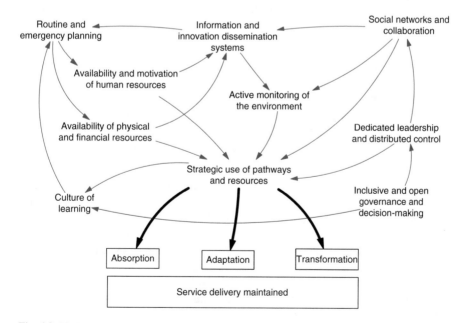

Fig. 6.3 UNRWA systems elements sustaining resilience capacities and service delivery

play a role in deploying resilience. While the former are clearly necessary for systems to function, the latter are particularly important in ensuring health systems and organisations deploy their resources strategically and make "resilient" decisions.

A second illustration on migration in Europe comes from our resilience analysis based on the paper published by Kotsiou et al. (2018). The Greek healthcare system has faced two severe shocks which have now transitioned to becoming chronic stressors. The first concerns the economic crisis and its effects on the country as a whole and the health system. Greece has experienced significant economic downturn, employment opportunities are rare and citizens face difficulties in securing their livelihood. Economic contraction has also implied limited investment in the health system: health facilities, particularly hospitals, are reported to lack equipment needed to deliver basic services; some health staff have migrated abroad or taken on multiple roles to secure a living, and human capacity needed for service delivery has therefore also depleted.

At the same time, the Greek system has had to cope with a second shock associated with the ongoing armed conflict in the Middle East: delivery of services to refugees crossing the Mediterranean as well as healthcare delivery to those refugees settling in Greece. The government has set up reception centres on its main islands and, within these, delivers a wide range of health services, including some that had never received priority within the Greek system (e.g. mental health). Fifty-seven thousand refugees resided in Greece in 2017/2018, with 60% settling on mainland Greece and the remainder residing in reception centres on Lesvos, Chios, Kos, Samos and Leros (UNHCR 2018b).

The above shocks have now resulted in considerable chronic strains on the health system, compromising the health of both host and refugee communities. Migrants particularly face:

- A high level and diversified profile of health needs: both communicable and non-communicable diseases are highly prevalent, and over 80% of refugees screened present with mental health needs that require treatment. Referrals to secondary care are high and this puts considerable strain on public services.
- Barriers to have access to healthcare: Registration with national social security authorities is a principal barrier to health access; transport and movement of refugees is additionally dependent upon the logging of an international protection applicant card. Linguistic and cultural barriers to care seeking also apply.

Examples of absorptive, adaptive and transformative resilience capacity are also evident across the Greek health system, though detailed resilience-oriented health systems assessments are likely needed to build on current crisis response:

Absorption: to mitigate the difficulties refugees face in accessing secondary care, some of the residence centres have used their own resources to provide organised transport (via bus and taxi travel) to other hospitals.

Adaptation: given the linguistic and cultural differences between Greek and refugee populations, it has been necessary for the Greek social workers to directly work inside primary healthcare settings; their role as a broker has been to create access for refugees to secondary and emergency services.

Transformation: inclusion of mental health services in Greek health facilities offered to refugees is notable; however, it is too early to state that mental health services have become routine practice in all hospitals although when delivered these services are now available to Greek patients.

To go further analysing the resilience of the Greek health system, capacities of the health system were analysed using Blanchet et al. (2017) framework.

Knowledge: only 11% of outpatient consultations are registered; the system thus does not have "live" information relating to the services it offers, nor their impact.

Uncertainty: it is unclear how the health system plans for emergencies; e.g. migration comes in ebbs and flows, but given gaps in knowledge cited above, it is unlikely the health system could predict service demand or project necessary resource allocation to meet unexpected needs.

Interdependence: it is clear that Greek authorities, NGOs as well as UNHCR collaborate in an intricate web of actors in order to secure the wellbeing of refugees. However, gaps in coordination are highlighted, particularly concerning referrals and access to secondary care.

Legitimacy: it is clear that both the refugee and economic crisis present substantive political challenges for the Greek government. Attention has largely shifted in the national discourse from addressing the needs of vulnerable Greek communities towards dealing with the challenges created by the migrant crisis—this risks alienating host communities and further may lead to difficulties in integrating refugee populations. Inter-sectoral responses—focused on both host and refugee communities and their integration efforts—are needed to meet such challenges.

Conclusion

In this chapter we put forwards a new framework for the analysis of health systems resilience, which is relevant to European countries who are trying to respond to migrants' health needs. This framework extends previously existing frameworks from ecological science to the study of health systems. Resilience is defined here as a measure of the amount of change a health system may experience and still retain control over its structure and functions. More specifically, health systems are resilient if they exhibit absorptive, adaptive or transformational capacity in the face of shocks such as a migration phenomenon. In our framework, managing health system resilience requires analysing (1) the mechanisms through which the variety of actors in the health system collect, organise, synthesise and interpret complex information, as well as the way this information feeds into complex decision-making processes; (2) the strategies health system actors may use to manage uncertainty and shocks in a very dynamic environment; (3) the interdependence of health systems with other systems (such as political and economic systems); and (4) the approaches through which health systems develop socially and contextually acceptable institutions and norms, which is very relevant when introducing the notion of migrants in some political spheres.

Large-scale migration movements may represent a "shock" to health systems and thus a test of resilient capacities, as well as a potential resource for their future strengthening. When trying to respond to migrant needs in Europe, this framework could be used by health systems researchers, health practitioners and policymakers to analyse the properties of resilient health systems and put forwards context-specific, evidence-based and comprehensive interventions to improve resilience and make sure that migrants' health can be covered with quality services.

Work on conceptualising resilience is now advancing; however, much work remains to be done on developing measurements of resilience in practice, integrating them within existing tools (such as health system assessments) and applying them in different contexts, including in European health systems in response to migratory flows. Most important of all from a policy perspective is building on early lessons in identifying determinants of resilience capacities and how to reinforce them in different contexts.

References

Adger, W. N., Brown, K., Fairbrass, J., Jordan, A., Paavola, J., Rosendo, S., et al. (2003). Governance for sustainability: Towards a 'thick' analysis of environmental decision making. *Environment and Planning A, 35*, 1095–1110.

Agani, F., Landau, J., & Agani, N. (2010). Community-building before, during, and after times of trauma: The application of the linc model of community resilience in kosovo. *American Journal of Orthopsychiatry, 80*, 143–149.

Ager, A., & Strang, A. (2008). Understanding integration: A conceptual framework. *Journal of Refugee Studies, 21*, 166–191.

Ajzen, J., & Madden, J. T. (1986). Prediction of goal directed behavior. *Journal of Experimental Social Psychology, 22*, 453–474.

Alameddine, M., Fouad, M., Diaconu, K., Jamal, Z., Gough, G., Witter, S., et al. (2018). Resilience capacities of health systems: Accommodating the needs of displaced Syrian refugees. *Social Science and Medicine, 10*, 18.

Albanese, J., Birnbaum, M., Cannon, C., Capiello, J., Chapman, E., Paturas, J., et al. (2008). Fostering disaster resilient communities across the globe through the incorporation of safe and resilient hospitals for community-integrated disaster responses. *Prehospital and Disaster Medicine, 23*, 385–390.

Almedom, A., & Tumwine, J. K. (2008). Resilence to disasters: A paradigm shift from vulnerability to strength. *African Health Sciences, 8*, 1–4.

Ben Farhat, J., Blanchet, K., Juul Bjertrup, P., Veizis, A., Perrin, C., Coulborn, R. M., et al. (2018). Syrian refugees in Greece: Experience with violence, mental health status, and access to information during the journey and while in Greece. *BMC Medicine, 16*, 40.

Berkes, F., Colding, J. F., & Folke, C. (2003). *Navigating nature's dynamics: Building resilience for complexity and change*. New York: Cambridge University Press.

Blanchet, K., Fouad, F. M., & Pherali, T. (2016). Syrian refugees in Lebanon: The search for universal health coverage. *Conflict and Health, 10*, 1–5.

Blanchet, K., & James, P. (2013). The role of social networks in the governance of health systems: The case of eye care systems in Ghana. *Health Policy and Planning, 28*, 143–156.

Blanchet, K., Nam, S. L., Ramalingam, B., & Pozo-Martin, F. (2017). Governance and capacity to manage resilience of health systems: Towards a new conceptual framework. *International Journal of Health Policy and Management, 6*, 431.

Blanchet, K., Palmer, J., Palanchowke, R., Boggs, D., Jama, A., & Girois, S. (2014). Advancing the application of systems thinking in health: analysing the contextual and social network factors influencing the use of sustainability indicators in a health system--a comparative study in Nepal and Somaliland. *Health Research Policy and Systems, 12*, 46.

Bloom, G., Edström, J., Leach, M., Lucas, H., Macgregor, H., Standing, H., et al. (2007). Health in a dynamic world. In *STEPS working paper 5*. Brighton: STEPS Centre.

Borgatti, S. P., Mehra, A., et al. (2009). Network analysis in the social sciences. *Science, 323*, 892–895.

Burt, R. S. (2003). The social capital of structural holes. In M. F. Guillen, R. Collins, P. England, & M. Meyer (Eds.), *The new economic sociology: developments in an emerging field*. New York: Russell Sage Foundation.

Campos-Matos, I., Zenner, D., Smith, G., Cosford, P., & Kirkbride, H. (2016). Tackling the public health needs of refugees. *BMJ, 352*, i774.

Carpenter, S., Walker, B., Anderies, J. M., & Abel, N. (2001). From metaphor to measurement: Resilience of what to what? *Ecosystems, 4*, 765–781.

Castleden, M., Mckee, M., Murray, V., & Leonardi, G. (2011). Resilience thinking in health protection. *Journal of Public Health, 33*, 369–377.

CCRIF. (2015). CCRIF Strategic Plan 2015 - 2018 Cayman Islands.

Da Rold, C. (2018). L'obbligo di non trascurare nuove realtà: il dramma dei migranti. *Recenti Progressi in Medicina, 109*, 413–416.

DARA. (2018). *Methodolgy of the risk reduction index*. Retrieved from https://daraint.org/wp-content/uploads/2012/01/How_does_the_RRI_work.pdf

de Savigny, D., & Adam, T. (2009). *System thinking for health systems strengthening*. Geneva: World Health Organisation, Alliance for Health Policy and Systems Research.

de Savigny, D., Blanchet, K., & Adam, T. (2017). *Applied systems thinking for health systems research: A methodological handbook*. New York: McGraw-Hill Education.

Delamou, A., Beavogui, A. H., Kondé, M. K., van Griensven, J., & de Brouwere, V. (2015). Ebola: Better protection needed for Guinean health-care workers. *The Lancet, 385*, 503–504.

DFID. (2011). *Defining disaster resilience: A DFID approach paper*. London: DFID.

Folke, C., Carpenter, S., Elmquist, T., Gunderson, L., Holling, C. S., & Walker, B. (2002). Resilience and sustainable development: Building adaptive capacity in a world of transformations. *Ambio, 31*, 437–440.

Folke, C., Hahn, P., Olsson, P., & Norberg, J. (2005). Adaptive giovernance of socio-ecological systems. *Annual Review of Environment and Resources, 30*, 441–473.

Giannoni, M., Franzini, L., & Masiero, G. (2016). Migrant integration policies and health inequalities in Europe. *BMC Public Health, 16*, 463.

Gieryn, T. (1999). *Cultural boundaries of science: Credibility on the line*. Chicago: Chicago University Press.

Gilson, L. (2005). Editorial: Building trust and value in health systems in low- and middle-income countries. *Social Science & Medicine, 61*, 1381–1384.

Grotti, V., Malakasis, C., Quagliariello, C., & Sahraoui, N. (2018). Shifting vulnerabilities: Gender and reproductive care on the migrant trail to Europe. *Comparative Migration Studies, 6*, 23.

Gunderson, L., & Holling, C. S. (2002). *Panarchy: Understanding transformations in human and natural systems*. Washington, DC, USA: Island Press.

Holling, C. S. (2001). Understanding the complexity of economic, ecological, and social systems. *Ecosystems, 4*, 390–405.

Hyder, A. A., Bloom, G., Leach, M., Syed, S. B., & Peters, D. H. (2007). Exploring health systems research and its influence on policy processes in low income countries. *BMC Public Health, 7*, 309.

ICRC. (2004). *World disasters report: Focus on community resilience*. Geneva: ICRC.

Janssen, M. A., Bodin, Ö., Anderies, J. M., Elmqvist, T., Ernstson, H., Mcallister, R. J., et al. (2006). Toward a network perspective of the study of resilience in social-ecological systems. *Ecology and Society, 11*, 15.

Juul Bjertrup, P., Bouhenia, M., Mayaud, P., Perrin, C., Ben Farhat, J., & Blanchet, K. (2018). A life in waiting: Refugees' mental health and narratives of social suffering after European Union border closures in March 2016. *Social Science & Medicine, 215*, 53–60.

Kasperson, R. E., Renn, O., Slovic, P., Brown, H. S., Emel, J., Goble, R., et al. (1988). The social amplification of risk: A conceptual framework. *Risk Analysis, 8*, 177–187.

Kieny, M. P., & Dovlo, D. (2015). Beyond Ebola: A new agenda for resilient health systems. *The Lancet, 385*, 91–92.

Kieny, M. P., Evans, D. B., Schmets, G., & Kadandale, S. (2014). Health-system resilience: Reflections on the Ebola crisis in western Africa. *Bulletin of the World Health Organization, 92*, 850.

Kotsiou, O. S., Kotsios, P., Srivastava, D. S., Kotsios, V., Gourgoulianis, K. I., & Exadaktylos, A. K. (2018). Impact of the refugee crisis on the greek healthcare system: A long road to Ithaca. *International Journal of Environmental Research and Public Health, 15*, 1790.

KPMG. (2018). *Change readiness index 2017*. Retrieved 30 October, 2018, from https://home.kpmg.com/xx/en/home/insights/2017/06/change-readiness-tool.html

Kruk, M. E., et al. (2017). Building resilient health systems: A proposal for a resilience index. *BMJ, j2323*, 357.

Lebel, L., Anderies, J. M., Campbell, B., Folke, C., Hatfield-Dodds, S., Hughes, T. P., et al. (2006). Governance and the capacity to manage resilience in regional social-ecological systems. *Ecology and Society, 11*, 19.

Lebel, L., Garden, P., & Imamura, M. (2005). The politics of scale, position and place in the management of water resources in the Mekong region. *Ecology and Society, 10*, 18.

Levine, S., & Mosel, I. (2014). Supporting resilience in difficult places. In *HPG commissioned report*. London: ODI.

Mackenzie, A., Abdulwahab, A., Sokpo, E., & Mecaskey, J. W. (2015). Building a resilient health system: Lessons from Northern Nigeria. In *IDS working paper*. Brighton: IDS.

Marin-Ferrer, M., Vernaccini, L., & Poljansek, K. (2017). Inform index for risk management Italy: Science for policy report by the Joint Research Centre (JRC).

McPake, B., Witter, S., Ssali, S., Wurie, H., Namakula, J., & Ssengooba, F. (2015). Ebola in the context of conflict affected states and health systems: Case studies of Northern Uganda and Sierra Leone. *Conflict and Health, 9*, 23.

Moon, S., Sridhar, D., Pate, M. A., Jha, A. K., Clinton, C., Delaunay, S., et al. (2015). Will Ebola change the game? Ten essential reforms before the next pandemic. The report of the Harvard-LSHTM Independent Panel on the Global Response to Ebola. *The Lancet, 386*, 2204–2221.

Nam, S. L., & Blanchet, K. (2014). We mustn't forget other essential health services during the Ebola crisis. *British Medical Journal, 349*, g6837.

Newman, L., & Dale, A. (2005). Network structure, diversity, and proactive resilience builiding: A response to Tompkins and Adger. *Ecology and Society, 10*, r2.

Nulden, U. (1996). Escalation in IT projects: Can we afford to quit or do we have to continue? In *The IEEE Computer Society Information Systems Conference* (pp. 136–142). Palmerston North, New Zealand: IEEE Computer Society Press.

O'neill, R. V., Johnson, A. R., & King, A. W. (1989). A hierarchical framework for the analysis of scale. *Landscape Ecology, 3*, 193–205.

Olsson, P., Gunderson, L. H., Carpenter, S. R., Ryan, P., Lebel, L., Folke, C., et al. (2006). Shooting the rapids: Navigating transitions to adaptive governance of social-ecological systems. *Ecology and Society, 11*, 18.

Permanand, G., Krasnik, A., Kluge, H., & Mckee, M. (2016). Europe's migration challenges: Mounting an effective health system response. *European Journal of Public Health, 26*, 3–4.

Plsek, P. E., & Greenhalgh, T. (2001). The challenge of complexity in health care. *British Medical Journal, 323*, 625–628.

Ramalingam, B. (2013). *Aid on the edge of chaos*. Oxford: OUP.

Raven, J., Wurie, S., & Witter, S. (2018). Fighting a battle': Health workers' experiences of coping with Ebola in Sierra Leone. *BMC Health Services Research, 18*, 251.

Ridde, V., Benmarhnia, T., Bonnet, E., et al. (2019). Climate change, migration and health systems resilience: Need for interdisciplinary research. *F1000Research, 8*, 22.

Rojek, A. M., Gkolfinopoulou, K., Veizis, A., Lambrou, A., Castle, L., Georgakopoulou, T., et al. (2018). Clinical assessment is a neglected component of outbreak preparedness: Evidence from refugee camps in Greece. *BMC Medicine, 16*, 43.

Rosenkotter, N., Brand, H., Mckee, M., Riley, N., Verma, A., & Verschuuren, M. (2014). The realisation of a European health information system--time to get the politicians involved. *European Journal of Public Health, 24*, 184–185.

Scoones, I. (2007). Sustainability. *Development in Practice, 17*, 589–596.

Senge, P., Scharmer, C. O., Jaworski, J., & Flowers, B. S. (2004). *Presence: Human purpose and the field of the future*. Cambridge: The Society for Organisational Learning.

Slovic, P. (2000). Perception of risk. In P. Slovic (Ed.), *The perception of risk*. Sterling, VA: Earthscan.

Streefland, P. H. (1995). Enhancing coverage and sustainability of vaccination programs - an explanatory framework with special reference to India. *Social Science & Medicine, 41*, 647–656.

Tadele, F., Manyena, S. B., & Adele, F. (2009). Building disaster resilience through capacity building in Ethiopia. *Disaster Prevention and Management, 18*, 317–326.

Thomas, S., Keegan, C., Barry, S., Layte, R., Jowett, M., & Normand, C. (2013). A framework for assessing health system resilience in an economic crisis: Ireland as a test case. *BMC Health Services Research, 13*, 450.

UNFPA & Options. (2015). *Rapid assessment of ebola impact on reproductive health services and service seeking behaviour in Sierra Leone*. Freetown, Sierra Leone: UNFPA.

UNHCR. (2018a). *Figures at glance*. Retrieved 30 October, 2018, from http://www.unhcr.org/figures-at-a-glance.html

UNHCR. (2018b). *Operational portal refugee situations*. Retrieved 24 June, 2018, from http://data2.unhcr.org/en/situations/mediterranean/location/5179

UNISDR. (2015). *Global assessment report on disaster risk reduction 2015*. Geneva: UNISDR.

Walker, B., Carpenter, S., Anderies, J., Abel, N., Cumming, G., Janssen, M., et al. (2002). Resilience management in social-ecological systems: A working hypothesis for a participatory approach. *Conservation Ecology, 6*, 14.

Westley, F., Zimmerman, B., & Patton, M. Q. (2006). *Getting to maybe: How the world is changed*. Toronto: Random House.

Wetzke, M., Happle, C., Vakilzadeh, A., Ernst, D., Sogkas, G., Schmidt, R., et al. (2018). Healthcare utilization in a large cohort of asylum seekers entering Western Europe in 2015. *International Journal of Environmental Research and Public Health, 15*, 2163.

WHO. (2008). *Sixty-first world health assembly - Resolutions and decisions*. Geneva: World Health Organisation.

Wilbanks, T. J., & Kates, R. W. (1999). Global change in local places: How scale matters. *Climatic Change, 43*, 601–628.

Wilkinson, A., & Leach, M. (2015). Briefing: Ebola - myths, realities and structural violence. *African Affairs, 114*, 136–148.

Wilson, F. (1992). Faust: The developer. *Working Paper*. CDR.

Chapter 7
Health Security in the Context of Forced Migration

Maike Voss, Katharina Wahedi, and Kayvan Bozorgmehr

Abbreviations

ECDC	European Centre for Disease Prevention and Control
GHS	Global health security
HIV/AIDS	Human immunodeficiency virus/acquired immune deficiency syndrome
IHR	International health regulations
NCD	Non-communicable disease
SDG	Sustainable Development Goal
UHC	Universal health coverage
UK	United Kingdom
UNDP	United Nations Development Program
US	United States
WHA	World Health Assembly
WHO	World Health Organization

Maike Voss and Katharina Wahedi: Joint first authorship.

M. Voss
Global Issues Division, German Institute for International and Security Affairs,
Berlin, Germany
e-mail: maike.voss@swp-berlin.org

K. Wahedi (✉)
Department of General Practice and Health Services Research, University Hospital
Heidelberg, Heidelberg, Germany

K. Bozorgmehr
Department of General Practice and Health Services Research, University Hospital
Heidelberg, Heidelberg, Germany

Department of Population Medicine and Health Services Research, School of Public Health,
Bielefeld University, Bielefeld, Germany
e-mail: kayvan.bozorgmehr@uni-bielefeld.de

© Springer Nature Switzerland AG 2020
K. Bozorgmehr et al. (eds.), *Health Policy and Systems Responses to Forced
Migration*, https://doi.org/10.1007/978-3-030-33812-1_7

Introduction

Rising numbers of migration to high-income countries and events of large-scale migration have triggered security concerns related to foreigners and disease. In the public debate, immigrants are frequently perceived, conceptualised, or framed as a threat. Such debates are often dominated by security concerns through health issues, resonating through public media in an "alarmist" way (Box 7.1) and implying that immediate (unexceptional) political action is required to reverse the threat.

> **Box 7.1: Quotes from the Media Related to Health and Security Concerns in the Context of (Forced) Migration**
>
> The Democrats […] do NOT want Border Security. They want Open Borders for anyone to come in. This brings large scale crime and disease […](Tweet by Donald J. Trump, Dec 11, 2018).
>
> Latin America's Zika virus is the latest undocumented immigrant to hit our shores (The National Review 2016).
>
> Risk of infection? Medical doctor fears danger of tuberculosis due to the massive influx of refugees – an expert disagrees (FOCUS 2016).

This process is known as "securitisation" and represents the opening up of the area of traditional security studies to the relatively new area of nontraditional or non-military security studies (Buzan et al. 1998). Its growing importance is attributed to the intellectual and policy space for non-military threats, which originated with the end of the Cold War (Lo Yuk-ping and Thomas 2010). The process of securitisation describes an extreme variant of politicisation by which a subject is identified as a threat to security, especially the security of a nation state. Through a more rational perspective, the securitised issue may not necessarily be the most urgent or threatening to survival but receives a disproportionate amount of attention and resources and broadens the political scope of action (Buzan et al. 1998). Issues of concern in the security agenda include climate change, natural disasters, and migration but also health aspects, such as infectious diseases. Security concerns in the context of health are reflected in the term "health security", which has become a prominent concept in global health policy. However, the tensions exist with other prominent global concepts, such as universal health coverage (UHC).

UHC means that all people receive the promotive, preventive, curative, rehabilitative, and palliative health services they need, of sufficient quality to be effective, while also ensuring that the use of these services does not expose the user to financial hardship (World Health Organization et al. 2010). Almost all definitions of UHC include three dimensions: universality (the whole population is included), access to services driven by demand, and protection from financial hardship when utilising the specified services. The concept is rooted in the human right to health, which is enshrined in international law as part of the International Covenant on Economic, Cultural, and Social Rights (UN Committee on Economic, Social and Cultural Rights 2000). The right to health regards inequalities in entitlements and access to health services based on, for example, race, ethnicity, nationality, or residence status as an undue violation of human rights. The right to health further requests that nation states refrain from actions that interfere with achieving the highest attainable state of health for individuals within their territory.

Countries have agreed to aim for achieving UHC by the year 2030 as part of the Agenda 2030 and the third Sustainable Development Goal (SDG 3) to "ensure health and well-being for all, at all ages; and in all settings, including humanitarian and fragile" (High Level Political Forum on Sustainable Development 2017). Conceptually, UHC focuses on reducing inequalities in health service provision and therefore tackles universal access for all people. It focuses on results and financing and takes the social determinants of health and population-level interventions into account.

As UHC and health security are prominent global health concepts which shape global health agendas and communities, debates have emerged whether the concepts collide or function synergistically with each other. While some policymakers and scholars have argued that promoting one agenda could benefit the other (Ooms et al. 2017), others have warned of the opposite effect: that promoting health security may limit and undermine UHC (Erondu et al. 2018).

One reason is that UHC is often considered a horizontal, comprehensive approach while health security is seen as a vertical, disease- or event-specific approach (Nicogossian et al. 2017). It has also been argued that health security is driven by political interests of governments of high-income countries and their national security concerns, while UHC is driven by civil society movements rooted in a sense of cosmopolitism (Ooms et al. 2017). UHC demands a bottom-up approach which assesses local needs, whereas health security is led by top-down interests (Ng and Ruger 2011). Additionally, in underfunded health systems with limited operational capacities, efforts towards UHC may conflict with the health security approach and vice versa (Ooms et al. 2017). This could be the case, for example, when investing in universal health-care access is pawned off against investing in infectious disease surveillance and control. Others have argued, however, that the health security agenda could raise awareness and as such additional funds for issues otherwise neglected, as was the case in the global HIV/AIDS epidemic at the turn of the millennium (Feldbaum et al. 2006).

This chapter provides an in-depth analysis of how health and security have been linked in the global debate and in the area of forced migration. Discussions around the meaning of global health security are commonly held by the global health community and in international relations, while health aspects of forced migrants tend to be addressed by domestic policies. Nevertheless, we argue both have been politicised and to some extent securitised, with important consequences for health policies among forced migrants. We start by examining the rising prominence of the concept of "global health security" and how it has come to be interpreted narrowly as "global infectious disease control". We then argue that through a similar process, health issues in the context of migration, especially among forced migrants, have been securitised. We provide examples from various countries and time periods, outlining how and why global infectious disease control and migrant health have been framed as security concerns. We proceed to analyse the consequences of the securitisation process in migrant health. The final section addresses the necessary political and conceptual changes required to make use of the benefits that come with the access of migrants to universal health care and infectious disease control for both the host population and forced migrants.

The Evolution of "Global Health Security"

The term "health security" is now widely used by both health-related security actors and the public health community. It has been introduced quite recently, but in order to fully grasp its history and the different meanings that have been attributed to it, we have to take into account the history of transborder security of infectious disease control.

In 1851, triggered by widespread cholera epidemics in Europe, the first international sanitary conference was the starting point for international health cooperation (Brown et al. 2006) and eventually led to the formation of the WHO. Since then, legally binding agreements in the form of "international health regulations" (IHR) (previously "international sanitary regulations") have been in place to combat the spread of a few infectious diseases.

The landmark document for the establishment of the term "health security" was the 1994 Human Development Report (United Nations Development Program (UNDP) 1994). It was themed around "human security" and identified seven dimensions of human security, health security being one. Overall, the report called for a transition from national security, with the nation state at its core, to a people-centred concept of protecting individuals. Based on the premise that security and peace are tied to development and human rights, the report describes health security as comprising two aspects: firstly, *collective* health security to reduce the vulnerability of societies to threats from cross-border health issues and secondly *individual* health security to promote access to safe and effective health services and medicines. This duality of addressing both individual and collective health aspects strongly characterises the comprehensive understanding advocated by UNDP. It explicitly includes anything relevant to individual health, both communicable and non-communicable disease, and links disease to poverty and vulnerability. However, the concept described in the report differs from the implementation of health security policies.

The understanding of health security has since been taken forward and changed by many actors, one of the most noteworthy being the World Health Organization (WHO). In 2001, the World Health Assembly (WHA) adopted a resolution on "Global Health Security: Epidemics Alert and Response" (WHA 2001). This was later described as the first step towards understanding global health security as compliance with the IHR (Aldis 2008) and called for a complete revision of the IHR. Subsequently, a comprehensive reform was undertaken in 2005, and one of the

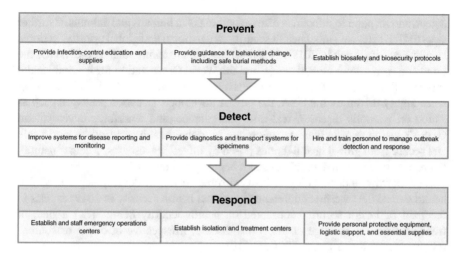

Fig. 7.1 Functions of the International Health Regulations (own illustration)

major changes was the abandonment of specifying diseases under the IHR (formerly yellow fever, cholera, and plague). While the revision broadened the scope using an all-risk approach, it neglected health inequalities and the social determinants of health. The IHR's scope now is to prevent, detect, and respond to the international spread of diseases that impose a risk to public health (see Fig. 7.1). Countries are compelled to notify the WHO in the case of infectious disease outbreaks with either serious public health impact, risk of international spread, or the possibility of travel and trade restrictions. The WHO can then proclaim a public health emergency of international concern ("PHEIC") and quickly initiate a coordinated global response in order to contain an outbreak where it occurs, minimising unnecessary interference on travel or trade (WHO 2008). Ever since the IHR revision, it has had an effect on the governance of health issues in the context of infectious diseases at the international, European, and national levels, by setting rules, norms, and mandates to react and respond to health threats.

The prominence of the concept of "health security" was further strengthened by the 2007 World Health Report. It confirms the necessity of compliance with the IHR in order to ensure global health security (Aldis 2008) but defines health security more broadly "as the activities required, both proactive and reactive, to minimise vulnerability to acute public health events that endanger the collective health of populations living across geographical regions and international boundaries" (WHO 2007). In addition to infectious disease, it also addresses issues such as poverty, violence, and chemical, biological, and nuclear attacks or accidents as important threats to achieving global health security.

In 2014, immediately preceding the 2014–2016 Ebola epidemic, the Global Health Security Agenda (GHSA) was launched as a new partnership in the global health security debate. Comprising over 64 states, international organisations and non-governmental organisations, it aims to support capacity building to prevent, detect, and respond to infectious disease outbreaks in humans and animals. It further aims to "[…] elevate global health security as a national and global priority" (Global Health Security Agenda 2019). Norm-setting organisations such as the WHO, the Food and Agriculture Organization, and the World Organization for Animal Health serve as advisors to the GHSA member states. Endorsed by the G7 in 2014 and ever since highly driven by the USA, the GHSA developed 11 action packages such as action on zoonotic diseases, real-time surveillance, and workforce development. GHSA's vision reveals their narrow scope in global health security: "a world safe and secure from global health threats posed by infectious diseases, whether natural, deliberate, or accidental"(Global Health Security Agenda 2019).

This narrow understanding is also mirrored in recent developments in global health debates. At the first conference on global health security in 2019, experts in the field of health security consented on health security being "[…] a state of freedom from the scourge of infectious disease, irrespective of origin or source" (Global Health Security Conference 2019).

Two polarising understandings of health security can be outlined: On the one hand, it has been described as addressing all possible threats to human health, both individually and collectively (UNDP definition). On the other hand, health security has been understood as freedom from those infectious diseases that may spread rapidly and therefore interfere with travel and trade.

These conflicting definitions have been addressed by scholars as "narrow" and "broad" definitions of health security (Ooms et al. 2017) or, with a slightly different connotation, as "statist" vs "global" (Rushton 2011). However, as in the case of the World Health Report 2007, definitions do not always fall neatly into these opposing categories, further complicating the discussion.

The term "health security", in its first interpretation by the UNDP, was promoted as "securing health" of individuals. It has then been used to refer to global infectious disease control and the international health regulations, coinciding with a complete reform of the international health regulations. It has been argued that through this shift "the dominant health security discourse captures only a very small proportion of the issues that threaten individual and population health worldwide—those which are of concern to the west" (Rushton 2011). High-income countries have therefore been identified as main actors in the process of securitising infectious disease control (Hwenda et al. 2011). Health security is now understood as security from ill health (as a threat mainly to high-income countries) instead of protecting individuals worldwide.

Securitisation of Health in the Context of Forced Migration

The growing emphasis on securing collective health over individual health needs, and the exclusive narrative of health security as security of selected populations, can also be identified in approaches to health among forced migrants. The securitisation of health in the context of forced migration, i.e. the process of considering migrants a threat to national public health, has a long history. This section provides a histori-cal example (Box 7.2) to outline how forced migrants' health has been identified

Box 7.2: The Case of Ellis Island: Systematic Exclusion of Persons Assumed to Suffer from Illness or Inability to "Make a Living"

Immigrants to late nineteenth-century USA, many of which were forced to leave their countries of origin due to fears of religious or political persecution, had to pass through the infamous "line" at Ellis Island. The "line" referred to a series of "gated pathways resembling cattle pens", where thousands of immigrants were examined rapidly by public health officials (Bateman-House and Fairchild 2008). Even though this procedure originally aimed at the detection of infectious disease, the responsible public health officers conducted a rather broad medical examination, focusing on the exclusion and classification of those who "would not make good citizens" (Bateman-House and Fairchild 2008).

Classification was realised in two categories: Those classified as A were either "dangerous contagious" (including, e.g. tuberculosis and syphilis) or suffering from a "loathsome disease" (including, e.g. "insane persons", "idiots", "feeble-minded", and "imbeciles") and denied entry. Category B consisted of conditions interfering with the ability to "earn a living", such as debility, senility, pregnancy, and "poor physique", and exclusion was up to the discretion of the responsible public health official (Fairchild 2003). When denied entry to the USA, migrants were either held captive in isolation on Ellis Island or deported directly. Some were granted hospital treatment, but on their own expenses. Often, this resulted in deportation due to pending medical bills (Bateman-House and Fairchild 2008).

Despite all restrictions, only a fraction of prospective migrants was effectively denied entry as demand for cheap labour force was high in the industrial era. Eventually, however, the labour market saturated and immigration procedures became more restrictive. In 1924, obligatory and privately paid medical examinations were introduced and had to be completed prior to departure (Bateman-House and Fairchild 2008). This so-called pre-entry screening is still in place, although the evidence suggests that only a small fraction of tuberculosis cases is identified pre-entry (Aldridge et al. 2016), and similar screening procedures are applied by many other high-income countries (e.g. Canada, Australia; see also Chap. 10). Remarkably, immigration regulations have not changed drastically since the nineteenth century: Prospective migrants to the USA are still categorized A or B, A implying infectious pulmonary tuberculosis and impeding admission to the country. Furthermore, current US law still lists under "inadmissible aliens on health-related grounds": anyone determined to have a communicable disease of public health significance and anyone with "a physical or mental disorder [...] that may pose, or has posed, a threat to the property, safety, or welfare of the alien or others".

and treated as a threat to the security of host populations over time. We argue that this not only happened in terms of infectious disease control but also included mental health and the public costs of disease. We continue to examine whether these approaches are still of importance today.

The example from Ellis Island (Box 7.2) serves as a particularly vivid case for the securitisation of migrants' health for three reasons: Firstly, it shows that contemporary screening programmes are often historically rooted and tend to persist. Secondly, it shows that the scrutiny of the screening depends on the political willingness to accept migrants. Thirdly, it illustrates the threats associated with the (ill) health of forced migrants: It is seen as a threat to population health through the importation and spread of infectious disease from high-endemic to low-endemic countries, a threat to overall security through mental illness, and a threat to prosperity and state budget through costly diseases. The significance of all three arguments and their (implicit or explicit) reflection in contemporary policy and practice will be examined briefly in the succeeding sections. To this end, we focus on current screening programmes, especially for tuberculosis, and discuss cost-containment policies and two case studies from Germany on mental health and vaccination among asylum seekers and refugees.

Screening for Infectious Disease: Security for Whom?

Besides the USA, many high-income countries screen asylum seekers for infectious disease through pre-entry screenings (e.g. Australia, Canada), directly at arrival, or in the scope of registration for the asylum process (e.g. Germany). Diseases screened for include tuberculosis, hepatitis B/C, and HIV (Kunst et al. 2017; ECDC 2018; see also Chap. 10 "Assessing the Health of Persons Experiencing Forced Migration: Current Practices for Health Service Organisations").

While the overall aim of screening programmes is to control infectious diseases, end transmission, and prevent infections, it remains unclear who or what they primarily intend to protect: migrants from the consequences of disease, migrants from other migrants in shared accommodation centres, native populations from migrants, or publicly financed health systems from costly treatments.

Public opinion tends to focus on protecting host populations (e.g. Die 2018). Nonetheless, most evidence shows that transmission of communicable disease rarely occurs between foreign-born and native-born populations. For tuberculosis, for example, molecular epidemiological studies show that even though in low-endemic settings migrant populations make up a relevant proportion of tuberculosis cases, transmission between foreign-born and native-born populations rarely occurs (Lillebaek et al. 2002; Sandgren et al. 2014). Migration may therefore be associated with rising incidence of tuberculosis in low-endemic countries, but the rising incidence stems from the reactivation of disease in migrants and not from transmission to the host population. Several studies even suggest that foreign-born patients with tuberculosis cases are less likely to transmit disease compared to native-born tuberculosis patients (Chin et al. 1998; Fok et al. 2008). If disease transmission does occur, this is far more likely to happen within migrant communities than to native populations (Sandgren et al. 2014). The same is true for many other infectious diseases, as is shown by the case example of disease outbreaks in shared housing facilities in Germany (Box 7.3). Better housing conditions, improved hygiene in reception centres (Bozorgmehr et al. 2016), social integration, and good access to primary care are measures to prevent such outbreaks. Although the evidence shows that structural factors and supply-side factors of the health system are the drivers of outbreaks and potential vaccination gaps, national policy responses have securitised the issue by passing legislation for mandatory vaccination programmes linked to financial penalties (Box 7.3).

Box 7.3: Gaps in Vaccination Coverage: A Demand-Side or a Supply-Side/Structural Problem?

A review of 10 years of infectious disease outbreaks for all shared housing facilities of asylum seekers in Germany (2004–2014) showed that outbreaks were related to vaccine-preventable and diarrhoeal disease (varicella, measles, scabies, rotavirus, influenza, salmonella, and norovirus) and in very few cases to tuberculosis. Only in 2 of 117 outbreaks over 10 years a transmission occurred to the population outside of the shelter. Both events were cases of measles (Kuehne et al. 2015).

These outbreaks are preventable through structural and individual preventive interventions, such as better vaccination services, which have been shown to be insufficient and poorly managed in the context of refugee shelters (Bozorgmehr et al. 2016). Experience from practitioners in refugee shelters, and evaluations of outreach vaccination programmes, shows that vaccination uptake is very high among asylum seekers and refugees (Brockmann et al. 2016). The evidence hence clearly shows that gaps in vaccination coverage among asylum seekers and refugees are a supply-side, rather than a demand-side, problem. Despite these facts, national legislation will be passed in 2019 making measles vaccination mandatory for asylum seekers and refugees in reception centres and shared accommodation facilities. Non-compliance will be penalised by high fines. The act of securitisation here addresses migrants' presumed denial of vaccinations, requiring the extraordinary measure of making vaccinations for asylum seekers mandatory.

If the rationale of screening was the protection of the individual from disease, we would expect to find the detection and treatment of disease to be consistent with the needs of forced migrants. Data about burden of disease of forced migrants is difficult to obtain due to intra-group heterogeneity, lack of reporting, and differences of social determinants in host countries (World Health Organisation Regional Office 2018). Despite these difficulties and uncertainties, however, overall trends show that even though migrants tend to have somewhat higher morbidity and mortality ratios for infectious disease than host populations (Aldridge et al. 2018), morbidity and mortality for non-communicable diseases (NCDs) are significantly higher: NCDs account for 86% of deaths and 77% of disease burden among migrants in the European region (World Health Organisation Regional Office 2018). Hence, from a population health perspective, the focus on screening for and treatment of infectious disease in forced migrants does not target the most important health needs of this very heterogeneous population. Nevertheless, forced migrants from countries with high prevalence of tuberculosis are at a higher risk of suffering from tuberculosis or being asymptomatically infected with the disease. Equally, extra-pulmonary tuberculosis poses a high risk (WHO 2018) but is not addressed by public health measures because it is not as infectious. An evidence-informed and needs-based rationale to screening for tuberculosis would therefore be (a) to explicitly target those at higher risk of having and developing tuberculosis (Bozorgmehr et al. 2019), (b) to take extra-pulmonary disease into consideration, and (c) to include screening for latent tuberculosis infection and offer treatment to those at risk of developing active tuberculosis (WHO 2018).

It seems reasonable to conclude that current programmes primarily serve to prevent the spread of disease in shared housing and migrant communities, therefore primarily protecting forced migrants themselves. However, it is not guaranteed that screening is accordingly perceived by migrants as being implemented for their own protection or that the aim of screening is communicated accordingly by public health authorities. Defining the target population is furthermore relevant for evaluating the effectiveness and cost-effectiveness of public health screening programmes (Wilson and Jungner 1968; Andermann 2008). A survey on screening measures for asylum seekers implemented in 28 European countries concluded that few experts considered the structure and implementation of screening measures in their countries to be sufficiently well executed (Kärki et al. 2014). The screening programmes in some regions of Germany, for example, have been criticised for being irrational, as screening is mandatory for very rare diseases, leading to low yields, a high number needed to screen, and high costs (Bozorgmehr et al. 2017).

We argue that these irrational and costly screening practices are the result of securitisation in the context of forced migration. As these investments are unlikely to translate into improved population health (of forced migrants or residents), they can be attributed as costs to suit the "security concerns" of authorities. What is more, parallel to the debate of "global health security", we see a strong focus on public health and collective security over ensuring the health of the individual. This is illustrated by more recent developments in the context of screening for and addressing mental diseases among asylum seekers and refugees (Box 7.4). While screening for mental illness, such as depression, has the potential to be cost-effective given appropriate follow-up care processes (Biddle et al. 2019), there are severe gaps in access to appropriate services (Satinsky et al. 2019). In Germany, these shortcomings can be attributed to limited capacities of the mental health-care system, but also to a lack of prioritisation in terms of health planning and budget allocation by policymakers. Well-intended attempts to raise awareness of this issue also

> **Box 7.4: Addressing Mental Illness Among Forced Migrants: Individual Need or Threat to Society?**
>
> Calls for addressing the mental health of forced migrants have been generally based upon a needs-based discourse, linking to human rights and equity arguments in providing psychosocial care for refugees or asylum seekers with a high burden of mental illness. Recently, however, a shift of the discourse towards securitisation can be observed. In a recent report on traumatised refugees, the National Academy of Sciences in Germany (Leopoldina) called for rapid measures to address the mental health needs of refugees in Germany. One of the main lines of argument is that a failure to address mental illness could pose a threat to German society, as refugees with untreated illness could potentially have a lower threshold for violence and aggression (Leopoldina - Nationale Akademie der Wissenschaften 2018). While the intention of this argument is to facilitate access and raise awareness among policymakers with regard to the potential consequences of untreated mental illness, the securitisation poses a slippery slope, potentially leading to a consideration of refugees themselves as a risk, motivating policymakers to impose even more restrictive immigration policies. This is particularly dangerous, as emerging evidence suggests that restrictive policies (i.e. securitisation of immigration) may increase mental illness among migrants (see Chap. 8 "Security over Health: The Effect of Security Policies on Migrant Mental Health in the UK").

make use of securitisation arguments in addition to needs-based ones, aiming to mobilise resources for identification and treatment of mental conditions (Box 7.4).

Even though in practice the aim of screening programmes is to protect the collective health of migrant and asylum-seeking populations, the public and medical debate seems to focus on the host population, a phenomenon which is described in more detail in Chap. 10 "Assessing the Health of Persons Experiencing Forced Migration: Current Practices for Health Service Organisations".

Restriction of Entitlements to Health-Care Services for Forced Migrants

Restriction of entitlements to health care for forced migrants are in place in many countries (International Organisation for Migration 2016). The act of restricting health-care entitlements for a certain population group is not commonly framed in the classic narrative of security theory because health-care utilisation is rarely explicitly named as threat to security. In this section, however, we argue that restrictions to health-care entitlements can actually be explained by classic security theory or by the resulting process of framing migrants themselves as a threat to society.

For refugees, the "Convention Relating to the Status of Refugees and its Protocol" explicitly guarantees the "same treatment with respect to public relief and assistance as is accorded with nationals" (United Nations High Commissioner for Refugees 2010). Nonetheless, national laws do not always endorse and respect international laws. Even though many countries, including all countries of the European Union, commit to UHC, this is often not realised for forced migrants (see also Chap. 5). For asylum seekers and especially irregular migrants, access is governed even more restrictively (Abubakar et al. 2018).

The reasoning behind restricting access is rarely stated explicitly by legislative authorities or bodies. However, there are two common readings, which may contribute to varying degrees to the decision to limit health-care entitlements: first, to protect the national health system from rising costs and, second, to discourage "health seeking migration", assuming that forced migrants may choose their destination based on considerations of where they might receive the best health care.

With respect to the first argument, the protection of the health system from costs arising as a result of disease treatment may be an especially relevant consideration for countries with premigration screening programmes. In the USA, for example, prospective migrants—including refugees—are required to complete screening and treatment for pulmonary tuberculosis at migrants' own expense before departure (Liu and Painter 2009). In Australia, applications for residency can be denied if "an applicant has a health condition for which treatment is likely to result in significant health care [...] costs to the Australian community" (Migration Regulations 1994 as cited by Abubakar et al. 2018). In Taiwan, migrants have been deported upon the detection of tuberculosis. This practice has recently been restricted to multidrug tuberculosis, which entails significantly longer—and therefore costlier—treatments (Kuan 2018).

Going back to the process of securitisation described by Buzan et al. (1998), they argue that the framing of an issue as threat to security serves not only to allocate an extraordinary budget but also *to use extraordinary measures* to respond to them: "to break the normal political rules of the game" or by "placing limitations on otherwise inviolable rights". This might be the reasoning behind restricting health care for specific groups, e.g. asylum seekers, despite committing to UHC, or behind infringing on the right to health despite having ratified the right to health. If the protection of public funds is the underlying motivation for entitlement restrictions as "extraordinary measure", adequate supranational health financing policies may help to overcome the security logic (see also Chap. 5).

In the case of the second argument, restricting health care is used as a political instrument to discourage migration. The same mechanism is applied, for example, in the UK, where "voluntary" repatriation is enforced by denying or charging for health services (United Nations High Commissioner for Refugees 2010) or when medical staff is required to report undocumented migrants (Abubakar et al. 2018). In these cases, health and access to care is used as an element of political control. In these processes, the object of securitisation is not migrants' health but the migrants themselves. These measures are thus repercussions of a broader context in which migrants have been securitised and the restrictions, denial, and charging for medical services are used as "extraordinary" mechanisms to respond to the threat migration poses to society (see also Chap. 8).

Negative Consequences of Securitising the Health of Forced Migrants

We have shown that forced migrants may be identified as a threat to population health by framing them as carriers of infectious disease, as a potential threat to security if (mentally) ill, and as causing costs rather than contributing to state-funded welfare systems. Reducing migrant health to infectious disease concerns has been called "the maybe most pervasive and powerful myth related to migrants and health throughout history" (Abubakar et al. 2018). We now examine three consequences of these security-based approaches on migrants' access to care and health-care provision.

The first consequence of securitisation is the effect on the allocation of resources. Budget allocation is directed towards those infectious diseases identified as threat to community health in host countries rather than the identification of needs and vulnerabilities of the individuals. While screening programmes for infectious disease are implemented in many high-income countries (ECDC 2018), very few have successfully implemented vulnerability assessments (despite existing legislative framework; see also Chap. 10). Another example is that access to vaccination against infectious disease is commonly recommended and provided for forced migrants, whereas, e.g. in Germany, vaccination against the human papilloma virus is not part of the package recommended for asylum seekers in reception centres (Robert Koch Institute 2015). Other potentially more important causes of disease to the individual, such as non-communicable diseases, may also be neglected.

The second consequence is the process of identifying the disease itself as threat, which may lead to discrimination and stigmatisation for the identified carrier of the disease. This process (shown for tuberculosis by Abarca Tomás et al. 2013) may cause asylum seekers to negate or deny symptoms of (infectious) disease or avoid accessing health services out of fear of negative repercussions for the asylum process. This can lead to the creation of additional barriers for migrants to access health services and may also dramatically undermine measures of effective disease control (see Chap. 11). This may result in the deterioration of health status and potentially avoidable health emergencies and hospitalisations (Lichtl et al. 2016).

The third consequence is that restriction of entitlements to health care may lead to difficulties in accessing UHC in all three of the dimensions mentioned previously: universality, services, and financial protection. Tying entitlements to health care to legal status and/or nationality clearly contradicts the concept of universality. Even though some countries generally grant access to health care for documented migrants, many countries limit them in their scope, granting access only to certain services, e.g. emergency care, acute conditions, or maternal services (see also Chap. 5). Financial protection, the third dimension, is also not guaranteed in many situations: with missing legal entitlements, as is often the case for undocumented migrants or transiting migrants, health expenses and necessary medication may need to be paid out of pocket or require co-payments (Abubakar et al. 2018). Furthermore, restricting health services to acute and urgent conditions has been shown to create exactly the opposite of the intended effect, leading to higher health-care expenditures among forced migrants through late diagnosis, preventable hospi-talisation, and a shift from primary care to tertiary care structures (Bozorgmehr et al. 2015). The consequences are even more detrimental for irregular migrants, as mandatory reporting of irregular migrant status by health-care workers may mean that health services are avoided at all costs (see also Chap. 8).

UHC for Forced Migrants: Benefits for Host Populations and Forced Migrants

Four mechanisms have been described and summarised by Wenham et al. (2019), describing the synergies of UHC and infectious disease control: Firstly, individuals suffering from disease may be detected and treated earlier under UHC (Jain and Alam, 2017). Secondly, when access to health services is assured, individuals are less likely to seek health care abroad, decreasing the risk of transnational spread of disease. Thirdly, UHC helps to build trust between citizens and (public) health insti-tutions, an essential prerequisite for effective cooperation in the case of an epidemic (Heymann et al. 2015). Finally, UHC protects people from poverty and therefore addresses the social determinants of infectious disease (Jain and Alam 2017). Positive effects operating the other way around have also been illustrated, as effec-tive infectious disease control reduces health inequities (Ooms et al. 2018). The conceptual convergences and divergences, synergies, and tensions are summarised in Fig. 7.2.

Even though the public health community tends to avoid the securitisation per-spective, in the context of migration securitising forced migrant's health may entail some benefits for host populations and forced migrants. In many countries where health entitlements are restricted, framing infectious diseases as threat has led to free provision of diagnostics and treatment for these diseases. In the UK, for exam-ple, tuberculosis treatment is exempted from the user fees imposed upon migrants who are denied asylum (United Nations High Commissioner for Refugees 2010). However, if implemented exclusively on a security rationale, this approach may also lead to the perception of forced migrants as vectors of infectious disease and deflect attention from the fact that forced migrants are a vulnerable population with indi-vidual health needs.

Lifting restrictions on health-care entitlements and ensuring UHC for all forced migrants, no matter their legal status, may be beneficial not only for migrants them-selves but also for infectious disease control. In the case of tuberculosis, data from national surveillance programmes in low-endemic countries shows that even though a growing proportion of detected cases is attributable to foreign-born patients, most of these cases cannot be detected by screening for active disease upon entry as they stem from the reactivation of latent disease and occur after migration (Aldridge et al. 2016). Avoiding stigmatisation and removing barriers to health service access contribute to a timely detection and lower cost of disease while decreasing risks for

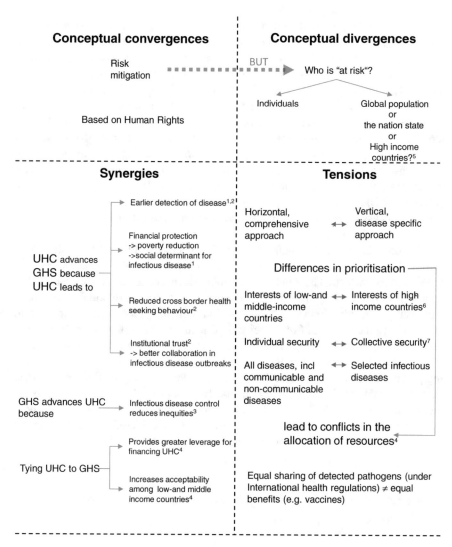

Fig. 7.2 Conceptual and empirical synergies and tensions between universal health coverage (UHC) and global health security (GHS), own illustration adapted from Wenham et al. (2019)

transmission (Lonnroth et al. 2017; Sreeramareddy et al. 2009). Additionally, adherence to treatment is essential in order to prevent the creation of drug-resistant bacteria. The accessibility of health information and positive experiences and interaction with health-care providers are thus of utmost importance (Abarca Tomás et al. 2013; Lonnroth et al. 2017), and this would be facilitated by providing UHC.

Ooms and Jahn (2017) state that "efforts to improve global health security contribute to global health equity, albeit only to a part of global health equity". The same is true in the context of forced migration. Combatting infectious disease in an evidence-based and cost-effective manner is in the best interest of everybody and ultimately contributes to migrants' health, despite being just one health concern among other, often more pressing issues. Acknowledging the heterogeneous nature of forced migrants requires the use of disaggregated data. This may then lead to targeted screening measures that increase effectiveness and cost-effectiveness of established screening programmes and help to tailor screening programmes to burden of disease (Bozorgmehr et al. 2019). Bringing current programmes in line with criteria for public health screening measures (see above Wilson and Jungner 1968; Andermann 2008) by explaining the procedure and consequences of outcomes and ensuring access to treatment may also increase the acceptability of screening programmes for migrants.

Tensions between individuals' rights and collective health are a classic public health dilemma and reinforce the need to carefully balance the harms to the individual against the actual benefits for the public. Beeres et al. (2018) suggest another approach to overcoming the ethical dilemma of restricting individuals' autonomy and liberty to decide whether to participate in a screening programme (Beeres et al. 2018). Using the concept of reciprocity, described as "to return good in the proportion to the good we receive, and to make reparations for the harm we have done" (Becker 2014), they argue that the participation of individuals in obligatory screening programmes creates the moral obligation of the executing institutions to assist "the individual (or the community) in the fulfilment of their health care needs, including identification of personal health needs and providing accessible treatment when needed". Such an approach, however, may be considered to collide with the notion of anchoring health services in the right to health.

How to Make Use of the Benefits: Necessary Conceptual and Political Changes

To make use of the benefits that come with migrants' access to universal health care and infectious disease control, practical and fast changes in health-care provision and policy are needed. In the following section, we provide three necessary steps for this:

Firstly, forced migrants' health needs to be de-securitised politically and in the public debate. Forced migrants do tend to have higher risks of suffering from infectious disease than the respective host populations, but transmission of infectious diseases between migrant groups and host populations rarely occurs. Rather, post-migration factors put forced migrants at higher risk of acquiring and suffering from infectious diseases. Acknowledging this and de-securitising migrants' health accordingly would help to remove associated stigma, benefitting both infectious disease control and access to services, while shifting the attention to post-migration social determinants which may favour the spread of infectious diseases among forced migrants. The securitisation process has further led to a discourse in which the rights and needs of the individual may be disregarded in order to ensure collective security. De-securitising migrants' health would help to equalise individual versus collective health aspects.

Secondly, in line with Heymann et al. (2015), we call for the acknowledgement that individual health security is an essential element for collective global health security and that effective risk reduction needs to address all levels—the individual, national, and global level. Successful collective health security and infectious disease control are therefore tied to UHC as a means to achieve individual health security.

Thirdly, and perhaps most importantly, both health security and UHC need to be interpreted inclusively and therefore truly anchored in the human right to health. Wenham et al. (2019) have argued that convergence between the two concepts of health security and UHC could "be found through the realization of the right to health, with both UHC and global health security requiring that states address inaction or regression in realizing the right to health to the mutual benefit of both […]".

Taking into consideration that Ooms et al. (2019) have demonstrated that the right to health has historically been considered a citizens' right, granting rights to those considered a citizen under the respective governments and excluding whoever was historically considered to be "non-citizens", such as women, slaves, or non-nationals—the common anchor in an inclusively interpreted right seems to be a crucial point to the discussion. The authors further argue that the "shift from citizens' rights to human rights has not been completed yet" and that moving beyond citizens' rights towards human rights requires citizens who challenge current policy narratives and who "elect governments that prioritize human rights in domestic and foreign policy" (Ooms et al. 2019). If both concepts are sustainably anchored in the right to health, inclusive health systems can promote health security efforts that respect the right to health and UHC for all, including forced migrants.

Conclusion

Linking health and security has triggered a process of securitising health. Over the years, the concept of "global health security" has been equated with infectious disease control. It has been implemented through the international health regulations and governed, to some extent, by high-income countries driven by their national rather than by global interests. At the same time, there has been a global movement advocating for the establishment of UHC. Its aim is to improve health care by ensuring universal access, essential services, and financial risk protection.

Both agendas, achieving UHC and global health security, have been promoted and advocated for sometimes by the same actors (e.g. WHO). This has caused a comprehensive discussion about whether the agendas complement or conflict with one another, by what means they could be aligned, and what positive or negative effects could be expected by such alignment.

The process of securitising health, especially infectious disease, has negatively affected forced migrants. Many high-income countries have installed comprehensive pre-entry screening measures for infectious diseases, while other countries have employed travel restrictions based on health status. At the same time, for reasons of containing costs or using access to health care as a political lever, forced migrants suffer from the exclusion from health systems, a limitation of services, and a lack of financial protection. Tendencies to use the denial of or charging for healthcare services as means to "disincentivise" forced migration or to enforce "voluntary" repatriation can be observed. To some extent, health security approaches have resulted in the creation of further barriers to health service access, resulting from stigmatisation and other negative repercussions of an infectious disease diagnosis.

Despite these current discrepancies, some synergetic potential for forced migration can be seen between the two seemingly contradicting agendas. We argue that a successful linkage of health security and UHC agendas to the benefit of both forced migrants and host populations is possible. However, three underlying conditions (political, practical, and conceptual) need to be fulfilled in order to achieve rational, effective, and cost-effective approaches to infectious disease control and UHC. This requires careful planning, disaggregated data, and a continuous evaluation of inclusive public health programmes which are anchored in the right to health.

References

Abarca Tomás, B., Pell, C., Bueno Cavanillas, A., Guillén Solvas, J., Pool, R., & Roura, M. (2013). Tuberculosis in migrant populations. A systematic review of the qualitative literature. *PLoS One, 8*(12), e82440.

Abubakar, I., Aldridge, R. W., Devakumar, D., Orcutt, M., Burns, R., Barreto, M. L., et al. (2018). The UCL–lancet commission on migration and health: The health of a world on the move. *The Lancet, 392*, 2606–2654.

Aldis, W. (2008). Health security as a public health concept: A critical analysis. *Health Policy and Planning, 23*(6), 369–375.

Aldridge, R. W., Nellums, L. B., Bartlett, S., Barr, A. L., Patel, P., Burns, R., et al. (2018). Global patterns of mortality in international migrants: A systematic review and meta-analysis. *The Lancet, 392*(10164), 2553–2566.

Aldridge, R. W., Zenner, D., White, P. J., Williamson, E. J., Muzyamba, M. C., Dhavan, P., et al. (2016). Tuberculosis in migrants moving from high-incidence to low-incidence countries: A population-based cohort study of 519 955 migrants screened before entry to England, Wales, and Northern Ireland. *The Lancet, 388*(10059), 2510–2518.

Andermann, A. (2008). Revisting Wilson and Jungner in the genomic age: A review of screening criteria over the past 40 years. *Bulletin of the World Health Organization, 86*(4), 317–319.

Bateman-House, A., & Fairchild, A. (2008). Medical examination of immigrants at Ellis Island. *Virtual Mentor, 10*(4), 235–241.

Becker, L. C. (2014). *Reciprocity*. London: Routledge.

Beeres, D. T., Cornish, D., Vonk, M., Ravensbergen, S. J., Maeckelberghe, E. L. M., Boele Van Hensbroek, P., et al. (2018). Screening for infectious diseases of asylum seekers upon arrival:

The necessity of the moral principle of reciprocity. *BMC Medical Ethics, 19*(1), 16. https://doi.org/10.1186/s12910-018-0256-7

Biddle, L., Miners, A., & Bozorgmehr, K. (2019). Cost-utility of screening for depression among asylum seekers: A modelling study in Germany. *Health Policy, 123*(9), 873–881.

Bozorgmehr, K., Preussler, S., Wagner, U., Joggerst, B., Szecsenyi, J., Razum, O., et al. (2019). Using country of origin to inform targeted tuberculosis screening in asylum seekers: A modelling study of screening data in a German federal state, 2002–2015. *BMC Infectious Diseases, 19*(1), 304.

Bozorgmehr, K., Schneider, C., & Joos, S. (2015). Equity in access to health care among asylum seekers in Germany: Evidence from an exploratory population-based cross-sectional study. *BMC Health Services Research, 15*(1), 502.

Bozorgmehr, K., Stefan, N., Thaiss, H. M., & Razum, O. (2016). Die gesundheitliche Versorgungssituation von Asylsuchenden Bundesweite Bestandsaufnahme über die. *Bundesgesundheitsblatt - Gesundheitsforschung – Gesundheitsschutz, 59*(5), 545–555.

Bozorgmehr, K., Wahedi, K., Noest, S., Szecsenyi, J., & Razum, O. (2017). Infectious disease screening in asylum seekers: Range, coverage and economic evaluation in Germany, 2015. *Eurosurveillance, 22*(40), 16-00677. https://doi.org/10.2807/1560-7917.ES.2017.22.40.16-00677

Brockmann, S., Wjst, S., Zelmer, U., Carollo, S., Schmid, M., Roller, G., et al. (2016). Public health initiative for improved vaccination for asylum seekers. *Bundesgesundheitsblatt, Gesundheitsforschung, Gesundheitsschutz, 59*(5), 592–598.

Brown, T. M., Cueto, M., & Fee, E. (2006). The World Health Organization and the transition from "international" to "global" public health. *American Journal of Public Health, 96*(1), 62–72.

Buzan, B., Wæver, O., & de Wilde, J. (1998). *Security: A new framework for analysis.* Boulder, CO: Lynne Rienner Pub.

Chin, D. P., Deriemer, K., Small, P. M., De Leon, A. P., Steinhart, R., Schecter, G. F., et al. (1998). Differences in contributing factors to tuberculosis incidence in U.S.-born and foreign-born persons. *American Journal of Respiratory and Critical Care Medicine, 158*(6), 1797–1803.

Die, W. (2018, April 30). Migration: Die Angst vor der eingeschleppten Tuberkulose. *Claudia Ehrenstein* [online]. Retrieved July 31, 2019, from https://www.welt.de/politik/deutschland/article175943319/Migration-Die-Angst-vor-der-eingeschleppten-Tuberkulose.html

ECDC. (2018). *Public health guidance on screening and vaccination for infectious diseases in newly arrived migrants within the EU/EEA* (p. 85). Solna, Sweden: ECDC.

Erondu, N. A., Martin, J., Marten, R., Ooms, G., Yates, R., & Heymann, D. L. (2018). Building the case for embedding global health security into universal health coverage: A proposal for a unified health system that includes public health. *The Lancet, 392*(10156), 1482–1486.

Fairchild, A. L. (2003). *Science at the borders: Immigrant medical inspection and the shaping of the modern industrial labor force.* Baltimore: Johns Hopkins University Press.

Feldbaum, H., Lee, K., & Patel, P. (2006). The National Security Implications of HIV/AIDS. *PLoS Medicine, 3*(6), e171.

Focus, F. (2016). Mediziner fürchtet Tuberkulose-Gefahr wegen Flüchtlingswelle - Experte widerspricht. *FOCUS Online* [online]. Retrieved July 31, 2019, from https://www.focus.de/gesundheit/ratgeber/seltenekrankheiten/steigendes-tuberkulose-risiko-mediziner-fuerchtet-bundesinstitut-verschweigt-ansteckungsgefahr-durch-fluechtlinge_id_5466971.html

Fok, A., Numata, Y., Schulzer, M., & Fitzgerald, M. J. (2008). Risk factors for clustering of tuberculosis cases: A systematic review of population-based molecular epidemiology studies. *The International Journal of Tuberculosis and Lung Disease, 12*(5), 480–492.

Global Health Security Agenda. (2019). *Global health security agenda.* Retrieved July 31, 2019, from https://www.ghsagenda.org/members

Global Health Security Conference. (2019). *Sydney statement on global health security.* Retrieved July 4, 2019, from https://www.ghs2019.com/sydney-statement.php

Heymann, D. L., Chen, L., Takemi, K., Fidler, D. P., Tappero, J. W., Thomas, M. J., et al. (2015). Global health security: The wider lessons from the west African Ebola virus disease epidemic. *The Lancet, 385*(9980), 1884–1901.

High Level Political Forum on Sustainable Development. (2017). *2017 HLPF thematic review of SDG3: Ensure healthy lives and promote well-being for all at all ages.* Retrieved June 30, 2019, from https://sustainabledevelopment.un.org/content/documents/14367SDG3format-rev_MD_OD.pdf

Hwenda, L., Mahlathi, P., & Maphanga, T. (2011). Why African countries need to participate in global health security discourse. *Global Health Governance, 4*(2), 24.

International Organisation for Migration. (2016). *Summary report on the MIPEX health strand and country reports.*

Jain, V., & Alam, A. (2017). Redefining universal health coverage in the age of global health security. *BMJ Global Health, 2*(2), e000255.

Kärki, T., Napoli, C., Riccardo, F., Fabiani, M., Grazia Dente, M., Carballo, M., et al. (2014). Screening for infectious diseases among newly arrived migrants in EU/EEA countries - varying practices but consensus on the utility of screening. *International Journal of Environmental Research and Public Health, 11*(10), 11004–11014.

Kuan, M. M. (2018). Nationwide surveillance algorithms for tuberculosis among immigrant workers from highly endemic countries following pre-entry screening in Taiwan. *BMC Public Health, 18*(1), 1151.

Kuehne, A., Huschke, S., & Bullinger, M. (2015). Subjective health of undocumented migrants in Germany - a mixed methods approach. *BMC Public Health, 15*(1), 926.

Kunst, H., Burman, M., Arnesen, T. M., Fiebig, L., Hergens, M.-P., Kalkouni, O., et al. (2017). Tuberculosis and latent tuberculous infection screening of migrants in Europe: Comparative analysis of policies, surveillance systems and results. *The International Journal of Tuberculosis and Lung Disease, 21*(8), 840–851.

Leopoldina - Nationale Akademie Der Wissenschaften. (2018). *Hilfe für traumatisierte Flüchtlinge. Wissenschaften veröffentlichen Stellungnahme.* Retrieved July 5, 2019, from https://www.leopoldina.org/presse-1/nachrichten/traumatisierte-fluechtlinge/

Lichtl, C., Gewalt, S. C., Noest, S., Szecsenyi, J., & Bozorgmehr, K. (2016). Potentially avoidable and ambulatory care sensitive hospitalisations among forced migrants: A protocol for a systematic review and meta-analysis. *BMJ Open, 6*(9), e012216.

Lillebaek, T., Andersen, Å. B., Dirksen, A., Smith, E., Skovgaard, L. T., & Kok-Jensen, A. (2002). Persistent high incidence of tuberculosis in immigrants in a low-incidence country. *Emerging Infectious Diseases, 8*(7), 679–684.

Liu, Y., & Painter, J. A. (2009). Overseas screening for tuberculosis in U.S.-bound immigrants and refugees. *The New England Journal of Medicine, 360*(23), 2406–2415.

Lo Yuk-Ping, C., & Thomas, N. (2010). How is health a security issue? Politics, responses and issues. *Health Policy and Planning, 25*(6), 447–453.

Lonnroth, K., Mor, Z., Erkens, C., Bruchfeld, J., Nathavitharana, R. R., Van Der Werf, M. J., et al. (2017). Tuberculosis in migrants in low-incidence countries: Epidemiology and intervention entry points. *The International Journal of Tuberculosis and Lung Disease, 21*(6), 624–637.

Ng, N. Y., & Ruger, J. P. (2011). Global health governance at a crossroads. *Global Health Governance, 3*(2), 1–37.

Nicogossian, A., Stabile, B., Kloiber, O., & Septimus, E. (2017). Global health security at the crossroads. *World Medical & Health Policy, 9*(1), 4–5.

Ooms, G., Beiersmann, C., Flores, W., Hanefeld, J., Müller, O., Mulumba, M., et al. (2017). Synergies and tensions between universal health coverage and global health security: Why we need a second 'maximizing positive synergies' initiative. *BMJ Global Health, 2*(1), e000217.

Ooms, G., Keygnaert, I., & Hammonds, R. (2019). The right to health: From citizen's right to human right (and back). *Public Health, 172,* 99–104.

Ooms, G., Ottersen, T., Jahn, A., & Agyepong, I. A. (2018). Addressing the fragmentation of global health: The Lancet Commission on synergies between universal health coverage, health security, and health promotion. *The Lancet, 392*(10153), 1098–1099.

Robert Koch Institute. (2015). Konzept zur Umsetzung frühzeitiger Impfungen bei Asylsuchenden nach Ankunft in Deutschland. *EpiBull, 41,* 439–445.

Rushton, S. (2011). Global health security: Security for whom? Security from what? *Political Studies, 59*(4), 779–796.

Sandgren, A., Sane Schepisi, M., Sotgiu, G., Huitric, E., Migliori, G. B., Manissero, D., et al. (2014). Tuberculosis transmission between foreign- and native-born populations in the EU/ EEA: A systematic review. *European Respiratory Journal, 43*(4), 1159–1171.

Satinsky, E., Fuhr, D. C., Woodward, A., Sondorp, E., & Roberts, B. (2019). Mental health care utilisation and access among refugees and asylum seekers in Europe: A systematic review. *Health Policy, 123*(9), 851–863.

Sreeramareddy, C. T., Panduru, K. V., Menten, J., & Van Den Ende, J. (2009). Time delays in diagnosis of pulmonary tuberculosis: A systematic review of literature. *BMC Infectious Diseases, 9*(1), 91.

The National Review. (2016, February 3). Chicken little Chuckie Schumer: America's disease-fighting phony. *National Review* [online]. Retrieved July 31, 2019, from https://www.national-review.com/2016/02/zika-virus-illegal-immigration/

UN Committee on Economic, Social and Cultural Rights. (2000). *General comment no. 14 (2000), The right to the highest attainable standard of health (article 12 of the International Covenant on Economic, Social and Cultural Rights)*. Retrieved from http://digitallibrary. un.org/record/425041

UNDP (Ed.). (1994). *Human development report 1994*. New York: Oxford Univ. Press.

United Nations High Commissioner for Refugees. (2010). *Convention and protocol relating to the status of refugees*. Retrieved July 4, 2019, from https://www.unhcr.org/3b66c2aa10

Wenham, C., Katz, R., Birungi, C., Boden, L., Eccleston-Turner, M., Gostin, L., et al. (2019). Global health security and universal health coverage: From a marriage of convenience to a strategic, effective partnership. *BMJ Global Health, 4*(1), e001145.

WHO (Ed.). (2008). *International health regulations: 2005* (2nd ed.). Geneva, Switzerland: WHO.

Wilson, J. M. G., & Jungner, G. (1968). *Principles and practice of screening for disease*. Geneva, Switzerland: World Health Organisation.

World Health Assembly. (2001). *Global health security: Epidemicalert and response* [online]. No. WHA 54.14. Retrieved July 4, 2019, from http://apps.who.int/medicinedocs/index/assoc/ s16356e/s16356e.pdf

World Health Organisation Regional Office. (2018). *Report on the health of refugees and migrants in the WHO European Region. No PUBLIC HEALTH without REFUGEE and MIGRANT HEALTH* [online]. World Health Organisation. Retrieved July 5, 2019, from https://apps.who. int/iris/bitstream/handle/10665/311347/9789289053846-eng.pdf?sequence=1&isAllowed=y

World Health Organization (WHO). (2007). *Global public health security in the 21st century: Global public health security*. Geneva, Switzerland: World Health Organization.

World Health Organization. (2010). In C. Etienne, A. Asamoa-Baah, & D. B. Evans (Eds.), *The World health report: Health systems financing: The path to universal coverage*. Geneva, Switzerland: World Health Organization.

Chapter 8
Security over Health: The Effect of Security Policies on Migrant Mental Health in the UK

Philipa Mladovsky

Abbreviations

AAR	Adults at Risk policy
BAME	Black, Asian, and minority ethnic
CAMHS	Child and Adolescent Mental Health Services
GP	General practitioner
IRC	Immigrant Removal Centre
NGO	Non-governmental Organisation
NHS	National Health Service
NICE	National Institute for Health and Care Excellence
PHE	Public Health England
PTSD	Post-traumatic stress disorder
UK	United Kingdom

Introduction: Conflicts Between Security and Health Agendas

The human right to health is, by definition, an inclusionary concept. Enshrined in the Human Rights Charter, it obliges nation states to ensure access to necessary preventive, promotive, and curative health resources irrespective of age, gender, social status, or migration history. Yet this concept is fundamentally at odds with migration policies, which are often exclusionary for forced migrants—concerned with determining the rights and responsibilities of certain individuals in contrast to others within the bounds of geopolitical nation states (Bozorgmehr and Jahn 2019).

This clash of concepts can be observed in many countries when considering restrictions in access to healthcare services based on citizenship or legal status.

P. Mladovsky (✉)

Department of International Development, London School of Economics and Political Science, London, UK

e-mail: p.mladovsky@lse.ac.uk

© Springer Nature Switzerland AG 2020

K. Bozorgmehr et al. (eds.), *Health Policy and Systems Responses to Forced Migration*, https://doi.org/10.1007/978-3-030-33812-1_8

Several countries in the European Union, for example, have foregone the right to health by providing only basic emergency care to undocumented migrants or by charging asylum seekers and refugees high out-of-pocket payments to receive care (Abubakar et al. 2018).

However, the clash is evident not only in the health sector. The human right to health requires intersectoral action between multiple institutions, as social determinants such as employment, housing, or legal aspects can have powerful influences on the distribution of illness and access to care. For migrants, decisions and discourses on migration made in policy spaces traditionally considered outside of the health realm have been shown to have a significant impact on health outcomes (Juárez et al. 2019). It is thus important to consider not only the securitisation of health issues that lie within the responsibility of the health sector (see also Chap. 7 "Health Security in the Context of Forced Migration") but also the effects of security discourses in the broader policy space. Recently, the Global Compact for Safe, Orderly and Regular Migration has encountered criticism for prioritising security concerns and sidelining the human right to health (Bozorgmehr and Biddle 2018). Yet the health effects of a shift of the political agenda towards security concerns have rarely been considered.

This chapter explores how the clash between security and health concerns has manifested through two case studies in the UK and considers the impact of security policies on the mental health of asylum seekers and refugees. The first case study is among asylum seekers in detention, while the second focuses on the asylum process and struggles for housing, employment, and experienced by forced migrants in their everyday lives. Using the UK as a pertinent example, this chapter finds evidence to support the argument that social policies targeting forced migrants not only fail to adequately treat mental health problems in forced migrants but also seem to create mental health problems in this population by prioritising security concerns over health.

Asylum Seeker and Refugee Mental Health in Detention

The first part of this case study concerns the treatment of mental health problems of migrants in detention centres. The UK is one of few countries that does not set a maximum time limit for holding asylum seekers in detention facilities and therefore holds people in these centres for longer than elsewhere in Europe (BMA 2017). The UK also has one of the largest immigration detention estates in Europe, holding up to 3500 individuals at any one time, in 11 immigration removal centres (IRCs) across the country. Decisions to detain are made by the Home Office and until very recently were not subject to automatic review by a court or other independent body (the Immigration Act 2016 brought in automatic bail hearings at the 4-month point). Individuals rarely know the term of their detention, meaning that immigration detention is often referred to as "indefinite" or "indeterminate" (BMA 2017).

Yet it is widely accepted that detention significantly negatively affects the mental health of asylum seekers; and the longer the length of time held in detention, the greater the deterioration (Priebe et al. 2016). International and UK evidence points to damaging effects of detention on asylum seekers' health, increasing the risk of conditions such as PTSD, anxiety, depression, and suicidal ideation, as well as suicide, with the negative effect of detention enduring long after release (BMA 2017; Priebe et al. 2016; von Werthern et al. 2018; Shaw 2016).

In 2010, the UK Border Agency changed the wording of its policy on detaining people with mental health problems, reversing the presumption against detaining mentally ill people. The previous policy provided that the mentally ill would "normally be considered suitable for detention in only very exceptional circumstances". The exclusion was amended to state: "those suffering from serious mental illness which cannot be satisfactorily managed within detention". The Secretary of State did not consult on this change of wording, nor did she undertake an equality impact assessment. There were successful legal challenges to this policy in the two years following its introduction, but the policy was not changed as a result (RCP 2013). As such, asylum seekers are treated for mental health conditions in parallel services in detention, provided separately from community services. These mental health services are co-commissioned by the National Health Service (NHS), the Home Office, and Public Health England.

The rationale for treating mental illness in detention is founded on security concerns. This was explained by Theresa May in 2015 when she was Home Secretary and commissioned an independent review into the Home Office policies and operating procedures that have an impact on immigration detainee welfare: "Immigration detention plays a key role in helping to secure our borders and in maintaining effective immigration control. The Government believes that those with no right to be in the UK should return to their home country and we will help those who wish to leave voluntarily. However, when people refuse to do so, we will seek to enforce their removal, which may involve detaining people for a period of time. But the wellbeing of those in our care is always a high priority and we are committed to treating all detainees with dignity and respect. I want to ensure that the health and wellbeing of all those detained is safeguarded" (Shaw 2016).

In her statement, the health and wellbeing of detainees is presented as a factor that needs to be traded off against the priority of national security. However, given the ongoing long period of chronic underinvestment into wider mental health in the NHS in England (Mental Health Taskforce 2016) (see below for further details), it is conceivable that the government's policy of safeguarding the health and wellbeing of detainees by providing parallel mental health services to migrants in detention could have resulted in relatively good access to care for this population.

The opposite appears to be true. The review commissioned by Theresa May, conducted by the former Prisons and Probation Ombudsman for England and Wales (Shaw 2016), in addition to other reports commissioned by the Home Office (Shaw 2018; Lawlor et al. 2015) and the NHS (Durcan et al. 2017), and reports by the HM Chief Inspector of Prisons all point to poor conditions in detention which lead to increased mental ill health among detainees, as well as poor-quality mental health-care in these settings.

For example, Shaw (2016) found that: "Detention worsened mental health because it diminished the sense of safety and freedom from harm, it was a painful reminder of past traumatic experiences, it aggravated fear of imminent return, it separated people from their support networks and it disrupted their treatment and care". In particular, he found that "most victims of torture experienced re-traumatisation, including powerful intrusive recall of torture experiences and a dete-rioration of pre-existing trauma symptoms".

In terms of quality of care in detention, the review noted poor mental health screening; the use of segregation (i.e. isolation) as the default location for those with serious mental health problems; insufficient provision of psychiatric care; and a lack of equivalence with mainstream community care, for example, due to the scar-city of cognitive-behavioural therapies in detention.

The various reports written over successive years all have similar findings, sug-gesting little has changed, although some tentative improvements were recently noted. For example, in a follow-up to his 2016 report, Shaw (2018) welcomes the Adults at Risk (AAR) policy that was introduced by the Home Office in response to his proposals to reduce the numbers of vulnerable people in detention but states that "while it is not clear that AAR has yet made a significant difference to those num-bers, it has engendered a genuine focus on vulnerability. The policy remains a work in progress and I have made recommendations to strengthen the protections it offers".

An interesting, but difficult, question considered in the wider health and securi-tisation literature is whether the prioritisations of security issues over health issues actually increases UK security. In the UK, in practice, most detainees are not deported, suggesting they were never a threat to security in the first place. Of the 14,062 asylum seekers who left detention during 2017, about a quarter (3171) were actually removed from the UK when they left detention. Eight thousand four hun-dred and sixty-two were granted temporary admission or released, and a further 2222 were released as a result of bail applications (Refugee Council 2018). Shaw finds that the argument justifying the provision of services in detention as protective of national security is probably incoherent and erroneous, as "evidence on compli-ance levels for alternative to detention programmes finds that well-funded, and well-supported case-management programmes offering legal advice, housing and access to social and health care have high levels of compliance with all stages of the immigration system, including removal" (Shaw 2018).

The findings outlined above suggest that in the UK, many asylum seekers are unnecessarily detained and that many of them are eventually returned into the com-munity with untreated, poorly treated, and/or exacerbated levels of mental ill health. The suggested causal link between detention and worsening of mental health in the UK is consistent with a limited number of international longitudinal studies and comparison studies which find that detention not only exacerbates existing mental health disorders but also contributes independently to the onset of new ones, although isolating the effects of detention alone remains a complex task (von Werthern et al. 2018). This is likely to create a greater burden of disease for mainstream community-based mental health services. As such, the prioritisation of security issues over migrant mental health in detention seems to promote inequitable, poor-quality, and inefficient care. However, ineffective policies and practices are not only found in the context of detention. Next, this chapter turns to the problems caused by further prioritisation of security over mental illness among forced migrants in the UK, in their everyday lives.

Security and Mental Health in the Everyday Lives of Asylum Seekers and Refugees

The anthropological analysis of securitisation has deconstructed the "securitisation" debate (see also Chap. 7 "Health security in the context of forced migration"), proposing an analysis of "security assemblages" to understand how security concerns manifest in the everyday lives of individuals (Samimian-Darash and Stalcup 2017). Security assemblages do not necessarily focus on security formations (such as detention centres) per se, and how much violence or insecurity they yield, but rather seek to identify and study security forms of action, whether or not they are part of the nation state. This approach is oriented towards capturing how these forms of action work and what types of security they produce. This means everyday forms of action outside official security formations can be analysed through a security lens.

Immigration policies and debates have been analysed as one such assemblage. In the UK, as in the EU more broadly, immigration is framed by some politicians and parts of the media and population as a threat to security. Forced and other types of migrants are seen not only as a threat to national internal security due to fears of terrorism (Huysmans and Buonfino 2008) but also as a threat to the supposed societal security conferred by a homogenous national communal identity and to economic security by supposedly creating a strain on employment and social welfare (Huysmans 2006).

In the UK, everyday forms of security action designed to deter immigration take place in the context of what until recently was officially termed by the government as the "hostile environment" policy (as a result of widespread criticism, since the summer of 2017 the government has used the term "compliant environment" instead) (Taylor 2018). The "hostile environment" policy refers to a range of government measures aimed at identifying and reducing the number of immigrants in the UK with no right to remain, including so-called failed asylum seekers. An overview of the policy has been set out by the House of Commons Home Affairs Committee, which stated: "Many of the measures designed to make life difficult for individuals without permission to remain in the UK were first proposed in 2012 as part of a 'hostile environment policy'. The aim of the policy is to deter people without permission from entering the UK and to encourage those already here to leave voluntarily. It includes measures to limit access to work, housing, healthcare, and bank accounts, to revoke driving licences and to reduce and restrict rights of appeal against Home Office decisions. The majority of these proposals became law via the Immigration Act 2014, and have since been tightened or expanded under the Immigration Act 2016" (House of Commons Home Affairs Committee 2018).

This policy has led to increased security concerns in many aspects of everyday life, both for migrants and the majority population. In the job market and housing, for example, employers and landlords are put in the position of internal border guards in order to police the implementation of immigration policies and detect undocumented migrants (Yuval-Davis et al. 2018). These policies accompany measures within the asylum system that seek to deter refugees and asylum seekers from entering or remaining in the UK by keeping access to employment and social welfare low. For example, compared to Spain, France, and Germany, Britain provides less financial support for asylum seekers to cover non-accommodation-related expenses. Compared to these three countries and Italy, the UK has the strictest restrictions on asylum seekers working as they are not allowed into paid employment unless they have been waiting to hear about their asylum claim for 12 months, and then they are only allowed to work in official "shortage occupations" for which there are not enough resident workers to fill vacancies (The Guardian 2017). Furthermore, 28 days after being granted refugee status, people stop receiving government support as an asylum seeker and must apply to receive mainstream benefits if needed, as stated in regulation 4 of the *Asylum Support Regulations 2002*. Although people granted status should have immediate access to the labour market and all key mainstream benefits, this transition can prove problematic and will often take longer than the prescribed 28 days. The last Labour government (1997–2010) provided support and advice to new refugees, so that they were better able to transition into mainstream society, funding both voluntary and local authority agencies to provide a package of support. However, this funding was cut in 2011 by the coalition government that came into power in 2010 (Carnet et al. 2014). Very few refugees are able to register for benefits in the 28-day "move on" period due to bureaucratic and administrative delays, and as a result, many become destitute or homeless (Smith 2019; Basedow and Doyle 2016; Carnet et al. 2014).

This process of securitisation, in which the government seeks to deter refugees and undocumented migrants through restricting their access to housing, employment, and healthcare, as well as prolonging and complicating the asylum process, has led to an increased risk of mental ill health in forced migrants. This is evidenced by a literature review on the impact of policies of deterrence on the mental health of asylum seekers in the UK and elsewhere (Silove et al. 2000). Deterrence measures covered by the study include confinement in detention centres, enforced dispersal within the community, the implementation of more stringent refugee determination procedures, and temporary forms of asylum. Additionally, in several countries including the UK, asylum seekers living in the community face restricted access to work, education, housing, welfare, and/or basic healthcare services. Allegations of abuse, untreated medical and psychiatric illnesses, suicidal behaviour, hunger strikes, and outbreaks of violence among asylum seekers in detention centres are reported. The study finds that despite methodological limitations due to sampling difficulties, there is growing evidence that salient post-migration stress facing asylum seekers adds to the effect of previous trauma in creating risk of ongoing post-traumatic stress disorder and other psychiatric symptoms. Indeed, an international review of the literature observed that adverse post-migratory socioeconomic conditions accounted for the larger burden of depression in settled refugees (>5 years) when compared to the host populations. The effect was not observed in refugees settled in the host country for <5 years (Priebe et al. 2016). This case study of the UK serves as an example of how such increases in mental ill health among refugees are actively shaped by policies of deterrence stemming from a process of securitisation.

In an example from the UK, a study of 84 Iraqi asylum seekers reports that low levels of social support and financial difficulties after migration were associated with heightened levels of depression (Gorst-Unsworth and Goldenberg 1998). In another study in which 138 refugees and asylum seekers were interviewed (Phillimore et al. 2007), the following post-migratory factors were reported by the interviewees to negatively impact their mental health: the length of time it took for an asylum decision to be reached; questioning of stories which were difficult to tell; uncertainty about the future; being detained; being criminalised, stigmatisation, and respondents developing a mistrust of the state; discrimination, feeling unwelcome, and being harassed or bullied; isolation, loss or separation from friends and family, and ethnic community; unemployment and skills downgrading and concerns around inability to be self-sufficient; culture shock and difficulties understanding how to conduct themselves in UK society; difficulties accessing services, in particular housing; and gender issues including isolation from traditional child rearing and social support networks, sexual and domestic violence, increased difficulties accessing services, English language classes and work, and the belief by some that women are inherently weak. Many, although not all, of these factors can be understood as policies of deterrence.

Another example comes from the housing sector. Individuals seeking asylum in the UK, and who can prove they are destitute, are eligible for support from the Home Office. Support can be financial and in the form of accommodation. However, a report by the House of Commons Home Affairs select committee (2017) highlighted that many properties in which asylum seekers were housed were characterised by substandard, unsanitary, or unsafe conditions, such as vermin infestation, and pointed to the failures of the inspection and compliance regimes to deal with these issues. Aside from the well-known negative effects poor housing has on mental health (Diggle et al. 2017), the report found specific conditions of the housing provided to be especially detrimental. Perhaps most notably, forced migrants were moved between housing facilities frequently and at very short notice, which often affected support networks, including losing vital access to Community Mental Health Team care as a result of the lack of effective onward referral.

A deterrence policy that has caused particular concern is the loss of asylum social welfare support for asylum seekers 28 days after they are granted status and the aforementioned cuts to the national programme that used to support new refugees during this 28-day "move on" period. The Refugee Council has documented the negative impact these cuts have had on the living conditions and mental health of refugees (Basedow and Doyle 2016). The report draws on interviews conducted with 11 newly recognised refugees who were interviewed up to four times during the year after they had been granted refugee status. The study found that all participants reported stress, anxiety, and depression (both clinically diagnosed and self-described) during their interviews. The initial 28-day "move on" period was the most stressful for participants, and the highest levels of anxiety were reported during this time.

Understanding the impact of specific post-migratory policies on the mental health of migrants can be difficult, however, as causes are likely to be multifactorial and cause and effect are often bidirectional. A study of refugees drawing on the Labour Force Survey in the UK illustrates this difficulty (Ruiz and Vargas-Silva 2018). The study finds those who migrated to seek asylum have worse labour market outcomes than natives and other types of migrants, including a lower likelihood of employment, lower weekly earnings, lower hourly salary, and lower number of hours worked. The study also finds that asylum seekers have worse mental health, but the authors are unable to determine the casual links between the two variables. The authors hypothesise that poor mental health (in the form of premigration trauma) may be a cause of lower employment, rather than vice versa. Indeed, the relationship between unemployment and poor mental health may work in both directions (Paul and Moser 2009). Another possible explanation they provide for their findings is evidence that refugee skills may be less readily transferable across countries than those of other migrants and that differences in the main motivation to migrate suggest that refugees may be less favourably selected for labour market success in the host country. They also consider the effect of policies of deterrence (i.e. lengthy legal restrictions to access the labour market while asylum claims are being evaluated) on refugee employment levels but recognise that these are unlikely to be the sole explanation.

It is difficult to determine exactly how and why policies of deterrence impact mental health. Meta-analytic evidence from international cross-sectional and longitudinal studies that demonstrate the negative effect of unemployment on mental health in general populations are unable to identify the specific mechanisms that mediate this association (Paul and Moser 2009). Qualitative research such as Phillimore's study of refugees (2007) is also limited in terms of providing robust evidence on causality, as it often relies on respondents' self-reports which may be unable to reliably unpack and explain causal chains.

Turning to the issue of whether deterrence policies are in fact an effective means of enhancing security, it seems this is difficult to assess in the UK. The UK's Independent Chief Inspector of Borders and Immigration has stated that "the Home Office does not have in place measurements to evaluate the effectiveness" of the "hostile environment provisions" (House of Commons Home Affairs Committee 2018).

Ostensibly, policies of deterrence may have been effective in reducing applications of asylum to the UK, which have decreased rapidly over recent years. Asylum applications declined sharply during the mid-2000s, compared to the peak in the early 2000s. They increased again from 2010 to 2015 (though well below the levels of the early 2000s) but have decreased again in 2016 and 2017 (The Migration Observatory 2019). However, this is unlikely to be caused by deterrence policies, as the causes of changes in asylum applications are complex and determined by multiple factors. Indeed, evidence from across the OECD suggests that rather than policies of deterrence, it is structural factors that largely lie beyond the reach of asylum policymakers, such as a country's prosperity, the unemployment rate, and historical ties, that determine asylum seekers' choice of host country (Thielemann 2003, 2004). It is also unlikely that the decrease in asylum seeking claims has in turn increased security in any sense of the word in the UK, as there is little evidence to suggest asylum seekers are in fact a threat to security (Innes 2010; United Nations General Assembly 2016).

However, regardless of the possible effects on security, what can be argued with confidence is that forced migrants are likely to have a relatively high level of need for mental health services compared to the majority population, given their past exposure to traumatic experiences and on ongoing stressors, and these needs are very likely be exacerbated by their experiences in detention and by policies of deterrence such as the "hostile environment". The next section looks in more depth at mental health services that are offered to forced migrants in the community.

Inadequate Mental Health Services for Forced Migrants

To what extent does the government in the UK provide or fund mental health services for forced migrants? In terms of eligibility, asylum seekers with an ongoing claim and refugees are entitled to the full range of NHS services. However, undocumented migrants and refused asylum seekers are charged for using the NHS, except for emergency care, discretionary acceptance by a GP to enrol in the primary care practice, and some specific services (infectious diseases, family planning, treatment of a physical or mental condition caused by torture, female genital mutilation, domestic violence, or sexual violence). As discussed above, some mental health services are also provided in detention.

Since 2015, as part of the "hostile environment" policy, fees charged for (non-emergency) secondary care to undocumented migrants increased to 150% of the actual cost. Hospitals are fined if fees are not recouped—they must therefore check patients' immigration status and chase the fee. Any immigration application from a person with more than £1000 debt for NHS services is automatically rejected.

These policies alone already severely limit access to needed health services, including mental health, for many forced migrants. However, under the "hostile environment" policy, the NHS has also been required to act as a form of border control, adding a further barrier to access. In the last few years, the Home Office gained permission to request non-clinical details from NHS Digital, including patients' names, dates of birth, and the individual's last known address. According to the Department of Health, the Home Office made 8127 requests for data in the first 11 months of 2016, which led to 5854 people being traced by immigration enforcement teams. Public Health England (PHE) warned that the sharing of personal information by NHS commissioners and healthcare providers risks undermining public confidence in the NHS and could have "unintended serious consequences" for patients. However, the Department of Health denied such claims, saying it had found "no evidence that this policy would deter migrants from seeking treatment", adding that it had weighed up privacy considerations and the "competing public interest in upholding the Government's immigration agenda". Fortunately, this damaging policy was recently officially overturned as a result of lobbying from multiple NGOs and stakeholders, but may still be ongoing in practice (Independent 2019).

In addition to these eligibility and privacy barriers, there is a general lack of provision of specialised mental health services for forced migrants. For example, a study found highly variable provision of mental health services for asylum seekers and refugees in London (Ward and Palmer 2005): only 5 of the 11 Mental Health Trusts provide specialist services that are specifically designed with the needs of refugees and asylum seekers in mind. Some services provided by the other Trusts provide specialist trauma services for refugees and asylum seekers (who make up about 50% of their client group), but do not have a team or an individual that works specifically with/specialises on asylum seekers and refugees.

Guidance on improving and commissioning mental healthcare for migrants in England is provided by the NGO MIND (Fassil and Burnett 2014; MIND 2009a, b, 2017). MIND points to some cases of best practice, but overall their reports suggest that mental health service provision for migrants in the community is inadequate and relies heavily on poorly funded voluntary organisations. They find that migrants' needs are not prioritised, in part due to a lack of understanding among these communities about how the health system works, including difficulties registering with GP practices. Even if migrants have accessible and supportive GPs, mental health services are spread very thinly, creating long waiting times for resource-poor services and therapies. MIND also finds that the stigma and taboo associated with mental illness can be harder to overcome in migrant populations, where cultural beliefs may perpetuate stereotypes and make it hard for families and communities to accept mental health problems. These problems accessing mental health services among forced migrants reflect the wider barriers to healthcare experienced by this population group in general (Mladovsky et al. 2012).

It is important to note that problems accessing mental health services among forced migrants in the UK also often reflect wider inequities in quality of mental healthcare experienced by black, Asian, and minority ethnic (BAME) groups. In the UK, there are wide ethnic inequalities in access to mental health services. Research over 50 years shows people from BAME backgrounds have worse mental healthcare access and outcomes compared to the majority UK population: they are over-represented in inpatient/psychiatric care and sectioned more often and under-represented in talking therapy (Joint Commissioning Panel for Mental Health 2014). Race equality legislation and policies to address discrimination have been introduced over the last several years, but racial discrimination remains an ongoing problem in the NHS. The Joint Commissioning Panel for Mental Health (2014) states this inequity is due to "socioeconomic factors, racism, and discrimination".

It is, however, difficult to generate robust evidence on inequities in access to mental health services among forced migrants in the UK, as the necessary data are rarely collected. The exact number of refugees living in local authority areas and their health status is generally unknown; and no routine information is collected at local authority level on the number of refused asylum seekers who remain in the UK or undocumented/illegal migrants and of their health status (Aspinall 2014).

In the UK there is no recording of asylum seeker, refugee, migrant/country of birth, or migrant subgroups data in Hospital Episode Statistics Datasets. The NHS Central (GP) Register only flags individuals where the previous address is outside the UK and the person enters England and Wales for the first time and registers with a GP, but not asylum- or refugee-specific data. By contrast, the Referral Route indicator in the Mental Health Minimum Data Set does include "asylum services" and the Child and Adolescent Mental Health Services (CAMHS) dataset has citizenship status and country of birth fields.

The lack of data means that an evidence base is lacking for the development of policy in the UK. For example, the *Mental Health: Migrant Health Guide* published by Public Health England (2017) contains advice and guidance on the health needs of migrant patients for healthcare practitioners, including refugees and asylum seekers. However, it mostly draws on international evidence from WHO and UNHCR, not evidence from the UK. Similarly, the National Institute for Health and Care Excellence (NICE) guidelines for the treatment of PTSD (NICE 2005) concerning refugees are based on samples of adult refugees from Kosovo in the UK, Cambodian adult refugees on the Thai border, Bosnian refugees living in Croatia, a community sample of Vietnamese adults in Australia, war-affected Tamil refugees and immigrants in Australia, tortured and non-tortured Bhutanese refugees living in Nepal and community samples in Algeria, Cambodia, Ethiopia, and Gaza. In the NICE (2009) guidelines for treatment of depression, ethnicity is discussed but there is no mention of asylum seekers or refugees at all.

Overall, then, the provision of mental health services to forced migrants in the community appears to be inadequate, data collection on this issue is poor, and the data that are available often do not seem to be used to inform policy. This situation is likely to be detrimental not only to forced migrants themselves but may also harm wider community relations, as poor mental health among forced migrants may hinder their successful integration (Phillimore 2011). Poor migrant integration in turn undermines the government's own security concerns, as successive governments in the UK over the last 20 years have portrayed poor migrant integration as a security threat, although the extent to which this is in fact the case is debatable (Garbaye and Latour 2016).

Bridging the Gap Between Security and Health Concerns

This chapter describes the contradictory nature of security concerns based on exclusionary principles and the right to health, which is inclusive. It also discusses how policy discourses have shifted in recent years towards security concerns, in terms of detaining mentally ill asylum seekers, providing mental health services in detention, and creating mental health problems in forced migrants through a process of securitisation of the wider asylum and immigration system. The prioritisation of security concerns has therefore increasingly led to a neglect of asylum seekers' right to health.

The UK case study highlights the mechanisms by which the mental health of forced migrants is created and exacerbated by policies intended to prioritise security concerns, both worsening the mental health status for these persons and further impeding access to necessary mental health services. The securitisation of migrant livelihoods through prolonged detention and deterrence measures, such as the difficult access of welfare benefits, employment, and education, exacerbates mental health problems by creating a lack of socioeconomic security, withdrawing social support networks and increasing discrimination (see also Chap. 11 "Discrimination as a Health Systems Response to Forced Migration"). At the same time, access to required mental health services is impeded through a number of securitising measures: through an active restriction of entitlements and increase in co-payments, by encouraging the "policing" of irregular migration in healthcare encounters and by failing to provide services which adequately cater to the needs of forced migrants (see also Chap. 12 "Health Systems Responsiveness to the Mental Health Needs of Forcibly Displaced Persons").

Ironically, this prioritisation of security issues seems to have provided neither health benefits nor benefits to security, whether national, economic, political, community, or individual. In the case of forced migrant mental health, however, according to the governments' own logic, securitisation may potentially ironically lead to greater insecurity, due to the poor social integration that may result from increased rates of forced migrant mental ill health.

The system is in need of major reform. The intersectoral approach enshrined in the right to health works both ways: not only can health be improved by adopting a human rights-based approach during the asylum process. The health of a society, safeguarded by an inclusionary right to health approach, can also arguably function as a resource enhancing the security of the nation state. Thus there is a need to cease to detain mentally ill asylum seekers; improve service provision to this population in the community; and adopt a more humane asylum system that does not actively create mental health problems, for example, by increasing access to work, housing, and healthcare.

References

Abubakar, I., Aldridge, R. W., Devakumar, D., Orcutt, M., Burns, R., Barreto, M. L., et al. (2018). The UCL–Lancet Commission on migration and health: The health of a world on the move. *The Lancet, 392*, 2606–2654.

Aspinall, P. J. (2014). *Hidden needs. Identifying key vulnerable groups in data collections: Vulnerable migrants, gypsies and travellers, homeless people, and sex workers.* Centre for Health Services Studies, University of Kent. Retrieved from https://assets.publishing.service.

gov.uk/government/uploads/system/uploads/attachment_data/file/287805/vulnerable_groups_data_collections.pdf

Basedow, J., & Doyle, L. (2016). England's forgotten refugees: Out of the fire and into the frying pan. *Refugee Council.* Retrieved from https://www.refugeecouncil.org.uk/wp-content/uploads/2019/03/England_s_Forgotten_Refugees_final.pdf

BMA. (2017). *Locked up, locked out: Health and human rights in immigration detention.* A report by the British Medical Association London.

Bozorgmehr, K., & Biddle, L. (2018). New UN compact for migration falls short on health. *British Medical Journal, 363,* k5327.

Bozorgmehr, K., & Jahn, R. (2019). Adverse health effects of restrictive migration policies: Building the evidence base to change practice. *The Lancet Global Health, 7,* e386–e387.

Carnet, P., Blanchard, C., & Apollonio, F. (2014). *The move-on period: An ordeal for new refugees.* London: British Red Cross.

Diggle, J., Butler, H., Musgrove, M., & Ward, R. (2017). *Brick by brick: A review of mental health and housing.* London: MIND.

Durcan, G., Stubbs, J., & Boardman, J. (2017). *Immigration removal centres in England. A mental health needs analysis.* London: Centre for Mental Health.

Fassil, Y., & Burnett, A. (2014). Commissioning mental health services for vulnerable adult migrants. Guidance for commissioners. *MIND.* Retrieved from https://www.mind.org.uk/media/1380137/Vulnerable-Migrants-guidance-for-commissioners-August-2014-FINAL.pdf

Garbaye, R., & Latour, V. (2016). Community and citizenship in the age of security: British policy discourse on diversity and counter-terrorism since 9/11. *Revue Française de Civilisation Britannique, XXI,* 867.

Gorst-Unsworth, C., & Goldenberg, E. (1998). Psychological sequelae of torture and organised violence suffered by refugees from Iraq. Trauma-related factors compared with social factors in exile. *The British Journal of Psychiatry, 172,* 90–94.

House of Commons Home Affairs Committee. (2018). *Immigration policy: Basis for building consensus, 15 January 2018, HC 500 of session 2017–19* (p. 20). London: House of Commons.

House of Commons Home Affairs Select Committee. (2017). *Asylum accomodation.* Retrieved from https://publications.parliament.uk/pa/cm201617/cmselect/cmhaff/637/63702.htm

Huysmans, J. (2006). *The politics of insecurity: Fear, migration and asylum in the EU.* London: Routledge.

Huysmans, J., & Buonfino, A. (2008). Politics of exception and unease: Immigration, asylum and terrorism in parliamentary debates in the UK. *Political Studies, 56,* 766–788.

Independent. (2019). *Home Office still using NHS patient data for immigration enforcement despite suggesting it would end practice.* Retrieved from https://www.independent.co.uk/news/uk/home-news/home-office-nhs-data-sharing-immigration-enforcement-a8761396.html

Innes, A. J. (2010). When the threatened become the threat: The construction of asylum seekers in British media narratives. *International Relations, 24,* 456–477.

Joint Commissioning Panel for Mental Health. (2014). *Guidance for commissioners of mental health services for people from black and minority ethnic communities.* Retrieved from https://www.jcpmh.info/wp-content/uploads/jcpmh-bme-guide.pdf

Juárez, S. P., Honkaniemi, H., Dunlavy, A. C., Aldridge, R. W., Barreto, M. L., Katikireddi, S. V., et al. (2019). Effects of non-health-targeted policies on migrant health: A systematic review and meta-analysis. *The Lancet Global Health, 7,* e420–e435.

Lawlor, D., Sher, M., & Stateva, M. (2015). *Review of mental health issues in immigration removal centres.* London: Immigration & Border Policy Directorate, The Home Office.

Mental Health Taskforce. (2016). *The five year forward view for mental health.* Mental Health Taskforce to the NHS in England.

MIND. (2009a). *A civilised society. Mental health provision for refugees and asylum-seekers in England and Wales.* London: MIND.

MIND. (2009b). *Improving mental health support for refugee communities – An advocacy approach.* Retrieved from https://www.mind.org.uk/media/192447/Refugee_Report_1.pdf

MIND. (2017). *Mental health commissioning with migrant communities. A guide for mental health service providers.* Retrieved from https://www.mind.org.uk/media/14259589/mental-health-commissioning-with-migrant-communities.pdf

Mladovsky, P., Ingleby, D., Mckee, M., & Rechel, B. (2012). Good practices in migrant health: The European experience. *Clinical Medicine, 12,* 248–252.

NICE. (2005). *Post-traumatic stress disorder: Management. Clinical guideline [CG26].* Retrieved from https://www.nice.org.uk/guidance/cg26

NICE. (2009). *Depression in adults: Recognition and management. Clinical guideline.* Retrieved from https://www.nice.org.uk/guidance/cg90/resources/depression-in-adults-recognition-and-management-pdf-975742638037

Paul, K. I., & Moser, K. (2009). Unemployment impairs mental health: Meta-analyses. *Journal of Vocational Behavior, 74,* 264–282.

Phillimore, J. (2011). Refugees, acculturation strategies, stress and integration. *Journal of Social Policy, 40,* 575–593.

Phillimore, J., Ergun, E., Goodson, L., & Hennessy, D. (2007). *They do not understand the problem I have: Refugee well-being and mental health.* York, UK: Joseph Rowntree Foundation.

Priebe, S., Giacco, D., & El-Nagib, R. (2016). *Public health aspects of mental health among migrants and refugees: A review of the evidence on mental health care for refugees, asylum seekers and irregular migrants in the WHO European Region.* Copenhagen, Denmark: WHO Regional Office for Europe; 2016 (Health Evidence Network (HEN) Synthesis Report 47).

Public Health England. (2017). *Mental health: Migrant health guide.* Retrieved from https://www.gov.uk/guidance/mental-health-migrant-health-guide#history

RCP. (2013). *Position statement on detention of people with mental disorders in immigration removal centres.* The Royal College of Psychiatrists. Retrieved from http://www.medicaljustice.org.uk/wp-content/uploads/2016/06/Appendix-A-The-Royal-College-of-Psychiatrists-Position-Statement-on-detention-of-people-with-mental-disorders-in-Immigration-Removal-Centres.pdf

Refugee Council. (2018). *Refugee Council information. When is detention used?* Retrieved from https://www.refugeecouncil.org.uk/wp-content/uploads/2019/03/Detention_in_the_Asylum_System_May_2018.pdf

Ruiz, I., & Vargas-Silva, C. (2018). Differences in labour market outcomes between natives, refugees and other migrants in the UK. *Journal of Economic Geography, 18,* 855–885.

Samimian-Darash, L., & Stalcup, M. (2017). Anthropology of security and security in anthropology: Cases of counterterrorism in the United States. *Anthropological Theory, 17,* 60–87.

Shaw, S. (2016). *Review into the welfare in detention of vulnerable persons: A report to the Home Office by Stephen Shaw. CM 9186.* London: HMSO.

Shaw, S. (2018). *Assessment of government progress in implementing the report on the welfare in detention of vulnerable persons. CM 9661.* London: HMSO.

Silove, D., Steel, Z., & Watters, C. (2000). Policies of deterrence and the mental health of asylum seekers. *JAMA, 284,* 604–611.

Smith, L. (2019). Mind the gap one year on. Continuation report on homelessness amongst newly recognised refugees. *The No Accomodation Network.* Retrieved from https://naccom.org.uk/wp-content/uploads/2019/06/NACCOM-Homelessnesss-Report_2019-06-18_DIGITAL.pdf

Taylor, R. (2018). *House of lords library briefing. 'Hostile environment' policy.* London.

The Guardian. (2017). *Britain is one of worst places in western Europe for asylum seekers.* Retrieved from https://www.theguardian.com/uk-news/2017/mar/01/britain-one-of-worst-places-western-europe-asylum-seekers

The Migration Observatory. (2019). *Migration to the UK: Asylum and refugees.* Retrieved from https://migrationobservatory.ox.ac.uk/resources/briefings/migration-to-the-uk-asylum/

Thielemann, E. R. (2003). *Does policy matter? On governments' attempts to control unwanted migration.* LSE European Institute Working Paper No. 2003–2. Retrieved from http://www.lse.ac.uk/collections/europeanInstitute/workingpaperindex.htm

Thielemann, E. R. (2004). Why asylum policy harmonisation undermines refugee burden-sharing. *European Journal of Migration and Law, 6*, 47–65.

United Nations General Assembly. (2016). *Report of the special rapporteur on the promotion and protection of human rights and fundamental freedoms while countering terrorism.* Retrieved from https://documents-dds-ny.un.org/doc/UNDOC/GEN/N16/285/61/PDF/N1628561. pdf?OpenElement

Von Werthern, M., Robjant, K., Chui, Z., Schon, R., Ottisova, L., Mason, C., et al. (2018). The impact of immigration detention on mental health: A systematic review. *BMC Psychiatry, 18*, 382.

Ward, K., & Palmer, D. (2005). Mapping the provision of mental health services for asylum seekers and refugees in London: A report. *ICAR.* Retrieved from https://lemosandcrane.co.uk/resources/ICAR%20-%20Mapping%20the%20provision%20of%20mental%20health%20services%20for%20asylum%20seekers%20and%20refugees%20in%20London.pdf

Yuval-Davis, N., Wemyss, G., & Cassidy, K. (2018). Everyday bordering, belonging and the reorientation of British immigration legislation. *Sociology, 52*, 228–244.

Chapter 9
Evidence on Health Records for Migrants and Refugees: Findings from a Systematic Review

Valentina Chiesa, Antonio Chiarenza, and Bernd Rechel

Abbreviations

HR	Health record
PHR	Personal health record
EMR	Electronic Medical Record
EHR	Electronic health record
IOM	International Organization for Migration
EC	European Commission
WHO	World Health Organization
UNRWA	United Nations Relief and Works Agency for Palestine Refugees in the Near East
VIA	Access to visitors' information [*visitantes información acceso*]
PANDA	The Pregnancy and Newborn Diagnostic Assessment
CARE	Common Approach for REfugees and other migrants' health
PRISMA	Prepared Items for Systematic Reviews and Meta-Analysis

V. Chiesa
Local Health Unit of Reggio Emilia, Reggio Emilia, Italy

London School of Hygiene & Tropical Medicine, London, UK

A. Chiarenza
Local Health Unit of Reggio Emilia, Reggio Emilia, Italy

B. Rechel (✉)
London School of Hygiene & Tropical Medicine, London, UK

European Observatory on Health Systems and Policies, Brussels, Belgium
e-mail: bernd.rechel@lshtm.ac.uk

© Springer Nature Switzerland AG 2020
K. Bozorgmehr et al. (eds.), *Health Policy and Systems Responses to Forced Migration*, https://doi.org/10.1007/978-3-030-33812-1_9

Introduction

This chapter describes the state of the art and the potential benefits of health records (HRs) for migrants and refugees worldwide, drawing on the findings of a systematic review of the literature.

Migrants and refugees face different barriers in accessing adequate health services, depending on the host country and the phase of the migration journey. These barriers are particularly problematic for undocumented migrants and asylum seekers with temporary protection (Winters et al. 2018). Severe travel conditions, including forced stops in detention centres or refugee camps, as well as their experience of conflicts, have adverse effects on the mental and physical health of migrants. Yet, restrictive policies and the lack of knowledge on entitlements and how and where to obtain health services often impede migrants' access to health services throughout their migration journey. In turn, health-care providers face challenges in providing optimal care for these vulnerable groups because of the lack of reliable information on the illness and health history of migrant patients.

One of the main challenges is the lack of access to medical records (Winters et al. 2018), for both migrant patients and health-care providers. Migrants and refugees are seen by different health professionals during the various phases of the migration process and often travel without any HRs.

Information on migrants' health history, their test results, vaccinations, diagnoses and medications are often dispersed (Schoevers et al. 2009), and this fragmentation results in the lack of reliable and timely data for health-care providers interacting with patients and for policymakers to improve health services. Health-care providers have to reconstruct the medical history at each phase of the migration process and across different health-care settings. This may comprise information on allergies, illnesses, surgeries, immunisations and results of physical exams and tests. It may also encompass information about medicines taken and health habits, such as diet and exercise, as well as family medical history. Consequently, migrant patients may have to undergo unnecessary consultations, repeated diagnostic and therapeutic interventions (e.g. vaccinations, blood tests and screening for HIV/AIDS or tuberculosis) and fail to gain proper access to emergency care.

In many countries, a national electronic health record is not available for the general population, and since there are no adequate systems for exchanging medical information between countries, this is even more of a problem for people on the move, such as migrants and refugees. In this context, the adoption of HRs for migrants and refugees offers several potential benefits (Socias et al. 2016), including improved health data collection and more efficient referral systems at local, national and international level. The effective implementation of a HR system allows health-care providers to learn about the medical history of newly arrived migrants and to establish more quickly and efficiently their health status and medical needs. It also facilitates data collection, analysis and transfer within the same country and also between countries. The use of HRs can improve the continuity and efficiency of health services for migrants and decrease costs, provided the HRs include all relevant medical information collected during the migration process, from origin to destination and in the different health-care settings involved (Socias et al. 2016).

The European Commission (EC) and the World Health Organization (WHO) have invested in the research and diffusion of electronic health records (EHRs) for the general population, partly in order to improve interoperability between national health systems. Despite these efforts, data sharing between countries remains a challenge, due to concerns about confidentiality, as well as technical and legal issues (WHO Global Observatory for eHealth 2012; Footman et al. 2014).

Another barrier is the lack of clear definitions regarding electronic health records (EHRs), Electronic Medical Records (EMRs) and personal health records (PHRs), even within the same country (Saavedra 2012).

EHRs, EMRs and PHRs have gained widespread use; most providers and patients, however, use the terms EHR, EMR and PHR interchangeably. It is therefore to clarify the terminology used, as this has an impact on implementation.

EMRs are digital versions of the paper records in the same health-care institutions; they contain the medical and treatment history of patients. The provider's portal may allow patients to access their EMRs.

EHRs collect data from all health workers involved in a patient's care, with entries from different health-care settings. All authorised health-care providers, including pharmacists and specialists, can access the EHRs (Saavedra 2012).

Finally, PHRs contain the same type of data related to diagnoses, medications, immunisations, family medical histories and provider contact information as EHRs but are designed to be set up, accessed and managed by patients. The PHR is a record that: '(1) contains all personal health information belonging to an individual; (2) is entered and accessed electronically by healthcare workers over the person's lifetime and (3) extends beyond acute inpatient situations including all ambulatory care settings at which the patient receives care' (World Health Organization 2006; Saavedra 2012).

In practice, the terms EMRs, EHRs and PHRs are often used synonymously, and their description may not coincide with their actual application.

The State of the Art and the Evidence on Health Records for Migrants and Refugees

According to M. C. Gibbons et al. (Gibbons and Rivera Casale 2010), the adoption of information technology systems in health care, in terms of impact and efficacy for under-resourced health structures and for disadvantaged populations, has not been adequately evaluated. In fact, very little research was available until a few years ago. A systematic review published in 2009 (Schoevers et al. 2009), which aimed to investigate the potential benefits of PHRs for undocumented migrants, was not able to identify a single relevant study. We therefore conducted a systematic review to assess the available evidence and state of the art concerning the implementation of HRs for migrants. *The systematic review focused on HRs implemented specifically for migrants and refugees following the Prepared Items for Systematic Reviews and Meta-Analysis (PRISMA) guidelines. The search was conducted in March 2018.*

The review focused on HRs implemented specifically for migrants and refugees; studies describing HRs in which migrants only represented one subcategory among many were excluded. Both the scientific and grey literature were searched; the reference lists of articles that met the inclusion criteria were checked and experts in the field consulted. The search was not limited in terms of date of publication, study design and type, and country of implementation.

Among the 33 articles that met the inclusion criteria, 20 different HRs were identified (Table 9.1). Some articles refer to the same HRs, as they were implemented by the same organisation/s or in the same country.

In addition, two multicentric studies by Giambi et al. (2017, 2018), in which several HRs were carried out across different countries, were included.

Among the different HRs realised for migrants, the following types of HRs were identified:

1. *PHRs* ($n = 12$):

   (a) Electronic Personal Health Records—e-PHRs ($n = 5$), including two PHRs with mobile applications (Borsari et al. 2017; Doocy et al. 2017a, b)
   (b) Non-electronic PHR ($n = 7$), which are usually defined as Patient-Held Personal Records; these are paper-based records.

2. *EMR* ($n = 3$).
3. *Mixed component HRs* ($n = 3$): electronic component (EMR or e-PHR) plus non-electronic component (held/paper record) (Solomon 2017; WHO Regional Office for Europe 2015; Letizia 1999; Bennett et al. 2000).
4. *Other HRs* ($n = 2$): these include two multicentre studies by Giambi et al. that could not be classified under a single HR as they describe national immunisation strategies implemented across different countries (Giambi et al. 2017, 2018).

The majority of the HRs identified were implemented in Italy, the United Kingdom (UK), Serbia and Greece. In the UK, they were exclusively Patient-Held Records, while in Italy, Greece and Serbia both Patient-Held Records and Electronic Personal Health Records were used. Some of these HRs identified in the UK and also the Netherlands (Goosen et al. 2013, 2014, 2015) were implemented at the national level, while other HRs were realised only in strategic spots or locally. Others, such as the Migrant Student Record Exchange Initiative (US Department of Education n.d.) and the Internet Medical Records for Migrant Workers (Solomon 2017), were available across the USA.

Importantly, some HRs were implemented internationally. These include: HRs realised in Jordan, Lebanon, Syria, the West Bank and the Gaza Strip by the United Nations Relief and Works Agency for Palestine Refugees in the Near East (UNRWA) and HRs implemented in Greece, Italy, Croatia, Slovenia, Cyprus, Romania and Serbia by the International Organization for Migration (IOM).

Table 9.1 Main characteristic of health records identified

Type of HR	Author organisation/s involved	Name of the HR organisation/s involved	Country/countries	Health-care setting	HR's target
1. Personal health record					
(a) *Electronic Personal Health Records—e-PHR*					
Electronic Personal Health Record with mobile application	Doocy et al. (2017a, b)	mHealth tool for NCDs—International Organization for Migration or the International Medical Corps	Lebanon	Ten primary care centre/s	Refugees with – Hypertension and/or DM type 2
Electronic Personal Health Record with mobile application	Borsari et al. (2017)	The Pregnancy and Newborn Diagnostic Assessment (PANDA)	Italy	Centre for asylum seekers	Migrants – During pregnancy
Electronic Personal Health Record stored into the USB device	CARE; user's manual (2017) (common approach for refugees and other migrants' health)	Health tracking and monitoring system—Consortium of the Common approach for refuges and other migrants' health (CARE) project	Italy and Greece	Hotspots	Migrants with – Multiple health conditions
Electronic Personal Health Record	Migrant Student Record Exchange Initiative (US Department of Education n.d.)	Migrant Record Exchange Initiative—Department of Education (ED), with direction from Congress	USA	Multiple settings	Migrant students with – Multiple health conditions
Electronic Personal Health Record	International Organization for Migration (IOM) (2018a, b)	Re-HEALTH[2]	Greece, Italy, Croatia, Slovenia, Cyprus, Romania and Serbia	Multiple: hotspots, reception or registration centres, hospitals or primary care centres	Newly arrived migrants and refugees with – Multiple health conditions

(continued)

Table 9.1 (continued)

Type of HR	Author organisation/s involved	Name of the HR organisation/s involved	Country/countries	Health-care setting	HR's target
(b) *Non-electronic Personal Health Record—Patient-Held Personal Record*					
Patient-Held Personal Record	Blackwell et al. (2002)	Health authorities and the National Asylum Support Service (NASS)	United Kingdom	Multiple settings	Asylum seekers with – Multiple health conditions
Patient-Held Personal Record	Schoevers (2011)	Exploratory study to assess the use and acceptability of a PHR (no specific name)	The Netherlands	Primary care centre/s and GPs	Undocumented women with – Psychosocial and gynaecological problems
Patient-Held Personal Record and advice booklet	McMaster et al. (1996)	Personal child health record and advice booklet—Ministry of Health, United Nations and non-governmental organizations (NGOs)	Bosnia	Multiple settings	Displaced children with – Multiple health conditions
Patient-Held Personal Record	Department of Health (2007)	Personal health record for asylum applicants and refugees—National Health System	United Kingdom	Multiple settings: · primary care, centres for asylum seekers and dental clinics	Asylum seekers and refugees with – Multiple health conditions
Patient-Held Personal Record	Martel et al. (2015)	Refugee Health Passport (RHP)—Refugee Health Initiative (RHI)	Canada	Acute care settings	Newly arrived migrants with – Acute encounters

Patient-Held Personal Record	International Organization for Migration (2015a, b)	Re-HEALTH	EU/EEA	Multiple: hotspots, reception or registration centres, hospitals or primary care centres	Newly arrived migrants and refugees with – Multiple health conditions
Patient-Held Personal Record	Campion et al. (2010)	Sheffield model of the personal health record—National Health System	United Kingdom	Dedicated service for asylum seekers	Asylum seekers with – Multiple health conditions
2. Electronic Medical Records—EMR					
Electronic Medical Record	Seth (2017)	CliniPAK Suite form VecnaCares—International Rescue Committee (IRC), NetHope Solutions, UNHCR	Kenya	Multiple settings: refugee camp with two inpatient hospitals, four clinics and several pharmacies	Refugees with – Multiple health conditions
Electronic Medical Record	Goosen et al. (2015) Goosen et al. (2014) Goosen et al. (2013)	MOA nationwide Electronic Medical Records database—the community health services for asylum seeker	The Netherlands	Centres for asylum seekers	Asylum seekers with – HIV during pregnancy Asylum seekers with – DM type 1/ type 2 Asylum seekers children with – Mental health distress

(continued)

Table 9.1 (continued)

Type of HR	Author organisation/s involved	Name of the HR organisation/s involved	Country/countries	Health-care setting	HR's target
Electronic Medical Record and health cards and identification numbers to trace the electronic data	Khader et al. (2012a, b) Khader et al. (2014) Shahin et al. (2015) United Nations Relief and Works Agency for Palestine Refugees in the Near East (2015) Ballout et al. (2017)	UNRWA—Electronic Medical Record system	Jordan, Lebanon, Syria, West Bank and the Gaza Strip	Primary care centre/s	Refugees with – DM type 1 – DM type 2 – DM type 2 and hypertension
3. Mixed component health records					
Patient-Held Personal Record ± Electronic Medical Record	WHO Regional Office for Europe (2015)	Commissariat for Refugees and Migration	Serbia	Centres for asylum seekers	Asylum seekers with – Multiple health conditions
Patient-Held Personal Record ± Electronic Medical Record	Bennett et al. (2000) Letizia (1999)	Safe Haven—The Kosovar Refugee Medical Surveillance Group	Australia	Multiple setting: a reception centre and eight haven centres in five states	Refugees with – Multiple health conditions
Electronic Personal Health Record with emergency photo-ID card with current medical conditions and primary care provider	Solomon (2017)	MiVIA/VIA: visitantes informatioń acceso (access to visitors' information)—St. Joseph's, Vineyard Worker Services and the Community Health Resource and Development Center	USA, California	Multiple settings: health clinics, the St. Joseph Health System's mobile medical units and hospital emergency rooms	Migrant farmworkers and their families with – Multiple health conditions

4. Other health records

Patient-Held Personal Record ± Electronic Medical Record	Giambi et al. (2018)	National immunisation strategies in European countries—National Health Systems	Croatia, Greece, Italy, Malta, Portugal and Slovenia	Multiple settings	Irregular migrants, refugees and asylum seekers – Immunisation status and vaccinations
Patient-Held Personal Record ± Electronic Medical Record	Giambi et al. (2017)	National immunisation strategies in non-European countries—National Health Systems	Albania, Algeria, Armenia, Bosnia and Herzegovina, Egypt, Georgia, Israel, Jordan, Kosovo, Moldavia, Palestine, Republic of Macedonia-FYROM, Serbia, Tunisia and Ukraine	Multiple settings	Newly arrived migrants – Immunisation status and vaccinations

Aim and Content of HRs

All HRs identified by this review had the aim to improve access to and utilisation of health services. In addition, 75% of HRs were also used for data collection, monitoring and reporting. Some HRs were specifically used for the initial health assessments, and a few others were specific for the surveillance of communicable diseases.

All the HRs identified in the review collected data on medical history (Fig. 9.1), except those described by Giambi et al. (2017, 2018) which focused exclusively on vaccinations and the verification of previous immunisations with a specific anamnesis or verification of immunisation cards. Other data frequently collected in HRs are related to vaccination uptake and immunisation status, child and obstetric care and medications. Notably, data related to follow-up or specialist care were rarely collected.

Setting and Target of HRs

More than half of HRs were realised in more than one health-care setting, encompassing hotspots, reception or registration centres, hospitals and primary care centres (Fig. 9.2). HRs were also implemented in primary care centres, such as those set up by UNRWA, and in centres for asylum seekers. HRs that were specifically used for asylum seekers, hotspots and acute care settings were limited (Fig. 9.3).

HRs mostly targeted asylum seekers and migrants in general, including a HR dedicated to migrant farmworkers and one dedicated to migrant students (US Department of Education n.d.; Solomon 2017). Importantly, the majority of HRs did not focus on a single or specific health condition (Fig. 9.4).

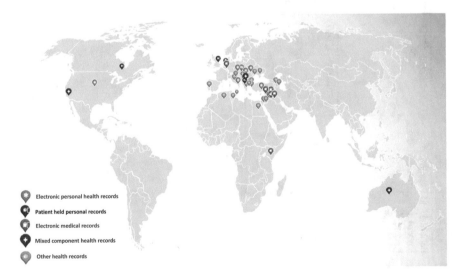

Fig. 9.1 Countries in which HRs have been implemented according to the type of records

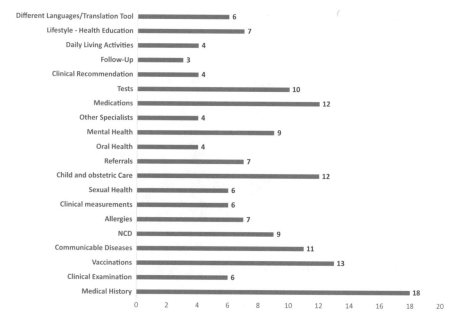

Fig. 9.2 Data collected in the health records

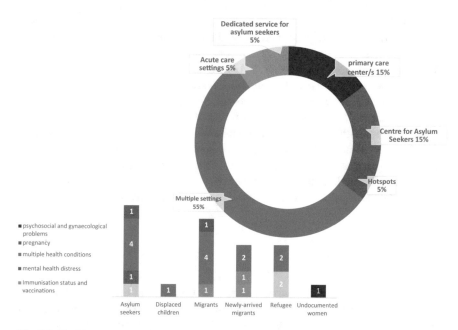

Fig. 9.3 Health-care settings in which HRs have been implemented

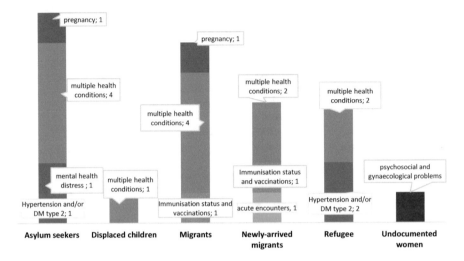

Fig. 9.4 Target of HRs according to migrant's category and health status

Accessing HRs

In general, Patient-Held Personal Records are controlled by the patients, and health-care providers can access them upon patients' consent, while electronic records can be controlled or accessed by both health workers and patients. Among the electronic records identified in our review, only four could be controlled or accessed by patients (Solomon 2017; Doocy et al. 2017a, b; US Department of Education n.d.).

Health-care providers can have different levels of permission in HR access and management. In some cases, specific training on the use of PHRs for health professionals and medical students has been organised (Martel et al. 2015).

Data sharing with other facilities or centres—in which the same HR was implemented—were mentioned in only 7 HRs, while information on the integration with other databases was identified in 10 HRs, including demographic data, reception data, referral hospital/s, maternal and child health services, mental health services, radiology databases, electronic databases of all asylum centres and police databases.

Successful Examples

HRs for migrants have been introduced for the first time in the USA for seasonal migrant workers. EHRs have been implemented in Colorado (Socias et al. 2016) in a Migrant Health Centre providing health services for low-income and medically underserved populations, including migrant and seasonal farmworkers. The Migrant Health Centre used EHRs also for surveillance of health and safety risks, e.g. injuries faced by these population groups.

The VIA, *visitantes información acceso* (access to visitors' information), has been implemented for migrant workers in Sonoma County, California (Solomon 2017). Migrant workers have their medical information stored in an Internet-based personal health record. The record can be downloaded by physicians of emergency rooms and clinics to quickly access information on an individual migrant worker's health history, medical conditions, allergies, medications and treatment plans. In the USA, records for migrant students and their families have been set up as part of the project 'Migrant Student Information Exchange' (US Department of Education n.d.). This medical record contains health information including immunisation status, thus reducing unnecessary immunisations of migrant children.

In Canada, the *Refugee Health Passport* (Martel et al. 2015) has been developed as a portable medical history tool for newly arrived refugees for acute care encounters. It 'is a held booklet, that includes: a streamlined medical history relevant to acute care situations, space for medical professionals to add new information, and a basic medical translation tool, for the language of the passport holder'.

Since 2009, the UNRWA has implemented an EHR (e-Health) system in primary health care, especially targeting patients with diabetes and hypertension, for five million Palestine refugees in Jordan, Syria, Lebanon, the West Bank and Gaza in 143 health centres (Ballout et al. 2017, 2018). The UNRWA e-Health system was evaluated by a panel of experts and health professionals, with the following findings:

- 'The daily medical consultations per doctor were reduced on average from 104 to 86 a day;
- The time needed to collect prescribed medication was reduced to 3 min;
- The antibiotics prescription rate was decrease from an average of 27.0–24.7%;
- The dashboard enabled managers and supervisors to remotely monitor all HCs daily operations and health care provided to patients;
- Comprehensive reporting and statistics on a daily basis;
- 89% of the physicians who were surveyed expressed satisfaction on e-Health, particularly on the fact of time-saving that allowed them to provide better and more attention to patients;
- Managing the crowds in a timely manner and with fairness' (Ballout et al. 2018).

Other positive examples include the e-PHRs realised for more than 4000 Kosovar refugees in Australia in the operation *Safe Haven* (Bennett et al. 2000; Letizia 1999). In this project, an e-PHR was provided to each refugee who attended the Haven Health Centre. The *Safe Haven* health records contained a photocopy of the immigration screening record, copies of other health records (such as dental examinations, radiology and pathology test results), data on immunisation status and a summary of the main issues with eventual indications for follow-up. The health data was shared between maternal and child health services, the mental health team and other staff.

In Sicily, Italy, a mobile health system (*m*Health) called *The Pregnancy and Newborn Diagnostic Assessment (PANDA)* was piloted in a migrant reception centre between 2014 and 2016, involving 150 migrant pregnant women (Borsari et al. 2017). This was an Electronic Personal Health Record with a mobile application, aiming to facilitate antenatal care among migrants. The mobile health system improved the collection of health data, the identification of at-risk pregnancies and health-care providers' adherence to antenatal care recommendations. In addition, the graphic interface of the *mobile* app facilitated the reminder of medical appointments and increased interest in health education modules. The PANDA system recorded a 91.9% patient satisfaction rate (Borsari et al. 2017).

Important results in the implementation of a PHR for migrants have been achieved by the IOM within the *Re-Health* and *Re-Health²* actions. In 2015, with funding from the European Commission, IOM implemented PHRs in several strategic EU spots. The action aimed at improving the capacity of EU member states under particular migratory pressure (International Organization for Migration 2015b). The 'Personal-Held Record' includes in a single document the patient's health data and information to help health professionals get a comprehensive view of patients. In addition, the project produced a Handbook for Health Professionals to help them to evaluate the health status and needs of refugees and migrants (International Organization for Migration 2015a).

In 2016, the *Re-Health²* action—*Implementation of the Personal Health Record as a tool for integration of refugees in EU health systems*—was launched. As part of this project, an electronic PHR and electronic platform were developed and piloted in four EU countries: Greece, Italy, Croatia and Slovenia. Subsequently, three additional countries were involved: Cyprus, Romania and Serbia. In Serbia, in 2018, after the first 2 months of the introduction of the EHR system, more than 400 electronic e-PHRs were collected in the Asylum Centre Krnjaca (Belgrade), including some migrants with e-PHRs initiated in Greece, and over 300 return visits were recorded.

Building on IOM's PHR, the EU Common Approach for Refugees and other migrants' health project (CARE) developed a new electronic system for tracking and monitoring the health status of migrants and refugees. This system includes a portable USB device to be delivered to migrants and refugees, containing their personal medical history, as well as information on any treatment provided. The software enables health-care providers to access the migrants' and refugees' PHR and to integrate it with follow-up examinations. This PHR has been introduced in the hotspots of Lampedusa and Trapani (Sicily, Italy), as well as Kos and Leros (Greece) in order to monitor and track migrants' and refugees' health status, with the aim of ensuring continuity of care, avoiding duplications in health treatment, reducing costs and establishing mechanisms of cooperation between countries of origin, transit and destination.

Strengths and Weaknesses of HRs for Migrants and Refugees

HRs seem to have great potential to improve health services for migrants. The evidence on electronic records, which include Electronic PHRs and EMRs, shows numerous benefits compared to Patient-Held Records (paper-based records).

Patient-Held Personal Records have several weaknesses compared to electronic records. These include: barriers due to low literacy of patients, privacy issues and additional time required for health workers to complete the records. In addition, the Patient-Held Record can be lost during the long migration process or destroyed on purpose to eliminate any document that might allow the identification of migrants or the countries they have passed through and may be sent back to.

In fact, the resistance by some health-care workers and migrants and refugees— especially for privacy issues—may be a problem to be solved. In order to guarantee data protection for migrants and refugees, a legal framework should be established in line with the International Health Regulations (19), consent and data sharing forms in compliance with national regulations, legislation on communicable diseases (such as reportable diseases) and national legislation with regard to data protection. In addition, cultural mediators and translational tools should be available in strategic spots and centres for asylum seekers in order to collect privacy consent appropriately.

A qualitative study conducted in six asylum seeker reception centres in five cities in Germany (Jahn et al. 2018) identified similar challenges with regard to Patient-Held Records. Health-care providers recognised the potential of Patient-Held Records to improve continuity and quality of care, but adherence and use was described as unsatisfactory.

Several articles included in our review reported advantages of electronic records, including improved quality and continuity of care, adherence to guidelines, patient and health worker satisfaction and patient education, with benefits including educational tools, data sharing, precision and reliability of statistical information. In addition, electronic records can be time-saving and reduce costs, as they avoid duplication of diagnostic and therapeutic interventions. Though, limitations identified include low provider uptake and frustration among health workers when the record does not perform as expected. Lack of financial resources and lack of time (due to migrants' short stay) to prescribe diagnostic or therapeutic interventions and for follow-up have also been reported.

However, in the systematic review, we did not retrieve articles with an experimental study design, and the majority of articles included had an observational study design, including cross-sectional studies (27%) and cohort studies (15%). Other articles included reports, official documents, opinion papers and webpages from non-governmental organisations (NGOs).

Conclusion

HRs can help to address some of the challenges that migrants face in terms of access to health services and continuity of care, as they often move within or between countries and consult different health-care providers and settings (Schoevers et al. 2009).

HRs, especially electronic records implemented in strategic spots, as in cross-border settings (World Health Organization 2006), can improve the quality of care (see also Chap. 12) and the quality of data recorded; provide access to health information anytime and anywhere; increase the efficiency of the health system; and avoid the duplication of diagnostic and therapeutic interventions such as vaccinations, blood tests and screening for infectious diseases (see also Chap. 10).

The HRs identified in our review can offer a tool for registering, monitoring and improving the health of refugees and migrants. They can be particularly effective when electronic and when they are applied in strategic spots and cross-border settings for migrants on the move.

Since the literature on this topic is scant and the HRs identified in this review are mostly based on observational studies, more research on this topic through studies with higher evidence is needed.

Despite the advantages in implementing HRs, there is large heterogeneity across countries in their definition and implementation: better coordination between countries and within the same country should be achieved in HR realisation.

References

Ballout, G., Al-Shorbaji, N., Abu-Kishk, N., Turki, Y., Zeidan, W., & Seita, A. (2018). UNRWA's innovative e-Health for 5 million Palestine refugees in the Near East. *BMJ Innovations, 4*, 128.

Ballout, G., Al-Shorbaji, N., Shishtawi, A., Abuzabaida, F., Shahin, Y., Khader, A., et al. (2017). Development and deployment of an e-Health System in UNRWA Healthcare Centers (HCs): The experience and evidence. *Studies in Health Technology and Informatics, 245*, 1212.

Bennett, C., Mein, J., Beers, M., Harvey, B., Vemulpad, S., Chant, K., et al. (2000). Operation Safe Haven: An evaluation of health surveillance and monitoring in an acute setting. *Communicable Diseases Intelligence, 24*(2), 21.

Blackwell, D., Holden, K., & Tregoning, D. (2002). An interim report of health needs assessment of asylum seekers in Sunderland and North Tyneside. *Public Health, 116*, 221–226.

Borsari, L., Stancanelli, G., Guarenti, L., Grandi, T., Leotta, S., Barcellini, L., et al. (2017). An innovative mobile health system to improve and standardize antenatal care among underserved communities: A feasibility study in an Italian hosting center for asylum seekers. *Journal of Immigrant and Minority Health, 20*, 1128–1136.

Campion, P., Brown, S., & Thornton-Jones, H. (2010). *After Wilberforce: An independent enquiry into the health and social needs of asylum seekers and refugees in Hull*. Hull: NHS Hull.

Common Approach for Refugees and Other Migrants' Health. (2017). *Health tracking and monitoring system - User manual*. European Commission. Start Date: 01/04/2016. End Date: 31/03/2017. JA2015 - GPSD [705038].

Department of Health. (2007). *Personal health record for asylum applicants and refugees*. Retrieved from www.dh.gov.uk/assetRoot/04/08/45/49/04084549.pdf

Doocy, S., Paik, K., Lyles, E., Tam, H. H., Fahed, Z., Winkler, E., et al. (2017b). Pilot testing and implementation of a mHealth tool for non-communicable diseases in a humanitarian setting. *PLoS Currents, 9*. https://doi.org/10.1371/currents.dis.e98c648aac93797b1996a37de099be74

Doocy, S., Paik, K. E., Lyles, E., Hei Tam, H., Fahed, Z., Winkler, E., et al. (2017a). Guidelines and mHealth to improve quality of hypertension and type 2 diabetes care for vulnerable populations in Lebanon: Longitudinal cohort study. *JMIR mHealth and uHealth, 5*, e158.

Footman, K., Cécile, K., Baeten, R., Ketevan, G., & Mckee, M. (2014). *Cross border health care in Europe*. Copenhagen: WHO Regional Office for Europe and European Observatory on Health Systems and Policies.

Giambi, C., Del Manso, M., Dalla Zuanna, T., Riccardo, F., Bella, A., Caporali, M. G., et al. (2018). National immunization strategies targeting migrants in six European countries. *Vaccine, 37*, 4610.

Giambi, C., Del Manso, M., Dente, M. G., Napoli, C., Montano-Remacha, C., Riccardo, F., et al. (2017). Immunization strategies targeting newly arrived migrants in non-EU countries of the Mediterranean Basin and Black Sea. *International Journal of Environmental Research and Public Health, 14*, 459.

Gibbons, M.C., Rivera Casale, C. (2010) Reducing disparities in health care quality: the role of health IT in underresourced settings. SAGE Publications Sage CA: Los Angeles, CA.

Goosen, S., Hoebe, C. J., Waldhober, Q., & Kunst, A. E. (2015). High HIV prevalence among asylum seekers who gave birth in the Netherlands: A nationwide study based on antenatal HIV tests. *PLoS One, 10*, e0134724.

Goosen, S., Middelkoop, B., Stronks, K., Agyemang, C., & Kunst, A. (2014). High diabetes risk among asylum seekers in the Netherlands. *Diabetic Medicine, 31*, 1532–1541.

Goosen, S., Stronks, K., & Kunst, A. E. (2013). Frequent relocations between asylum-seeker centres are associated with mental distress in asylum-seeking children: A longitudinal medical record study. *International Journal of Epidemiology, 43*, 94–104.

International Organization for Migration (IOM). (2018a). *Re-Health2. Electronic personal health record proves its efficiency*. 27 February 2018 Belgrade, Serbia (Online). Retrieved from http://serbia.iom.int/node/305

International Organization for Migration (IOM). (2018b). *Re-Health2. Migration's health – A multisectoral challenge*. 27 February 2018 Belgrade, Serbia (Online). Retrieved from http://re-health.eea.iom.int/migration's-health---multisectoral-challenge-27-february-2018-belgrade-serbia

International Organization for Migration, & European Commission. (2015a). *Handbook for health professionals. Health assessment of refugees and migrants in the EU/EEA*. Luxembourg: Publications Office of the European Union. https://doi.org/10.2875/450321

International Organization for Migration, & European Commission. (2015b). *Personal health record*. Luxembourg: Publications Office of the European Union. https://doi.org/10.2875/08133

Jahn, R., Ziegler, S., Nost, S., Gewalt, S. C., Strassner, C., & Bozorgmehr, K. (2018). Early evaluation of experiences of health care providers in reception centers with a patient-held personal health record for asylum seekers: A multi-sited qualitative study in a German federal state. *Globalization and Health, 14*, 71.

Khader, A., Ballout, G., Shahin, Y., Hababeh, M., Farajallah, L., Zeidan, W., et al. (2014). Treatment outcomes in a cohort of Palestine refugees with diabetes mellitus followed through use of E-Health over 3 years in Jordan. *Tropical Medicine & International Health, 19*, 219–223.

Khader, A., Farajallah, L., Shahin, Y., Hababeh, M., Abu-Zayed, I., Kochi, A., et al. (2012a). Cohort monitoring of persons with diabetes mellitus in a primary healthcare clinic for Palestine refugees in Jordan. *Tropical Medicine & International Health, 17*, 1569–1576.

Khader, A., Farajallah, L., Shahin, Y., Hababeh, M., Abu-Zayed, I., Kochi, A., et al. (2012b). Cohort monitoring of persons with hypertension: An illustrated example from a primary healthcare clinic for Palestine refugees in Jordan. *Tropical Medicine & International Health, 17*, 1163–1170.

Letizia, T. (1999). Setting up and managing the Safe Haven Health Information Services. A health information manager's experience. *Health Information Management, 29*, 131–132.

Martel, N., Franco-Lopez, H. D., Snyder, E., Cheskey, S., Fruchter, L., Ahrari, A., et al. (2015). The refugee health passport: A portable medical history tool that facilitates communication for newly arrived refugees in interpretation-limited, acute care settings. *Annals of Global Health, 81*, 115.

Mcmaster, P., Mcmaster, H. J., & Southall, D. P. (1996). Personal child health record and advice booklet programme in Tuzla, Bosnia Herzegovina. *Journal of the Royal Society of Medicine, 89*, 202–204.

Saavedra, J. F. (2012). *Development and evaluation of a web-based electronic medical record system without borders*. University of Washington.

Schoevers, M. A. (2011). *"Hiding and seeking": Health problems and problems in accessing health care of undocumented female immigrants in the Netherlands*. S.l.: s.n.

Schoevers, M. A., Van Den Muijsenbergh, M. E., & Lagro-Janssen, A. L. (2009). Patient-held records for undocumented immigrants: A blind spot. A systematic review of patient-held records. *Ethnicity & Health, 14*, 497–508.

Seth, O. (2017). *NetHope. Webinar recap: Electronic medical solutions in low-resource settings* (Online). Retrieved from https://solutionscenter.nethope.org/resources/webinar-recap-electronic-medical-solutions-in-low-resource-settings

Shahin, Y., Kapur, A., & Seita, A. (2015). Diabetes care in refugee camps: The experience of UNRWA. *Diabetes Research and Clinical Practice, 108*, 1–6.

Socias, C., Liang, Y., Delclos, G., Graves, J., Hendrikson, E., & Cooper, S. (2016). The feasibility of using electronic health records to describe demographic and clinical indicators of migrant and seasonal farmworkers. *Journal of Agromedicine, 21*, 71–81.

Solomon, C. (2017). Internet medical records for migrant workers. *Sonoma Medicine*. The magazine of the Sonoma County Medical Association.

United Nations Relief and Works Agency for Palestine Refugees in the Near East. (2015). *Department of health. Annual report 2014*. UNRWA.

US Department of Education. (n.d.). *Migrant student record exchange initiative*. Retrieved from https://msix.ed.gov/msix/#!/login

WHO Global Observatory for Ehealth. (2012). *Management of patient information: Trends and challenges in Member States: Based on the findings of the second global survey on eHealth*. World Health Organization. Retrieved from http://www.who.int/iris/handle/10665/76794

WHO Regional Office for Europe. (2015). *Serbia: Assessing health-system capacity to manage sudden large influxes of migrants. Joint report on a mission of the Ministry of Health of Serbia and the WHO*. Regional Office for Europe with the collaboration of the International Organization for Migration.

Winters, M., Rechel, B., de Jong, L., & Pavlova, M. (2018). A systematic review on the use of healthcare services by undocumented migrants in Europe. *BMC Health Services Research, 18*, 30.

World Health Organization. (2006). *Electronic health records: Manual for developing countries*. Manila: WHO Regional Office for the Western Pacific.

Chapter 10
Assessing the Health of Persons Experiencing Forced Migration: Current Practices for Health Service Organisations

Dominik Zenner, Kolitha Wickramage, Ursula Trummer, Kevin Pottie, and Chuck Hui

Abbreviations

WHO	World Health Organization
MIPEX	Migration Policy Index
IOM	International Organization for Migration
EU	European Union
EEA	European Economic Area
UNGA	United Nations General Assembly
GCM	Global Compact for Safe, Orderly and Regular Migration
WHA	World Health Assembly
UNHCR	UN High Commissioner for Refugees
CEAS	Common European Asylum System
EC	European Commission
CEA	Cost-effectiveness analysis

D. Zenner (✉)
International Organization for Migration, Brussels, Belgium
e-mail: dzenner@iom.int

K. Wickramage
International Organization for Migration, Manila, Philippines
e-mail: kwickramage@iom.int

U. Trummer
Center for Health and Migration, Vienna, Austria
e-mail: ursula.trummer@c-hm.com

K. Pottie
Bruyere Research Institute, University of Ottawa, Ottawa, ON, Canada
e-mail: kpottie@uottawa.ca

C. Hui
University of Ottawa, Ottawa, ON, Canada
e-mail: chui@cheo.on.ca

© Springer Nature Switzerland AG 2020
K. Bozorgmehr et al. (eds.), *Health Policy and Systems Responses to Forced Migration*, https://doi.org/10.1007/978-3-030-33812-1_10

GDPR   General Data Protection Regulation (EU)
GP   General Practitioner
HIS   Health information system

Introduction

The objective of this chapter is to review the current evidence and practice regarding health assessments and linkage to care for populations who experience forced migration. After embedding the chapter in a historical and legal framework and background, it will discuss the health, health assessments and linkage to care for persons who experience forced migration and review some of the practical and ethical issues around it, identify gaps in evidence and research and conclude with a summary.

The term 'forced migration' is often used to distinguish acute, crisis-driven, 'forced' migrant movements, sometimes including asylum seekers and undocumented migrant groups such as trafficked or smuggled persons from 'voluntary', long-term, economic movements including migrant groups such as registered labour migrants. Defining mobility trajectories based on a person's agency, 'forced' versus 'voluntary' migration can be simplistic, and in reality, a continuum of agency exists (Erdal and Oeppen 2018), and IOM regularly reports on mixed migration (International Organization for Migration 2018), which can be defined as 'complex population movements including refugees, asylum seekers, economic migrants and other migrants' (International Organization for Migration 2008). However, the term 'forced migration' is often used in political, policy and research discourse and will be used here. The chapter is designed to cover health assessments and care linkage amongst all who experience forced migration, although a lot of relevant evidence is from refugee resettlement programmes and large asylum centre reception centres, as evidence and practice is not as readily available for other, more irregular forms of migration.

Refugee Health Access and Health Assessments

There is a long history of global refugee movements and coordinated health assessments, the latter often mandated by receiving country governments. Health assessments, defined here as formal health assessment carried out in relation to international borders, have been part of immigration and visa regulations at least since the early twentieth century, often as extension to quarantine regulations and implemented by port health departments (Taylor 2016). However, the magnitude of movements, and with it the interest in health assessments, has changed over time. In 2017, it was estimated that there were about 258 million (United Nations Population Division, Department of Economic and Social Affairs n.d.) international migrants globally, of which approximately 25.4 million were refugees and 3.1 million asylum seekers (United Nations High Commissioner for Refugees n.d.-a). This overall volume of global migrants has significantly increased over the last 10 years. The routes of migration and recipient countries have also changed (International Organization for Migration 2019), not least because of the changing nature of conflicts and border control factors and also in line with potential receiving country preferences (case study 1 in Box 10.1). This means that the context, scope and reach of health assessments for refugees is almost constantly changing and leading to a decrease of resettlement-related health assessments in some countries, whilst others have only recently initiated or significantly increased their resettlement intake and with it often the number of health assessments. There is, therefore, a significant interest in these health assessments and to identify best practice and ensure coordination and standardisation of these efforts, particularly from receiving countries, who recently experienced increased inward migration. There also now appears to be general agreement at international level of the value of access to relevant health services for migrant populations.

Box 10.1 The ePHR to Assess Health Status and Needs of Arriving Refugees/Migrants

The ePHR is a tool to assess the health status and related health needs of refugees and migrants arriving in Europe including specifically vulnerable groups and to store health data in a database to make it available in transit and destination countries. It is built on three components: a personal health record (PHR) which is held by the individual migrant in paper or electronic form, a handbook for professionals and an electronic health database.

The ePHR helps to (re)construct the medical history of arriving migrants and provides an opportunity to record subsequent provision of treatment, including vaccinations, and to offer counselling and health education services. It is a personal document that migrants and refugees should keep with them and that contains the individual's health data. It offers the unique possibility of a health record that can be stored and shared across borders and that facilitates continuity of medical care for individuals and surveillance relevant for public health.

The accompanying handbook for health professionals supports the systematic health assessment and also seeks to ensure that health assessment and preventive and health promotion measures are provided via the employment of health mediators and interpreters.

The ePHR was developed and implemented in selected European countries in two consecutive actions by the International Organization for Migration (IOM)—Migration Health Division—and co-funded by the European Union (EU), starting in 2016, in the 'Re-Health' and 'Re-Health2' projects (http://

re-health.eea.iom.int/). Re-Health/Re-Health2 aims at improving the capacity of EU member states under particular migratory pressure to address the health-related issues of migrants arriving at key reception areas whilst preventing and addressing possible communicable diseases and cross-border health events.

A feasibility study was conducted by the Center for Health and Migration, Vienna, during the initial testing phase, assessing the acceptability, feasibility and transferability of the ePHR. The ePHR was well-received by migrants with 91% ($n = 2.838$ of 3.125) giving informed consent. Reasons for non-consent were fear of use of information against the migrant's interest and that migrants couldn't see any benefits.

Acceptability by staff was measured with effort and payoff of using the ePHR. Ideally, high payoff can be achieved with low effort. Those staff members who see high payoff will be more willing to take high efforts; staff members who experience high effort and low payoff will not favour the ePHR. A majority of staff reports high payoff with high effort (66%; $n = 23$), and 26% ($n = 9$) report high payoff with low effort. Named efforts are mainly connected to explaining the ePHR to migrants to get informed consent and to overcome technical barriers. Payoffs are seen in the systematic collection of data and in the possibility to share data electronically.

Feasibility of the on-site use of ePHR was seen as mainly related to mediation services available and the technical quality and user-friendliness.

Most important elements for further development were seen in training of staff; information for migrants about scope, purpose and benefits of ePHR, about data safety and that the ePHR is not connected to the asylum procedure; provision of sufficient technical equipment; and availability of medical staff on site.

Predeparture health assessments have been the preferred model for a number of countries such as the USA, Canada, Australia or New Zealand for humanitarian entrants through refugee resettlement programmes (Douglas et al. 2017). These pre-entry assessments have been particularly attractive for specific target groups (such as vulnerable refugees) or specific disease groups and have been integrated in the resettlement process. As resettlement has become more targeted, the role of predeparture assessment has increased in importance. It is worth noting that many countries with resettlement programmes also have a separate system to assess asylum seekers.

Health assessments can be done at various points in the refugee's journey: predeparture, on arrival or post arrival. Health assessments are often determined by trajectories of migration routes, including irregular migration. For example, in some Southern European border states, who recently experienced a higher number of informal arrivals, post arrival health assessments, often carried out in reception centres, were more common. More recently, some countries of origin (such as Sri

Lanka) have started performing health assessments amongst specific types of emigrants (e.g. labour migrants). Nevertheless, the landscape of health assessments is constantly changing, and there has been a recent political interest for stronger support of migration management in transition countries (European Council 2018), and this may make pre-entry health assessments more attractive and feasible for these receiving countries.

The objectives and the scope of health assessments are highly variable and not always known to the migrant (see also Chap. 7). Some countries appear to screen exclusively for public health reasons and to prevent excessive demand on their healthcare system, and this can lead to a policy of exclusion, so that persons with certain illnesses, especially infectious diseases or mental health conditions are prevented from entry.

The objective of other health assessment programmes includes a check for medical conditions to facilitate care of patients in the receiving country and to detect conditions which require urgent treatment and linkage to care, such as tuberculosis (TB) and human immunodeficiency virus (HIV) (UK Home Office et al. 2017). These preferences are often informed by the context—for example, states which take refugees with the United Nations Refugee Agency (UNHCR) vulnerability criteria may choose the latter. Screening in reception centres can have similar objectives, but its processes can be more dependent on the acuteness of situation and the logistics on the ground, and on occasion, a stronger emphasis is placed on protecting public health or on detecting vulnerabilities. Pragmatism and logistics can also be important factors influencing process on the ground.

A key component of health assessments and detecting vulnerabilities should be linkage to appropriate care along with the ability to access this care (Pareek et al. 2018). However, this significantly varies according to circumstances and receiving countries. In their analysis of health systems, the health strand of the Migrant Integration Policy Index (MIPEX) (International Organization for Migration 2017) provides a good overview of some of the difficulties and barriers faced by migrants and refugees (including undocumented migrants) to access to 38 different receiving countries' health systems (EU/EEA, Bosnia and Herzegovina, Macedonia, Turkey, Australia, Canada, New Zealand and the USA) across the dimensions of entitlement and access of healthcare. It is obvious that both not only vary by receiving country but also by legal status of the migrant.

The Policy Context of Health Assessment and Linkage to Care

Within the context of forced migration, there is consensus to ensure that basic provisions in terms of food, shelter and social security should be made by receiving countries (see also Chap. 13). In declaring solidarity with and acknowledging responsibility for people who are faced with forced migration, the United Nations General Assembly (UNGA) adopted the New York Declaration in September 2016 (United Nations General Assembly n.d.), pledging that basic health needs of refugee communities are met, particularly those of vulnerable populations, including women and children.

The New York Declaration also commits member states to working towards the Global Compact for Safe, Orderly and Regular Migration (GCM) (United Nations General Assembly n.d.), setting out to provide a framework for international cooperation for all types of migration, including forced migration. The GCM provides much more detail on addressing vulnerabilities in migration (objective 7); strengthening procedures for screening, assessment and referral (objective 12); and providing access to basic services for migrants (objective 15). Objective 7 is particularly concerned with ensuring early recognition of vulnerabilities and appropriate response and referral mechanisms, especially for vulnerable women, and minors, including healthcare and psychological services. Objective 12 commits to improving predictability and legal certainty of migration procedures but also seeks to ensure that assessments and screening procedures are appropriate, standardised and aimed at detecting vulnerable populations, such as unaccompanied minors. Objective 15 aims to ensure that the human right of access to basic services can be exercised by refugees, and this includes non-discriminatory access to appropriate and responsive services including accessible information about the services and a mandate for human right organisations to monitor (or if necessary) help mitigate access issues.

Based on previous resolutions, including the one on the health of migrants (WHA 61.17), member states through the World Health Assembly have endorsed a resolution on 'Promoting the Health of Refugees and Migrants' in May 2017, which calls on member states to promote a framework of guiding priorities and guiding principles for migrant health, including the right to enjoy the highest principles of physical and mental health, the principle of equality and non-discrimination, equitable access to health services and the promotion of people-centred and migrant-sensitive health systems, amongst others (World Health Organization n.d.).

Within the EU/EEA, minimum standards for asylum seekers have been adopted in Directive 2013/33/EU (European Commission n.d.), and article 17 recommends that, on reception, basic needs of asylum seekers, including those pertaining to physical and mental health should be provided for, and article 10 mandates that persons in detention should have access to appropriate medical treatment and psychological counselling. Provision of healthcare is further specified in article 19, detailing that all asylum applicants should have access to at least essential healthcare as well as treatment of mental health conditions and that there should be appropriate services for those with special needs.

In fact, there is a specific obligation on national authorities to identify and monitor vulnerable persons to ensure appropriateness of reception conditions. The minimum standards for asylum seekers discourage the detention of vulnerable migrants, particularly children (article 11), although it allows medical screening on public health grounds. Persons with special needs are defined as those who are vulnerable; this includes minors, unaccompanied minors, disabled people, elderly people, pregnant women, single parents with minor children, victims of trafficking, victims of female genital mutilation, persons with mental health problems and persons who have been subjected to torture, rape or other serious forms of psychological, physical or sexual violence (article 22). There is a requirement to identifying and specifying the exact nature of these vulnerabilities and to adequately support these persons throughout the asylum process.

In summary, there now appears to be a general agreement at international level that culturally and medically appropriate healthcare access, including for urgent and mental health conditions should be accessible to all migrants, including for those suffering forced migration. Special efforts should be made to identify persons and circumstances of vulnerability to ensure that circumstances and care can be tailored appropriately. However, as described in the Migration Policy Index (MIPEX), entitlements and access to care can be highly variable, even between European Union member states, and frequently, those affected by forced migration, including asylum seekers, and those uncertain legal status are the least likely to be able to efficiently access the receiving countries' health system (see also Chap. 5). It is currently not entirely clear to what extent persons with vulnerabilities are systematically and effectively identified and their care appropriately adapted. This chapter seeks to look at health assessments and in-country examples to examine this question.

Health Assessments and Health Access of Persons Experiencing Forced Migration: Current State of Affairs

Here, we aim to provide a comprehensive picture on the current knowledge of the health, health assessments and health access of persons who experienced forced migration. It is important to recognise that persons in these circumstances are a very heterogenous group—because of age and gender, socio-economic and geographical determinants, and not least because of their variable legal status in transit and receiving countries. The health, health access and health assessments (if any) will significantly vary depending on whether they have recognised refugee status, are asylum seekers, are failed asylum seekers or are undocumented. There are still a lot of variations in the use of the terminology, and this has been shown to affect health policy and ultimately access to care (Hannigan et al. 2016). The chapter also has a specific focus on the identification and linkage to care for the subgroup with vulnerability criteria. Literature is scarce, particularly on the latter issue, so this chapter brings together case studies from specific contexts with a narrative literature review.

A recent WHO-commissioned review on the health of refugees and asylum seekers in the European region found a very mixed picture across the region and was limited by the fact that settings are not always comparable and that most studies came from few receiving countries, including Scandinavia and the United Kingdom (UK) (Bradby et al. 2015). This finding of practice variabilities has been corroborated in other reviews (Hvass and Wejse 2017). However, and acknowledging the limitations, the WHO review found evidence for increased prevalence of specific infectious diseases and some mental health conditions. A systematic review on current diagnoses of mental illness indicated that refugees resettled in Western countries could be about 10 times more likely to have post-traumatic stress disorder than age-matched general populations in those countries (Fazel et al. 2005). However, there is considerable heterogeneity of prevalence rates in studies, and comparability to the nonmigrant population is contested. Depending on the particular circumstances of their forced migration, non-communicable diseases, including prevalent respiratory or heart diseases, musculoskeletal conditions or diabetes may be undermanaged not least due to financial and access barriers particularly in transit and may require attention and appropriate care in receiving countries (Amara and Aljunid 2014). Some of the vulnerabilities amongst persons who experience forced migration have been well-documented—for example, there is good evidence of adverse perinatal and maternal health outcomes amongst refugees (Bollini et al. 2009; Gagnon et al. 2009) or mental health (Porter and Haslam 2005).

The vulnerability not only of children and adolescents exposed to violence but also protective factors such as social support in the receiving countries has been equally well-documented (Fazel et al. 2012). Complexities in healthcare provision owing to cultural-linguistic barriers, healthcare provider capacity issues and legality concerns have been well-described (Suphanchaimat et al. 2015).

Central to the concept of the European Commission (EC) directive on asylum seekers in the EU and the Common European Asylum System (CEAS) is the notion of vulnerability. This is one of the key reasons why its legislation mandates the systematic identification of vulnerabilities, which would then be translated into procedural safeguards for protection of the individual (European Commission n.d.; European Union n.d.). The concept is not new in Europe, being recognised by the European Court of Human Rights, and not unique to the EU setting, with a number of other available legal instruments, such as the UN Convention on the Rights of the Child or the UN Convention on the Rights of Persons with Disabilities, providing legal context, adopted by a number of non-European countries. It should be noted that detecting vulnerabilities is primarily an immigration function, not a health function, and ill physical and mental health is just a subset to vulnerability criteria at large.

The concept of health risks and vulnerability and its safeguards appear intuitive; it is reasonable to prioritise those who have specific needs, either by virtue of their demographic characteristics, health or welfare concerns, or protection needs. There is a considerable amount of literature, including tools describing how to screen or elicit these concerns, but there is no uniform agreement on what is included in refugee health risks and vulnerabilities, with marked differences across countries (United Nations High Commissioner for Refugees n.d.-b) and some authors arguing that the asylum seeking status itself can be regarded as vulnerabilities.

In addition to these country- and setting-specific differences, the tools, capacity and training to screen for vulnerabilities are also highly heterogenous. There may be a risk of recall and observer bias when trying to elicit vulnerabilities not readily recognisable, and such assessments may be setting, client and provider dependent. Whilst robust training and legal support networks may risk over-ascertainment, the lack of these together with stigma and cultural-linguistic barriers may risk under-ascertainment. Such decreased sensitivity and specificity can be highly consequential to the migrant and the society of the receiving country. There is therefore a legitimate concern about the current over-reliance on identification of vulnerabilities to define migrants worthy of protection in the European context. Health equity has emerged as a principle that can help us with this assessment of refugees who are at risk to the medical system.

Since the majority of vulnerability criteria (which emerged from a human right perspective) are not directly health related, the responsibility of assessments thereof does not usually lie with health professionals. The link to health assessments, which initially evolved from a traditional quarantine perspective, is variable but can be relatively loose. Information from health assessments, if carried out well, can be used to corroborate a narrative from the vulnerability assessment, and this may take the form of expert witness statements. Yet the extent to which information from health assessments is systematically used to inform the detection or validation of criteria informing a vulnerability assessment is variable. More information and better targeted research about optimising the link between health and vulnerability assessments and their use to inform each other may be urgently needed.

Refugees may have poor or deteriorating health, because of conditions experienced before, during or after arrival to new country. A healthcare system that is poorly adapted to their needs compounds this situation, resulting in further marginalisation and health inequities. It is critical to identify preventable and often unrecognised clinical care gaps that can result from such majority-system biases (Pottie et al. 2011).

The nature and extent of health assessments is inevitably determined by the setting. Health, access and assessments are probably best documented for recognised refugees, and a significant body of literature is set in the resettlement context, and a number of countries run programmatic health assessments or screenings for refugees awaiting resettlement prior to departure to the receiving country (case study 2 in Box 10.2). Many of these programmes are well-established, have clear guidelines and often are quality assured and monitored (UK Home Office et al. 2017; Immigration Refugees and Citizenship Canada 2013; Centers for Disease Control and Prevention (CDC) 2017). In this context, health assessments are often part of a more comprehensive process, including security-related assessments, and can take place considerable time before resettlement takes place. These health examinations can include a general assessment of health status, including a physical examination, routine bloods and urine and often include multiple specific disease areas, including screening for mental health conditions or an assessment of drug and alcohol use, an assessment of disabilities and infectious disease screening. The latter often depends on the epidemiology in the country of origin and receiving country, for example, for active tuberculosis, hepatitis B and C, HIV, helminths or malaria. In addition, many programmes offer vaccination for common vaccine-preventable diseases, including diphtheria and tetanus, meningococcal disease, polio, measles or rotavirus amongst others.

Box 10.2 Health Assessments for UK-Bound Refugees

The UK has a number of refugee programmes, including for those arriving from Sub-Saharan Africa, such as the Gateway Protection Programme, and those arriving from the Middle East through the Syrian Vulnerable Person Resettlement Programme (VPRS). Until relatively recently, the UK programme included a few hundred refugees each year. However, following an announcement of the (then) prime minister David Cameron on 7 September 2015, the VPRS was expanded to take 20,000 Syrian refugees between 2015 and 2020.

The UK prioritises resettlement according to the UNHCR vulnerability criteria. Criteria include persons who have demonstrated legal and physical protection needs—such as being survivors of violence and torture, elderly refugees, women-at-risk, children and adolescents, those seeking family reunification, those with medical needs and those who lack local integration prospects. All UK-bound refugees undergo a standardised health assessment prior to departure, guided by technical instructions on refugee screening and covering a wide range of general and specific disease topics. Noting aforementioned vulnerability criteria, the primary objectives of these health assessments are to identify health conditions for which treatment is recommended before the individual travels to the UK (including fitness to travel), to ensure the individual is settled in a location that has appropriate facilities to meet their health and social care needs and to use the opportunity to bring their vaccinations up to date and in the singular case of active pulmonary TB for public health reasons.

The health assessment is therefore very broad and includes determining the general health status as well as screening for specific diseases of which screening for a number of them, including tuberculosis, hepatitis B and C or malaria, is informed by receiving country epidemiology. In addition, vaccinations are provided to ensure they are up to date with the UK vaccination schedule. A basic mental health assessment is also performed, and more recently, the more extensive Global Mental Health Assessment Tool (GMHAT) has been piloted amongst a Syrian refugee population in Lebanon. Health assessments for refugees are carried out by qualified doctors and nurses in the field, mostly through the International Organization for Migration.

Treatment is provided prior to departure or organised post arrival, depending on specific disease area, circumstances and individual or public health need; and with the help of the receiving local authority and health authority, refugees are provided with good access to required key services, including health.

The objectives of these assessments can vary and include receiving country public health considerations (as justification for infectious disease screening, such as tuberculosis) but can also include considerations about costs to the receiving country healthcare system or society (Immigration Refugees and Citizenship Canada 2013; Centers for Disease Control and Prevention (CDC) 2017). However, the aim can also be to ensure that resettlement circumstances are optimised to meet the refugee's health needs (UK Home Office et al. 2017). In the latter scenario, screening for health-related vulnerabilities is included in the assessment in order to aid matching local facilities to the need of the refugee (case study 2 in Box 10.2). Practical barriers, which may impede the full implementation of such objectives, can include resource pressures, competing objectives and, not least occasionally suboptimal, often hierarchical information flows (Fig. 10.1). The latter can arise because of the challenge to provide to each of the multiple agencies involved in resettlement the needed and appropriate context-specific information about the refugee whilst adhering to relevant data protection regulations (such as the EU General Data Protection Regulation, GDPR (European Commission 2016)). There can be barriers and delays if, for example, the local health economy or, if relevant, the local healthcare providers do not receive appropriate and complete health information in a timely manner. Much progress has been made in ensuring that refugee health data is captured in confidential, transferable and accessible databases, but competing systems and slow implementation has been a barrier to this process. The feedback mechanism, including information from providers about the appropriateness, usefulness, timeliness or completeness of such information, is often narrative, and published literature on such questions is scarce. In a desire to improve mental health-related information, the Global Mental Health Assessment Tool (GMHAT) (GMHAT 2019) was recently piloted amongst UK-bound refugees in Lebanon. An audit amongst UK General

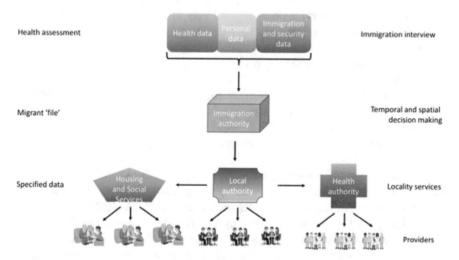

Fig. 10.1 Country example of hierarchical framework for sharing health information

Practitioners (GPs) found that the information was not always received by them in a timely fashion (author communication).

Health assessments in immediate reception or transit centres are now very common but highly variable. The population in reception centres tends to be socioeconomically, culturally, linguistically and legally more heterogenous than in a pre-migration setting and to a large extent includes persons applying for protection (asylum seekers), rather than those who have been granted protection (refugees), and applying meaningful health assessment and screening processes can therefore be more challenging. Health screens are often focused on the detection of immediate conditions of concern, particularly if conducted in a setting including persons whose health may be immediately affected by their journey (e.g. by boat through the different Mediterranean routes). They often include screening for infectious disease conditions, such as active tuberculosis. Assessing people with vulnerabilities, as well as assessing the vulnerabilities themselves can be very complex and requires thorough understanding and embedding within the sociocultural context (Raghavan 2018). Equally, the assessment of mental health morbidities may be hampered by cultural and linguistic barriers for which recent computer-based solutions may be a helpful adjunct (Morina et al. 2017).

In settings with large secondary migration (facilitated by contiguous landmass) or scheduled onward movements, it is possible for health assessments to take place in more than one location, making duplication of such efforts likely, especially if health conditions are not well-recorded or records are not shared. In many instances and apart from conditions or diseases requiring immediate attention, it is unclear to what extent information from health assessment, including assessment of vulnerabilities is utilised for the benefit of the migrant. Screening even for infectious diseases such as tuberculosis is not always well-recorded, which can lead to considerable uncertainties about calculating screening yields (Bozorgmehr et al. 2018). This could hinder targeted service provision and may affect wider health policy decisions. Conversely, there is good evidence that well-ascertained and recorded information can be helpful even within initial settings, such as refugee camps, for example, in the recording and early detection of infectious disease outbreaks (Rojek et al. 2018).

A number of different health record systems have been tried, and a key challenge seems to be balancing the need for readily available information with data protection considerations. It is possible that electronic systems have an advantage, compared to systems which rely on the migrant to bring a paper or electronic mobile storage device (Jahn et al. 2018). The need for accurate, timely and appropriate health information for healthcare providers in the immediate reception setting and further on in the migrants' journey has been well-recognised and has resulted in several initiatives, including the establishment of an electronic health record, funded by the European Commission (case study 1 in Box 10.1) (European Commission and Directorate-General for Health and Food Safety 2015) (see also Chap. 9).

Amongst undocumented migrants, the entitlement and access to healthcare provision can be severely limited, and alternative systems can be overwhelmed and health problems amplified, whilst additional barriers occur due to fear (often justified) and stigma (Hacker et al. 2015). This pattern of differential healthcare access stratified by legal status in the receiving country and often caused by bureaucratic barriers has been recently confirmed and well-described in the MIPEX (International Organization for Migration 2017). It has been noted in various European projects concerned with healthcare for undocumented migrants that, in absence of legal access to regular public health services, NGOs act as healthcare providers for undocumented migrants and in this role also take over health assessments. However, this information is rarely made available to the public health system and for further development of services, as NGOs often act in parallel to the country's healthcare system. This can create a situation where data is there, but not used and/or synthesised for public health purposes. Benchmarking country health information systems (HIS) with respect to the ability to assess the health status and healthcare situation of forced migrants is important. Bozorgmehr and colleagues developed a HIS Tool for Asylum Seekers (HIATUS) and applied the tool to the HIS in Germany and Netherlands (Bozorgmehr et al. 2017a). HIATUS revealed substantial limitations in HIS capacity to assess the health situation of asylum seekers in both countries and allowed for intercountry comparisons.

The urgent need for also including undocumented migrants into electronic health information systems, coupled with the complete absence thereof, has been documented in a systematic review (Schoevers et al. 2009).

Ethical Considerations

There are inherent ethical challenges associated with the health assessment of migrants. Many programmes are set up with the objective of population health and national health security (public policy and country laws), whilst it is an individual's health that is being assessed. Indeed, in some situations, the primary user of this health information is not a healthcare worker, but the government. Many migrants do not understand this difference which may lead to health-related consequences and further costs (Pacheco et al. 2016). A new migrant could also consider screening tests a threat to their migration status. The lack of linkage to care or intention of treatment or lack of informed consent in migrant health screening are ethical dilemmas (Denholm et al. 2015; Beeres et al. 2018) that have not been addressed in many national policies. The healthcare practitioners may have conflicting and dual loyalties and obligations providing care in limited settings and not able to optimally advocate for their patients (Hui and Zion 2018).

It also has to be considered that health assessments have the potential to be misused as instruments of migration control. From an ethical, human right and public health perspective, health assessment should not be constructed as instruments of discrimination, but rather instruments of public health good. Additionally, programmes without sufficient evidence base or without adequate epidemiological rationale particularly if diagnostic yield is low or diagnostic tests expensive, such as those focussing primarily on health security issues, may risk inappropriate use of resources (Bozorgmehr et al. 2017b). In this context, there may be issues around detection of conditions and linkage to care in settings where access to care is restricted.

There are additional challenges concerning data protection when undertaking health assessments and formulating health information systems of forced migrant populations, not least because of the numerous actors involved. Finally, it must be understood that health assessments are also a snapshot in time, whereas health needs are dynamic and dependent on many variables (Schoretsanitis et al. 2018), and that the occupational health particularly of migrant workers is not addressed in most health assessments.

What Are the Gaps for Policy and Research?

A recent bibliometric analysis demonstrated that the field of migration health is severely under-researched, particularly in international collaboration and specific topic and disease areas and by developmental or income gradients of countries (Sweileh et al. 2018). A small number of systematic reviews have explored the topics of mental health status (Amara and Aljunid 2014), maternal health, infectious disease and non-communicable disease (Amara and Aljunid 2014) status of various refugees and asylum seekers. These studies have also indicated major gaps in the evidence landscape by country, migrant category and migration corridor. Many disease areas also remain uncovered, and most of the underlying studies have been carried out in specific contexts and amongst specific populations, making generalisability difficult. The best data come from well-structured refugee programmes often within the health assessment context (Crawshaw et al. 2018) or with standardised medical record systems (Kane et al. 2014). Data on health of migrants and refugees via irregular migration pathways and with lesser legal entitlements or access, such as asylum seekers or undocumented migrants, are particularly scarce. A key finding of the bibliometric analysis was also the scarcity of research data on international migrant workers which comprised of only 6% of totally research despite the total number of migrant workers being seven times higher than refugees. Despite their economic contributions, migrant workers, and in particular those low-skilled from lower-income nations, are 'left behind' in global migration health research. The fact that many migrant workers undergo a health assessment as part of visa issuance and travel is significant, and analysis of such data is critical for both labour-sending and labour-receiving countries (Wickramage and Mosca 2014). Particular attention needs to be focused on gender dimensions, the human rights and health vulnerabilities of female migrant workers.

Equally, healthcare entitlements and access have been reasonably well-documented for a number of countries in the EU/EEA (International Organization for Migration 2017). However, such output has also been temporal and geographically restricted, with uncertainty about entitlements and access for asylum seekers and undocumented migrants, particularly in a rapidly changing policy environment.

Similarly, health assessment procedures are well-documented for highly structured and quality-assured programmes in the context of resettlement programmes (Centers for Disease Control and Prevention (CDC) 2017), with considerable uncertainty around context, content, transmission and use of health assessment information in other contexts, such as reception centres or even unregulated camp situations. In addition, traditionally, health assessments have been created as part of immigration procedures, often informed by public health aspects (including prevention of transmission), and sometimes to identify and exclude individuals whose conditions may be regarded as 'cost pressures' to the receiving country health system. Such assessments are therefore often designed to maximise disease detection sensitivity and less to benefit individuals, and much more evidence is required to assess and inform which health assessments and in which contexts and point in the migration journey would have a positive impact for the individual and society (Crawshaw et al. 2018). Recent systematic reviews carried out for European migrant infectious disease screening guidelines demonstrated that robust studies on some of the key questions around health assessments, such as effectiveness and cost-effectiveness or even target populations, are scarce, although, more recently, significant progress has been made with a series of systematic reviews, including for tuberculosis (Greenaway et al. 2018b), hepatitis B and C (Greenaway et al. 2018a; Myran et al. 2018), HIV (Pottie et al. 2018) or vaccine-preventable diseases (Hui et al. 2018). There is a scarcity of routine data for monitoring health assessments, as has recently been described in the case of tuberculosis screening amongst asylum seekers in Germany (Bozorgmehr et al. 2018). The screening and detection of vulnerabilities and their link to care are equally under-researched.

This scarcity of research for significant parts of population groups who experienced forced migration including their health assessments and linkage to care has important policy implications in several aspects. Firstly, the absence of reliable figures can have adverse effects on planning for accessible, culturally appropriate health services, which in turn could generate health service pressures and a risk of knock-on effects such as perception of or actual under-provisions for the population in the receiving country. Secondly, an in-depth understanding of the demography, health status and epidemiology of such groups is important for healthcare provider and public health training purposes. Thirdly, although a number of studies, including the MIPEX (International Organization for Migration 2017) or specific member state papers, have provided reasonable attempts to demonstrate evidence of cost-effectiveness for universal healthcare access for all groups of migrants who experienced forced migration into the receiving country healthcare system (Bozorgmehr and Razum 2015), the debate has not been sufficiently settled to convince policymakers of the merits of this, and more robust cost-effectiveness analyses are needed. Conversely, more evidence is needed about the health and social impact as well as the long-term economic costs of restricted access to health and social care. Fourthly, there is an urgent need for a better understanding of how to optimise health assessments to ensure effectiveness and cost-effectiveness and maximise the benefits for the individual and society and how to best integrate and use resulting information for healthcare planning in the receiving country and to address any individual healthcare needs. The current situation risks missing a valuable tool for targeting and optimising care (including addressing vulnerabilities) for those who need it most.

Conclusions

Health and vulnerability assessments of migrants all have a long history but have evolved significantly. They started from very different origins and with different foci; health assessments stem from quarantine arrangements and vulnerability assessments from a human right perspective although they are still frequently used for immigration control purposes. More recently, they have been developed significantly, and there are increasing tendencies to utilise these tools for the benefit of the migrant and his/her integration in the receiving country. However, even with a clear legislative framework, both internationally and at EU level (including a mandatory requirement to screen for vulnerabilities and ensure appropriate services to meet the needs), the reality is highly heterogenous, and the implementation of EU directives to protect vulnerable migrants is still sketchy. Despite the recognition of health as a human right and notwithstanding numerous international resolutions and documents, the linkage to care is at best variable and in the current political climate potentially worsening in many settings. Much remains to be done to ensure that these instruments, some of which were initially implemented as instruments of immigration control, are used for the benefit of the migrants themselves and ultimately their integration into the receiving country. Ultimately, healthy migrants are in the best interest of receiving countries and global health at large (Abubakar et al. 2018).

Acknowledgments We would like to express our special thanks to Prof. Michael Knipper, University of Giessen, Germany, for his helpful review and suggestions towards this manuscript.

Disclaimer The opinions expressed in this book chapter are those of the author and do not necessarily reflect the views of the International Organization for Migration (IOM). The designations employed and the presentation of material throughout the articles do not imply the expression of any opinion whatsoever on the part of IOM concerning the legal status of any country, territory, city or area, or of its authorities, or concerning its frontiers or boundaries.

References

Abubakar, I., Aldridge, R. W., Devakumar, D., Orcutt, M., Burns, R., Barreto, M. L., et al. (2018). The UCL–Lancet Commission on Migration and Health: The health of a world on the move. *The Lancet, 392*(10164), 2606–2654. https://doi.org/10.1016/S0140-6736(18)32114-7

Amara, A. H., & Aljunid, S. M. (2014). Noncommunicable diseases among urban refugees and asylum-seekers in developing countries: A neglected health care need. *Globalization and Health, 10*, 24. https://doi.org/10.1186/1744-8603-10-24

Beeres, D. T., Cornish, D., Vonk, M., Ravensbergen, S. J., Maeckelberghe, E. L. M., Boele Van Hensbroek, P., et al. (2018). Screening for infectious diseases of asylum seekers upon arrival: The necessity of the moral principle of reciprocity. *BMC Medical Ethics, 19*, 16. https://doi.org/10.1186/s12910-018-0256-7

Bollini, P., Pampallona, S., Wanner, P., & Kupelnick, B. (2009). Pregnancy outcome of migrant women and integration policy: A systematic review of the international literature. *Social Science & Medicine, 68*, 452–461. https://doi.org/10.1016/j.socscimed.2008.10.018

Bozorgmehr, K., & Razum, O. (2015). Effect of restricting access to health care on health expenditures among asylum-seekers and refugees: A quasi-experimental study in Germany, 1994–2013. *PLoS One, 10*, e0131483. https://doi.org/10.1371/journal.pone.0131483

Bozorgmehr, K., Goosen, S., Mohsenpour, A., Kuehne, A., Razum, O., & Kunst, A. E. (2017a). How do countries' health information systems perform in assessing asylum seekers' health situation? Developing a Health Information Assessment Tool on Asylum Seekers (HIATUS) and piloting it in two European countries. *International Journal of Environmental Research and Public Health, 14*. https://doi.org/10.3390/ijerph14080894

Bozorgmehr, K., Wahedi, K., Noest, S., Szecsenyi, J., & Razum, O. (2017b). Infectious disease screening in asylum seekers: Range, coverage and economic evaluation in Germany, 2015. *Eurosurveillance, 22*, 16–00677. https://doi.org/10.2807/1560-7917.ES.2017.22.40.16-00677

Bozorgmehr, K., Stock, C., Joggerst, B., & Razum, O. (2018). Tuberculosis screening in asylum seekers in Germany: A need for better data. *The Lancet Public Health, 3*, e359–e361. https://doi.org/10.1016/S2468-2667(18)30132-4

Bradby, H., World Health Organization, Regional Office for Europe, & Health Evidence Network. (2015). *Public health aspects of migrants health: A review of the evidence on health status for refugees and asylum seekers in the European Region.* Copenhagen: World Health Organisation, Regional Office for Europe.

Centers for Disease Control and Prevention (CDC). (2017). Panel physicians technical instructions. Immigrant and refugee health. *CDC.* Retrieved August 18, 2018, from https://www.cdc.gov/immigrantrefugeehealth/exams/ti/panel/technical-instructions-panel-physicians.html

Crawshaw, A. F., Pareek, M., Were, J., Schillinger, S., Gorbacheva, O., Wickramage, K. P., et al. (2018). Infectious disease testing of UK-bound refugees: A population-based, cross-sectional study. *BMC Medicine, 16*, 143. https://doi.org/10.1186/s12916-018-1125-4

Denholm, J. T., Matteelli, A., & Reis, A. (2015). Latent tuberculous infection: Ethical considerations in formulating public health policy. *The International Journal of Tuberculosis and Lung Disease, 19*, 137–140. https://doi.org/10.5588/ijtld.14.0543

Douglas, P., Posey, D. L., Zenner, D., Robson, J., Abubakar, I., & Giovinazzo, G. (2017). Capacity strengthening through pre-migration tuberculosis screening programmes: IRHWG experiences. *The International Journal of Tuberculosis and Lung Disease, 21*, 737–745. https://doi.org/10.5588/ijtld.17.0019

Erdal, M. B., & Oeppen, C. (2018). Forced to leave? The discursive and analytical significance of describing migration as forced and voluntary. *Journal of Ethnic and Migration Studies, 44*, 981–998. https://doi.org/10.1080/1369183X.2017.1384149

European Commission. (2016). Regulation (EU) 2016/679 of the European Parliament and of the Council of 27 April 2016 on the protection of natural persons with regard to the processing of personal data and on the free movement of such data, and repealing Directive 95/46/EC (General Data Protection Regulation) (Text with EEA relevance).

European Commission. (n.d.). Directive 2013/33/EU of the European Parliament and of the Council of 26 June 2013 laying down standards for the reception of applicants for international protection, p. 21.

European Commission, & Directorate-General for Health and Food Safety. (2015). *Handbook for health professionals health assessment of refugees and migrants in the EU/EEA.* Luxembourg: Publications Office.

European Council European Council Conclusions. (2018, June 28). *Consilium.* Retrieved September 10, 2018, from http://www.consilium.europa.eu/en/press/press-releases/2018/06/29/20180628-euco-conclusions-final/

European Union. (n.d.). Minimum standards for the reception of asylum seekers (recast) ***I. European Parliament legislative resolution of 7 May 2009 on the proposal for a directive of the European Parliament and of the Council laying down minimum standards for the reception of asylum seekers (recast) (COM(2008)0815 – C6-0477/2008 – 2008/0244(COD)). Retrieved from https://eur-lex.europa.eu/legal-content/EN/TXT/?uri=CELEX:52009AP0376

Fazel, M., Reed, R. V., Panter-Brick, C., & Stein, A. (2012). Mental health of displaced and refugee children resettled in high-income countries: Risk and protective factors. *The Lancet, 379*, 266–282. https://doi.org/10.1016/S0140-6736(11)60051-2

Fazel, M., Wheeler, J., & Danesh, J. (2005). Prevalence of serious mental disorder in 7000 refugees resettled in western countries: A systematic review. *The Lancet, 365*, 1309–1314. https://doi.org/10.1016/S0140-6736(05)61027-6

Gagnon, A. J., Zimbeck, M., Zeitlin, J., ROAM Collaboration, Alexander, S., Blondel, B., et al. (2009). Migration to western industrialised countries and perinatal health: A systematic review. *Social Science & Medicine, 69*, 934–946. https://doi.org/10.1016/j.socscimed.2009.06.027

GMHAT. (2019). *Global mental health assessment tool*. Retrieved from www.gmhat.org

Greenaway, C., Makarenko, I., Chakra, C. N. A., Alabdulkarim, B., Christensen, R., Palayew, A., et al. (2018a). The effectiveness and cost-effectiveness of hepatitis C screening for migrants in the EU/EEA: A systematic review. *International Journal of Environmental Research and Public Health, 15*. https://doi.org/10.3390/ijerph15092013

Greenaway, C., Pareek, M., Chakra, C. N. A., Walji, M., Makarenko, I., Alabdulkarim, B., et al. (2018b). The effectiveness and cost-effectiveness of screening for active tuberculosis among migrants in the EU/EEA: A systematic review. *Euro Surveillance, 23*. https://doi.org/10.2807/1560-7917.ES.2018.23.14.17-00542

Hacker, K., Anies, M., Folb, B. L., & Zallman, L. (2015). Barriers to health care for undocumented immigrants: A literature review. *Risk Management and Healthcare Policy, 8*, 175–183. https://doi.org/10.2147/RMHP.S70173

Hannigan, A., O'Donnell, P., O'Keeffe, M., & MAcFarlane, A. (2016). *Health evidence network synthesis report 46: How do variations in definitions of "migrant" and their application influence the access of migrants to health care services?* Copenhagen: WHO Regional Office for Europe.

Hui, C., Dunn, J., Morton, R., Staub, L. P., Tran, A., Hargreaves, S., et al. (2018). Interventions to improve vaccination uptake and cost effectiveness of vaccination strategies in newly arrived migrants in the EU/EEA: A systematic review. *International Journal of Environmental Research and Public Health, 15*. https://doi.org/10.3390/ijerph15102065

Hui, C., & Zion, D. (2018). Detention is still harming children at the US border. *BMJ, 362*, k3001. https://doi.org/10.1136/bmj.k3001

Hvass, A. M. F., & Wejse, C. (2017). Systematic health screening of refugees after resettlement in recipient countries: A scoping review. *Annals of Human Biology, 44*, 475–483. https://doi.org/10.1080/03014460.2017.1330897

Immigration Refugees and Citizenship Canada. (2013). *Panel members' handbook 2013*. AEM. Retrieved August 18, 2018, from https://www.canada.ca/en/immigration-refugees-citizenship/corporate/publications-manuals/panel-members-handbook-2013.html

International Organization for Migration. (2008). Challenges of irregular migration: Addressing mixed migration flows. *Discussion note*. International Dialogue on Migration.

International Organization for Migration. (2017). *Summary report on the MIPEX health strand and country reports*. https://doi.org/10.18356/c58c11aa-en

International Organization for Migration. (2018, April). *Mixed migration flows in the Mediterranean compilation of available data and information*. DTM Europe, Reports.

International Organization for Migration Missing Migrants Project: Mixed Migration routes to Europe. https://missingmigrants.iom.int/mixed-migration-routeseurope. Accessed 17 Nov 2019

Jahn, R., Ziegler, S., Nöst, S., Gewalt, S. C., Straßner, C., & Bozorgmehr, K. (2018). Early evaluation of experiences of health care providers in reception centers with a patient-held personal health record for asylum seekers: A multi-sited qualitative study in a German federal state. *Globalization and Health, 14*, 71. https://doi.org/10.1186/s12992-018-0394-1

Kane, J. C., Ventevogel, P., Spiegel, P., Bass, J. K., van Ommeren, M., & Tol, W. A. (2014). Mental, neurological, and substance use problems among refugees in primary health care: Analysis of the Health Information System in 90 refugee camps. *BMC Medicine, 12*, 228. https://doi.org/10.1186/s12916-014-0228-9

Morina, N., Ewers, S. M., Passardi, S., Schnyder, U., Knaevelsrud, C., Müller, J., et al. (2017). Mental health assessments in refugees and asylum seekers: Evaluation of a tablet-assisted screening software. *Conflict and Health, 11*, 18. https://doi.org/10.1186/s13031-017-0120-2

Myran, D. T., Morton, R., Biggs, B.-A., Veldhuijzen, I., Castelli, F., Tran, A., et al. (2018). The effectiveness and cost-effectiveness of screening for and vaccination against hepatitis B virus among migrants in the EU/EEA: A systematic review. *International Journal of Environmental Research and Public Health, 15*. https://doi.org/10.3390/ijerph15091898

Pacheco, L. L., Jonzon, R., & Hurtig, A.-K. (2016). Health assessment and the right to health in Sweden: Asylum seekers' perspectives. *PLoS One, 11*, e0161842. https://doi.org/10.1371/journal.pone.0161842

Pareek, M., Noori, T., Hargreaves, S., & van den Muijsenbergh, M. (2018). Linkage to care is important and necessary when identifying infections in migrants. *International Journal of Environmental Research and Public Health, 15*, 1550. https://doi.org/10.3390/ijerph15071550

Porter, M., & Haslam, N. (2005). Predisplacement and postdisplacement factors associated with mental health of refugees and internally displaced persons: A meta-analysis. *JAMA, 294*, 602–612. https://doi.org/10.1001/jama.294.5.602

Pottie, K., Greenaway, C., Feightner, J., Welch, V., Swinkels, H., Rashid, M., et al. (2011). Evidence-based clinical guidelines for immigrants and refugees. *Canadian Medical Association Journal, 183*, E824–E925. https://doi.org/10.1503/cmaj.090313

Pottie, K., Lotfi, T., Kilzar, L., Howeiss, P., Rizk, N., Akl, E. A., et al. (2018). The effectiveness and cost-effectiveness of screening for HIV in migrants in the EU/EEA: A systematic review. *International Journal of Environmental Research and Public Health, 15*. https://doi.org/10.3390/ijerph15081700

Raghavan, S. S. (2018). Cultural considerations in the assessment of survivors of torture. *Journal of Immigrant and Minority Health, 21*, 586. https://doi.org/10.1007/s10903-018-0787-5

Rojek, A. M., Gkolfinopoulou, K., Veizis, A., Lambrou, A., Castle, L., Georgakopoulou, T., et al. (2018). Clinical assessment is a neglected component of outbreak preparedness: Evidence from refugee camps in Greece. *BMC Medicine, 16*, 43. https://doi.org/10.1186/s12916-018-1015-9

Schoevers, M. A., van den Muijsenbergh, M. E. T. C., & Lagro-Janssen, A. L. M. (2009). Patient-held records for undocumented immigrants: A blind spot. A systematic review of patient-held records. *Ethnicity & Health, 14*, 497–508. https://doi.org/10.1080/13557850902923273

Schoretsanitis, G., Bhugra, D., Eisenhardt, S., Ricklin, M. E., Srivastava, D. S., Exadaktylos, A., et al. (2018). Upon rejection: Psychiatric emergencies of failed asylum seekers. *International Journal of Environmental Research and Public Health, 15*, 1498. https://doi.org/10.3390/ijerph15071498

Suphanchaimat, R., Kantamaturapoj, K., Putthasri, W., & Prakongsai, P. (2015). Challenges in the provision of healthcare services for migrants: A systematic review through providers' lens. *BMC Health Services Research, 15*, 390. https://doi.org/10.1186/s12913-015-1065-z

Sweileh, W. M., Wickramage, K., Pottie, K., Hui, C., Roberts, B., Sawalha, A. F., et al. (2018). Bibliometric analysis of global migration health research in peer-reviewed literature (2000–2016). *BMC Public Health, 18*, 777. https://doi.org/10.1186/s12889-018-5689-x

Taylor, B. (2016). Immigration, statecraft and public health: The 1920 aliens order, medical examinations and the limitations of the state in England. *Social History of Medicine, 29*, 512–533. https://doi.org/10.1093/shm/hkv139

UK Home Office, Public Health England, & International Organization for Migration. (2017). *Health protocol: Pre-entry health assessments for UK-bound refugees.*

United Nations General Assembly. (n.d.). Resolution adopted by the General Assembly on 19 September 2016: 71/1 The New York Declaration for Refugees and Migrants.

United Nations High Commissioner for Refugees. (n.d.-a). *Figures at a glance*. UNHCR. Retrieved September 10, 2018a, from http://www.unhcr.org/figures-at-a-glance.html

United Nations High Commissioner for Refugees. (n.d.-b). *UNHCR-IDC vulnerability screening tool - Identifying and addressing vulnerability: A tool for asylum and migration systems*. UNHCR. Retrieved September 10, 2018b, from http://www.unhcr.org/protection/detention/57fe30b14/unhcr-idc-vulnerability-screening-tool-identifying-addressing-vulnerability.html

United Nations Population Division. Department of Economic and Social Affairs. (n.d.). *International migrant stock: The 2017 revision*. Retrieved September 10, 2018, from http://www.un.org/en/development/desa/population/migration/data/estimates2/estimates17.shtml

Wickramage, K., & Mosca, D. (2014). Can migration health assessments become a mechanism for global public health good? *International Journal of Environmental Research and Public Health, 11*, 9954–9963. https://doi.org/10.3390/ijerph111009954

World Health Organization. (n.d.). *Promoting the health of refugees and migrants: Draft framework of priorities and guiding principles to promote the health of refugees and migrants*. WHO. Retrieved October 14, 2018, from http://www.who.int/migrants/about/who-response/en/

Chapter 11
Discrimination as a Health Systems Response to Forced Migration

Yudit Namer, Canan Coşkan, and Oliver Razum

Abbreviations

MIPEX   Migrant Integration Policy Index
IOM   International Organization for Migration

Introduction: Forced Migration and Health Systems

Health systems' responses to migration can be conceived in terms of entitlement and access to health care. Entitlements and access to health care vary considerably between countries, as shown by the health strand of the Migrant Integration Policy Index (MIPEX) developed by the International Organization for Migration (IOM). Across Europe, 'legal' migrants (those with a residence status) either have analogous health coverage as taxpayers in tax-based health systems or their entitlement is dependent on their residence (they pay into a system they cannot benefit from, should they leave the country). Asylum seekers, on the other hand, have restricted entitlements in most of Europe. Undocumented migrants are invisible to systems and structures, and in many European countries, they risk detention and deportation when seeking care or are covered only with an emphasis on emergency care (Ingleby et al. 2018). As Crawley and Skleparis (2017) put it: "Migration regimes, like all other ordering systems, create hierarchical systems of rights" (p. 51).

Forced migrants have been globally met with punitive measures, from denial of entry or detention upon entry to denied access to services secured by international right-based conventions, as the UCL-Lancet Commission on Migration and Health

Y. Namer (✉) · O. Razum
Department of Epidemiology and International Public Health, School of Public Health, Bielefeld University, Bielefeld, Germany
e-mail: yudit.namer@uni-bielefeld.de

C. Coşkan
Institute for Interdisciplinary Research on Conflict and Violence, Bielefeld University, Bielefeld, Germany

© Springer Nature Switzerland AG 2020
K. Bozorgmehr et al. (eds.), *Health Policy and Systems Responses to Forced Migration*, https://doi.org/10.1007/978-3-030-33812-1_11

points out (Abubakar et al. 2018) (see also Chap. 13). Several country-based examples illustrate the wide spectrum in entitlement and access: In Germany, 'legal' migrants (as long as they maintain their residency) have analogous entitlements to health care as citizens. Asylum seekers, however, have restricted entitlements in the first 15 months of their arrival, comprising emergency care in the case of acute pain, maternity care and select vaccinations (Razum and Bozorgmehr 2016; Ingleby et al. 2018). In Norway, 'legal' migrants with more than a year's residency permit, as well as asylum seekers, are entitled to health care once they become members of the national insurance system. Undocumented migrants receive only emergency and 'absolutely essential' care with the requirement to pay after care, and health systems may be obligated to report them to the authorities (Huddleston et al. 2015). Spain, on the other hand, has recently reintroduced universal health care for asylum seekers and undocumented migrants (analogous to citizens) and ensures specialised treatment for survivors of trauma among forced migrant groups. Although full access to health care exists in Belgium, Greece, Ireland, Italy and Serbia as well, access is severely complicated by the barriers of language, delayed asylum registration processes, remoteness of refugee accommodations and/or other administrative issues (Asylum in Europe 2017). Overall, politically constructed categories of migration ('legal migrant', 'refugee', etc.) mostly determine the type and extent of entitlements, and access barriers complicate these responses almost everywhere.

Social exclusion, as a result of processes such as discrimination, is considered among the social determinants of health (Wilkinson et al. 2003). Discrimination and social exclusion are in mutual reproduction with poverty, lack of access to education, employment and social and political participation (e.g. Gordon et al. 2017). The duration of exposure to social exclusion is linked to the range and severity of health disadvantages (Wilkinson et al. 2003). Depending on the policy environment, being a migrant limits an individual's choices in the social, economic, political and health-related spheres and thus is also considered a social determinant of health on its own (Castãneda et al. 2015). The two social determinants of health—social exclusion and migration—are intertwined in creating layers of health inequities through discrimination. We follow Crawley and Skleparis' (2017) argument that categories of migrants are political constructs and not necessarily representations of actual migratory accounts. The various labels based on artificial boundaries (e.g. involuntary vs voluntary migration or refugee vs migrant) may serve to homogenise and atomise migration experiences. Moreover, the categories themselves may prepare the ground for 'othering' (the social construction of people as the 'other'), and as such, they are used in health systems as a tool for discrimination.

Discrimination against multiple minority groups lies at the centre of exclusionary and oppressive practices which exist even in today's supposedly multicultural societies. Specifically, discrimination against forced migrants in health care systems constitutes an underspecified example of such exclusionary practices: forced migrants may be subjected to various forms of discrimination in their country of origin (depending on their reason to migrate), during transit (depending on the nature of the journey and the borders crossed) and in the country of destination (depending on the migration policies of the host country). We now consider how certain constructions of others are institutionalised in ways that perpetuate disadvantage, such as in the case of health systems response to the needs of forced migrants.

First, we discuss discrimination as a health systems response from a sociopsychological and biopolitical perspective emphasising critical approaches that have developed recently. Several empirical contributions in social and political psychology offer intra- and interpersonal as well as intergroup explanations to systematically uncover the dynamics of discrimination. However, few of these contributions provide a macro level analytical frame which also accounts for the politics of life. Biopolitical approaches fill this gap by highlighting power dynamics, sovereignty and population control or discipline. Therefore, in the first two sections, we provide a sociopsychological account of discrimination based on social and political psychological theories and complement the major gap with current explanations from theories of biopolitics and biopower. We then present infrahumanisation, a mechanism employed to derogate and to delegitimise a group perceived as less than human and to justify discrimination of that group (Leyens et al. 2007) and its health care counterpart 'health-based deservingness', as a point of juncture to explain the intertwined dynamics of social exclusion. Next, we provide case examples of how European health systems response to forced migration, and the broader societal response reflected upon its operations have been characterised by discrimination and infrahumanisation. Finally, we suggest an updated ethics of care to counter the social exclusion of forced migrants.

Sociopsychological Perspectives on Discrimination

Stereotyping and Prejudice

Stereotypes are pictures in our heads, beliefs and opinions about the characteristics and behaviours of members of various groups (Hilton and von Hippel 1996). For instance, the stereotype content model (Fiske et al. 2002) suggests that the social strategy of regulating the interactions with the outgroup depends on the ingroup's perception of the outgroup's warmth and competence, which also influences their practices of inclusion and exclusion as well as type and degree of discrimination. Prejudice, on the other hand, is an *attitude* directed toward people because they are members of a specific social group (Allport 1954; Brewer and Brown 1998). Finally, discrimination consists of *treating people differently* from others based primarily on membership in a social group (Sue 2003).

In many instances of social exclusion (such as forced migrants' exclusion from some health systems), these processes are intertwined. Through stereotypes, prejudices and discrimination, social realities are constructed or dismantled by providing them with meaning and consequence; as such, they become embedded in the reproduction of relations of power, inequality and resistance. They mutually amplify each other through several factors, including perceived threat from the outgroup. Therefore, Dixon (2017) proposes to consider "stereotypes in their wider discursive, historical and political contexts and to recognise their status as forms of social action designed to justify how we treat one another" (p. 21). This also requires acknowledging how certain constructions of others are institutionalised in ways that perpetuate disadvantage, as might be the case in health systems' response to the needs of forced migrants.

From this perspective, categorisations adopted by health systems play a significant part in discrimination against migrants (Scott et al. 2017; Abubakar et al. 2018; Wenner et al. 2019). Migration categories are deeply rooted in states' unique historical representations of immigration and are reproduced in the society even though they do not reflect lived experiences (Scott et al. 2014; Crawley and Skleparis 2017). In Europe, labelling the labour migrants as 'guest workers' implied that host health systems were not responsible for the long-term health of these individuals and their families (Razum and Wenner 2016). The distinction between voluntary and forced migrants or between economic migrants and 'real refugees' prompted the prejudices about the assumed intentions of migrants and served the questioning of the legitimacy of the right to protection from persecution (Crawley and Skleparis 2017). Differentiating between regular, legal and irregular or undocumented migrants and the illegality stereotype used to represent the latter reflect the criminalisation of the act of crossing a border and connote that one group is more deserving of accessing regular services than others (Willen and Cook 2016). Rather than focusing on the unique circumstances of individuals along with the contextual and cultural dynamics of human movements, health systems became fixated on legal status and categories, which often grossly neglect ethics of care discussed later in the chapter.

(Inter-)Group and Social Identity Processes

Intergroup conflicts could be rooted in concerns over collective identity and competition over material resources in social hierarchies (Tajfel and Turner 1979; Turner et al. 1987). For instance, the actions or even the existence of outgroups often lead ingroups to feel as though their group's status is threatened (Branscombe et al. 1999). Intergroup threat is experienced when members of one group perceive another group as intending to cause them harm, thereby inducing a sense of realistic threat (i.e. concern about physical harm or a loss of resources) and/or symbolic threat (i.e. concern about the integrity or validity of the ingroup's meaning system). Accordingly, intergroup threats have destructive effects on intergroup relations, such as between 'host' society members and migrants (Stephan et al. 1999).

Mummendey and Wenzel (1999) suggested that social discrimination results from an ingroup's practices of inclusion and exclusion: Based on superordinate category (e.g. humans with dignity) which would include both the ingroup and the outgroups, the ingroup generalises its attributes to that inclusive category and create 'criteria' for judging the outgroup (e.g. ethnocentrism). If the difference perceived from the outgroup is judged to be non-normative and inferior, devaluation, discrimination and hostility are likely responses toward that homogenised outgroup, as can increasingly be seen in many European societies' relationship with migration (see also Simon 1992; Fein and Spencer 1997; Brewer 1999).

Social Dominance and Power

The discriminatory practices are themselves mutually constitutive with group-based social hierarchy. According to social dominance theory (Sidanius 1993), discrimination across multiple levels (institutions, individuals and collaborative intergroup processes) is coordinated to favour dominant groups over subordinate groups (such as through providing selectively accessible health services) by legitimising myths or societal, consensually shared social ideologies (Pratto et al. 2006). Hence, hierarchy is normalised to maintain the status quo via asymmetric distribution of values and discrimination (Sidanius and Pratto 1999). The *normalisation of hierarchy* in societal systems also leads the way to discrimination against more than one group.

More elaborate approaches, such as by Turner (2005), reject an understanding of power as the capacity for influence based on the control of resources valued or desired by others (i.e. dependency). They argue that the control of resources (such as access to health care) produces power which is the basis of influence and that mutual influence leads to the formation of a psychological group, also offering a distinction between individual power and group power. The UCL-Lancet Commission on Migration and Health argues that, in their most just interpretation, international conventions protecting the rights of migrants necessitate the signatory countries to secure that no governmental or non-governmental body interferes with migrants' right to health through discrimination. Not only do most nation-states neglect this responsibility; they become the agents of discrimination through restricting entitlements and imposing barriers to accessing existing limited services, thereby constructing a legitimate ground for the social exclusion by controlling the health care resources (Abubakar et al. 2018). Health systems response to forced migration is framed within a discourse of solving the problem (Nyers 2006), which positions refugees "as an anomaly that needs a solution" and connotes the representation of realistic threat (Turner 2015, p. 140). The framing of such a solution implies, however, that any services provided for refugees are "exceptional, temporary and often in legal grey zones" (Turner 2015, p. 140). The emergency-focused, restricted and anomaly-oriented structure of health services provided, coupled with access barriers most migrants face (e.g. in terms of language), suggests that the national priorities are imposed at the expense of needs and rights, thereby creating a hierarchy of rights (as suggested by Crawley and Skleparis 2017) within health systems.

Recently, Sindic (2015) argued that identity is essential to political power, and the latter constitutes the means through which identity and the vision of social life it entails are actualised in practices and institutions. Accordingly, the system of social relations determines powerfulness/powerlessness of individuals and groups and regulates the dynamics of social inclusion and exclusion. Therefore, not only examining the intergroup relations per se but also considering the cultural and structural settings in which they occur is needed to better account for the interplay between psychological and societal processes of dominance and discrimination without reductionism and to create scientific roads for taking sides and producing strategies for counter-dominance (Reicher 2004).

Biopolitical Perspectives on Discrimination

While intrapersonal, interpersonal or (cross-)cultural conceptualisations of norm construction and normalisation in psychology generally underestimate *institutionalised* relations of power, biopolitical approach explains how norms and normalcy as the regulatory mechanisms of the governing powers set the ground for discrimination: the norm determines the normal. The culture is recreated and reproduced on different levels, including the macro level constituted by the sovereign controlling and/or disciplining state. Foucault (2003) ties the norm to *disciplinary power* and argues that the norm "brings with it a principle of both qualification and correction. The norm's function is not to exclude and reject. Rather, it is always linked to a positive technique of intervention and transformation, to a sort of *normative project*" (p. 50). Health is one major area where nation-state politics and sovereignty discourses crystallise through institutionalisation and surveillance.

Current updates on Foucault's conceptualisation of biopolitics slightly diverge from his original formulation (Lemke et al. 2011; Lemke 2016). According to Fassin (2001, 2006), the biopolitics based on *biolegitimacy*, which recognises biological life as the highest (moral) value, simultaneously prioritises human life and includes some groups (e.g. refugees with temporary residence for treatment of diseases untreatable at their home countries) as having (right to) biological life (humanitarian project) and excludes some groups (e.g. political asylum seekers) as not having (a right to) political life. Such a selective permeability of right to life through border politics as well as the praxis of mutating citizenships (e.g. Ong 2006) articulated and regulated by the states create multiple layers of inclusion and exclusion which surpass the lines between the biological/medical, the political and the moral. These layers are frequently intertwined with racism, and the practices of racism in the daily realm of social and health politics constitute an excessive *immunitarian project* of conserving life at the expense of (others' as well as own) life (Esposito 2008).

In Esposito's (2008) formulation, the self and the other's point of contact is the immune system. It has been suggested that migrants, that is, those who have crossed external borders, remind one of the permeability of internal boundaries and are thus perceived as uncanny and threatening (Bohleber 1995). As discussed in the previous section, this is also supported by the sociopsychological account of negative stereotypes constructed upon an imagined threat on the well-being of the 'host' society, which fuels intergroup conflict (Stephan and Stephan 2000). According to Esposito (2008), when communities are formed on the basis of biologically determined ethnonational terms, defence is conceptualised in terms of immunity against outside threats. In other words, "to affirm the lives of insiders, in terms of the cultural and biological integrity of their identity and the quality of their lives, they must be immunized from foreign contamination" (Bird and Short 2017, p. 308). The health status of forced migrants is used as a rationale for discrimination by the normative and immunitarian project of regulating life through several mechanisms such as surveillance and screening, reproduced through the existing international politics of borders and the health care system, both Foucauldian disciplinary power apparatuses, and its instruments such as humanitarian workers and health professionals (see also Chaps. 7 and 8).

Point of Juncture: Infrahumanisation and Health-Based Deservingness

The simultaneous dynamics of governing life and death are always in play in the discrimination of oppressed minority groups via *infrahumanisation* and *dehumanisation* processes. Dehumanisation is denying victims' identity and community, thereby erasing, respectively, their distinct individuality and their belonging to a network of caring interpersonal relations (Haslam and Loughnan 2014). Infrahumanisation specifically involves considering outgroups 'less human and more animal-like' than the ingroup, which is perceived, in essence, as fully human (Leyens et al. 2007). Both dehumanisation and infrahumanisation delegitimise the social category, the beliefs, the behaviours and the very existence of an outgroup while also legitimising the stereotypes, prejudices and discrimination against that group.

The distinction between dehumanisation and infrahumanisation, despite being blurry, lies on the intensity, or magnitude, and the quality (Leyens et al. 2007). The processes of dehumanisation are representatively coupled with crimes against minority groups, with a dimension of ultimate moral exclusion, including genocide (Opotow 1990), while those of infrahumanisation are generally coupled with many (implicit and explicit) exclusionary and discriminatory practices embedded in daily societal life. To illustrate, racism, which includes ethnocentric discriminatory practices, is socially prohibited in many societies. Anti-migrant attitudes, however, which include stereotypical and prejudicial social stances of not only denial but also neglect of the other, are not met with such prohibition (Abubakar et al. 2018). While overtly racist treatment within health systems would perhaps cause public indignation, anti-migrant treatment by health systems, which endorses social exclusion, perhaps provokes outrage only in some segments of society due to this distinction. As such, the model of infrahumanisation hypothesises that attributed degrees of humanity differ with group membership, and it helps us explain better possible consequences of the wide spectrum of entitlement and access for migrants, hence the *deservingness* conceptualisation much used in academic work explaining the discrimination of migrants in health systems.

Health-Based Deservingness

Willen (2012) introduced the concept of 'health-based deservingness' as a factor intervening with provision of rights. In her conceptualisation, deservingness interferes with right-based approaches and places conditional moral evaluations before the principles of universality and equity. Migrants who are unauthorised, she posits, are portrayed as undeserving in current global political discourses, with labels such as 'parasites', 'freeloaders' and 'criminal aliens' (Newton 2012) used to describe those deemed undeserving.

Often generated by negative stereotypes (e.g. migrants perceived and depicted as less warm—cold—and incompetent and hence labelled as 'less grateful'), enhanced with an imagined 'realistic threat' on the 'host' society's health care resources (e.g. Stephan et al. 1999), such deservingness-based discourses ascribe diverse motives and moral character to those who migrated, meditate on their legality of entry and degree of vulnerability and assess migrants' social closeness to citizens of the host society which are continuously suspected (Willen and Cook 2016). The suspicion and the constant questioning of the legitimacy of migrants' right to health are fuelled by and further contribute to infrahumanisation: As the recipient of humanitarian aid (or of the 'generosity' of host nations), that is, in return of their biological needs being cared for, forced migrants are imposed to be politically undemanding in order to be deserving (Turner 2015). Hence, "by focusing on the correspondence between individual beliefs and the supposedly 'objective' characteristics of others", one risks neglecting the discursive practices through which the social realities, including structural disadvantages are constructed and reproduced (Dixon 2017, p. 4). Deservingness debates maintained by stakeholders, filled with commonly held negative stereotypes, fail to acknowledge the structural disadvantages experienced by migrants. This lack of recognition then serves the purpose of recreating these structural disadvantages and social hierarchies (Willen and Cook 2016), removing health systems even more from an ethics of care.

Health-based deservingness discourses are in turn internalised or utilised by migrants. Huschke (2014) showed that, even when undocumented migrants access health care provided by humanitarian organisations (which will not report them to the authorities), they felt the need to display performative expressions of deservingness. These expressions included lengthy explanations of pain and demonstration of suffering, appearing in poverty when seeking care while performing 'normalcy' in everyday life or silence when faced with disrespectful treatment in order to overcome infrahumanisation by themselves and to justify access.

Discrimination as Health Systems Response to Forced Migration: Case Examples

Hostile Environments

Health services themselves assume the role of discriminating agents by building hostile environments through the implementation of legal entitlement restrictions and the failure of removing barriers to access (recreating the hierarchy of rights) even if this violates the principles of ethics of care. This affects forced migrants in different ways: They may choose not to seek care when in need of care, because of fear of deportation, criminalisation and/or institutionalisation, or they may need to prove at length that they deserve health care. In many places, separation of children from parents, detention and deportation are real threats for undocumented migrants (Doctors of the World 2017). The burden of living with such fear, anxiety and the real adverse consequences often lead to negative physical and mental health, which exacerbate the vicious circle of barriers to access, ill health and barriers complicated by worsened health status (Abubakar et al. 2018) (see also Chap. 8).

In the United Kingdom (UK), the 'hostile environment policy', which was implemented through the Immigration Acts of 2014 and 2016, became known to larger communities in 2017, when access to health care was denied to the Windrush generation, who arrived in the UK from the Caribbean countries in the 1950s (Liberty 2018). This policy also affected migrants without an explicit right to remain and asylum seekers whose cases were deemed 'complicated', since the passing of the Immigration Acts. Such service users were billed up front for health care and were denied continued and emergency care unless they could pay for services beforehand (Bulman 2017; Abubakar et al. 2018). Following the Immigration Acts of 2014 and 2016, the UK's National Health System further agreed to share confidential personal data with the Home Office, which meant that the immigration enforcement could contact people suspected to be undocumented or whose application for asylum was rejected, if they were to seek health care (Liberty 2018). Considering the care with which citizens' personal data are protected across Europe, as reflected by the Data Protection Act of 2018, such lack of concern regarding non-citizens' data implies first a normalisation of hierarchy and second an infrahumanising stance based on the sovereign's assumed legitimacy of control and discipline.

Surveillance

Surveillance characterises nation-states' relationship to forced migration. Health systems play a crucial role in surveillance, specifically when they classify "migrants as potential sources of infection and disease" (Scott et al. 2014, p. 11), that is, as infrahumanised subjects who are biopolitical threats to the immunitarian project. Scott et al. (2014) argue that migrants are classified in order to keep the national boundaries impermeable and thus invulnerable. The discourse of forced migrants as carriers of disease serves the purpose of reinstating nation-states as holders of (bio) power and promoting immunity, thereby justifying the existing hierarchy and social dominance relations through legitimising myths. There is empirical evidence supporting the mechanism: Murray et al. (2017) documented a positive relationship between perception of disease threat and moral vigilance, an increased sensitivity to moral violations. This relationship was not only correlational; when the threat of diseases was made salient to participants, they made harsher judgments regarding moral violations.

Denial of entry or deportation on the grounds of infectious diseases, non-communicable illnesses and/or cost of care is not performed in Europe. However, some high-income countries such as the USA and Canada have health-related eligibility criteria for entry and/or residency (see also Chap. 7). In the USA, persons with communicable disease considered to have 'public health significance' are denied entry. In Canada, permanent residency is dependent on a health status that does not pose a threat to public health or safety, or the nation's immunity (Abubakar et al. 2018). Such residency restrictions, which do not apply to citizens, and entry restrictions which apply to select countries communicate that migrants are less (human) than citizens or that bodies are threatening to the ingroup's immunity only when they come from certain parts of the world, contributing to the infrahumanising discourse.

Harper and Raman (2008) further argue that public health research contributes to the infrahumanising 'foreign body' discourse of migration and disease. They posit that epidemiological research continues to utilise the phrase 'foreign born' as an epidemiological signifier in tuberculosis research, which then leads to health systems efforts in the forms of pre-migration and border screenings to keep the foreign bodies out. Within the already prejudicial and infrahumanising discourse, forced migrants are considered as not only a danger to themselves but a threat to society.

Screening

Surveillance and thus implementation of biopower also take the form of screening. Screening of asylum seekers for tuberculosis is performed in all European states in one way or another with the rationale of protecting the majority population (Dara et al. 2016) despite evidence that prevalence of tuberculosis in subpopulations born outside of Europe has no significant impact on native-born subpopulations in Europe (Sandgren et al. 2014) (see also Chap. 10). The effectiveness of some existing screening policies is further questionable, missing latent infection with no systematic follow-up (Pareek et al. 2011; Aldridge et al. 2016; Dara et al. 2016). Health workers in Germany involved in mandatory tuberculosis screening of asylum seekers and refugees residing in mass accommodation solely cited the disease control law when justifying screenings (Kehr 2012). In other words, they used legalism to normalise the social hierarchy. Kehr (2012) argues that screening, done superficially, based on administrative categories or without attention to the social and political realities of the individuals, misses the complex health needs of forced migrants, complicating their access to the care needed. This may function as providing rational basis for reinforcing the prejudices against forced migrants by homogenising the outgroup.

The relationship between biopower and infrahumanisation is illustrated by another example Kehr (2012) provides: Roma patients diagnosed with tuberculosis in France are at risk of deportation upon hospitalisation despite negotiations between public health professionals and immigration enforcement. They are then forced to abandon treatment due to the threat of or actual deportation, running the danger of multi-resistance. This then leads to the doctors' decision of not treating Roma patients in the first place as they are likely not to complete treatment, deeming Roma patients more vulnerable to be seen as 'disease holders'. Surveillance then becomes problematic when it serves the immunitarian conceptualisations of who should be inside and who should be outside.

If diagnosed following screening, "the same body that is subject to a systematic colonisation by bio-medicine and the state often seems to be one of the very few tools left through which protest, resistance and despair can be articulated" (van Ewijk and Grifhorst 1998, p. 255). When treatment is refused, and the bodies are used as sites of resistance (by negotiating privileges within accommodation in return of treatment adherence), health professionals morally ascribed patients' refusal to ignorance, irresponsibility or deviance. These ascribed qualities were in turn attributed to refugees' 'culture', such as a relative ease with the concept of dying, an infrahuman quality in the age of biolegitimacy (van Ewijk and Grifhorst 1998). In line with the establishment of health-related prejudices against migrants, Taylor (2013) argues that migrant non-compliance and moral irresponsibility especially in the case of multidrug-resistant tuberculosis as assigned to migrants are part of the disease identity of tuberculosis in Europe.

Depending on state policies, health status could be utilised to document that a person's existing health status puts them at even further risk in detainment conditions, that their health status has deteriorated in detainment or that their experiences of torture or mistreatment in their country of origin are medically valid. Medical professionals at such facilities increasingly voice the ethical dilemma they find themselves in: their refusal to intervene would mean people in need may not receive care, whereas their participation in documenting health status enables such practices. Avoiding to ascribe uniquely complex human emotions to patients, that is, one form of infrahumanisation, is a strategy also employed by health professionals to protect themselves. Those more likely to infrahumanise patient suffering (in terms of ascribing basic emotions not uniquely human) were less likely to report exhaustion or decreased work engagement and professional inefficacy (Vaes and Muratore 2013). Christoff (2014), however, strongly questions the ethics of 'effective' infrahumanising and dehumanising strategies and argues that a more acceptable strategy would be "to relieve the person in power of the decision-making responsibility and to place it where it rightfully belongs", with the patient: a clear sign of relational autonomy (p. 4).

Strategy for Social Inclusion: An Updated Ethics of Care

Discrimination is first legitimised by the border politics of nation-states; this legitimisation is further reproduced in health systems. This chapter presents only a limited snapshot of this legitimisation in health systems on both structural and individual (intergroup or interpersonal) levels. Specifically, we suggest that using migrant status and health status in health systems as a rationale for discrimination contributes to societal infrahumanising discourses, discrimination and social exclusion in mutual reproduction. Both statuses exist in contrast to the biolegitimised social identity of the 'healthy citizen', thereby serving the twofold function of 'protecting and defending' the citizens by the nation-state. Based on the sociopsychological and biopolitical literature reviewed, we propose to consider the discursive, historical and political context of discrimination (Dixon), to remember that identity is constructed through institutionalised power (Sindic) and to take sides by reflecting on how to produce strategies for counter-dominance (Reicher). We acknowledge that those who work in the health care systems or in voluntary organisations in relation to forced migrants are first and foremost care workers. As structural and individual levels are intertwined, we also argue that social change could and should be pushed forth by those who are within the (health) system and that health care workers could be the agents of this change. We accordingly suggest an updated account of ethics of care integrated with intersectional and anarchist approaches for health care workers and diverse parties in the health system as a possible strategy for the elimination of infrahumanisation and discrimination and the prevention of social exclusion of migrants in health systems, on both structural and individual levels.

We mainly follow Hankivsky (2014) who has critically elaborated on the feminist ethics of care approach (Tronto 1993) and suggested an intersectional understanding of care ethics. Intersectional ethics of care considers perspectives of gender, race, sexual orientation, geographic location, immigrant status, ability and class "and a more expansive and accurate portrayal of the interlocking and mutually enforcing axes of power that affect the operationalisation of care on a global level" (Hankivsky 2014, p. 255). Efforts to apply intersectional ethics of care can create space for self- and group reflexivity upon the master statuses which built the dominating social identities (Reicher 2004). Seeing through the eyes of the other (Hurtado 2018), thereby, can allow to overcome tendencies of social dominance and act in solidarity (not for but) with the oppressed. Still, as neither the nation-states nor the private sectors are willing to prioritise intersectionality in providing the most equitable and efficient distribution of health needs and resources of forced migrants, the intersectional ethics of care can be complemented with values of autonomy, responsibility, solidarity and community (anarchistic values, according to Scott 2018). This approach to health care can reclaim health as a common good that cannot be subject to instrumentalisation or compromise (Rogers 2006; Harvey 2007). This would entail counteracting the commodification of health, a consequence of excessive immunitarian project which excludes the other even to the point of self-/group destruction in Esposito's terms, through corporeal relation of care as a form of political relatedness (Hoppania and Vaittinen 2015).

The dismantling of infrahumanisation, discrimination and thus social exclusion of migrants can be possible by rejecting commodification (of health) in health systems and by recognising the crucial role of health workers as *homines curans* (caring people, Tronto 2017). On the structural level, this would require a framework of laws and regulations that avoids entitlement restrictions and actively removes access barriers to health care (Razum and Bozorgmehr 2016). Informed by a descriptive and transformative intersectionality-based policy analysis, such a framework also needs to emphasise developing non-hierarchy within and consensus among all parties and participants of the care relationship, practicing reflexivity and prioritising social justice and equity (Hankivsky et al. 2012).

On the individual level, we suggest understanding responsibility through continuous self-reflexivity, enhancing autonomy, creating solidarity and empowering community. This would firstly require all care workers and potential agents of social change to engage in continuous self-reflection upon one's own privileges, social advantages and critical roles in the system and to recognise the specificities of needs in those intersecting axes of power. Second, Scott (2018) proposes conceiving "autonomy …[as] truly self-determining and support[ing] an individual in pursuit of that person's life projects and health as a good" (p. 219). Applying this to the health needs of migrants would mean co-creating space for the capacity of migrants' self-determination of movement as well as of health care along with an attempt to redefine the relationship with the other, hence mutually developing relational autonomy (Braidotti 2006). More importantly, health care workers who engage in daily interaction with forced migrants can adopt a patient-centred approach which would enable care workers to avoid the dehumanising effects of institutionalisation and infrahumanising tendencies of dominating social identities by thinking more creatively about patient need (Scott 2018). Finally, as also suggested by Dutt and Kohfeldt (2018), a liberatory care for the community can be built which would help care workers and community members to interrogate the power relations and to redefine health needs in terms of common goods for the inhabitants of this world (instead of individual or group commodification). This does not only build a line of solidarity and prepare the ground for mutual empowerment, but it also establishes care as the centre of a new definition of the economy (Schmitt et al. 2018).

References

Abubakar, I., Aldridge, R. W., Devakumar, D., Orcutt, M., Burns, R., Barreto, M. L., et al. (2018). The UCL–Lancet Commission on Migration and Health: The health of a world on the move. *Lancet, 392*, 2606. https://doi.org/10.1016/S0140-6736(18)32114-7

Aldridge, R. W., Zenner, D., White, P. J., Williamson, E. J., Muzyamba, M. C., Dhavan, P., et al. (2016). Tuberculosis in migrants moving from high-incidence to low-incidence countries: A population-based cohort study of 519 955 migrants screened before entry to England, Wales, and Northern Ireland. *Lancet, 288*, 2510–2518. https://doi.org/10.1016/S0140-6736(16)31008-X

Allport, G. W. (1954). *The nature of prejudice*. Reading, MA: Addison-Wesley. https://archive.org/details/TheNatureOfPrejudice

Asylum in Europe. (2017). *Reception conditions*. Retrieved April 3, 2019, from https://ec.europa.
   eu/home-affairs/what-we-do/policies/asylum/reception-conditions_en
Bird, G., & Short, J. (2017). Cultural and biological immunization: A biopolitical analysis of
   immigration apparatuses. *Configurations, 25*, 301–326.
Bohleber, W. (1995). The presence of the past - Xenophobia and Right-wing extremism in the
   Federal Republic of Germany: Psychoanalytic reflections. *The American Imago, 52*, 329–344.
Braidotti, R. (2006). Affirmation versus vulnerability: On contemporary ethical debates.
   Symposium: Canadian Journal of Continental Philosophy, 10, 1–18. https://doi.org/10.5840/
   symposium200610117
Branscombe, N. R., Ellemers, N., Spears, R., & Doosje, B. (1999). The context and content of
   social identity threats. In N. Ellemers, R. Spears, & B. Doosje (Eds.), *Social identity: Context,
   commitment, content* (pp. 35–58). Oxford: Blackwell.
Brewer, M. B. (1999). The psychology of prejudice: Ingroup love and outgroup hate? *Journal of
   Social Issues, 55*, 429–444.
Brewer, M. B., & Brown, R. (1998). Intergroup relations. In D. T. Gilbert, S. T. Fiske, & G. Lindzey
   (Eds.), *The handbook of social psychology* (pp. 554–594). New York: McGraw-Hill.
Bulman, M. (2017). Thousands of asylum seekers and migrants wrongly denied NHS healthcare.
   Independent.
Castañeda, H., Holmes, S. M., Madrigal, D. S., Young, M. E. D., Beyeler, N., & Quesada, J.
   (2015). Immigration as a social determinant of health. *Annual Review of Public Health, 36*,
   375–392. https://doi.org/10.1146/annurev-publhealth-032013-182419
Christoff, K. (2014). Dehumanization in organizational settings: Some scientific and ethical consid-
   erations. *Frontiers in Human Neuroscience, 8*, 748. https://doi.org/10.3389/fnhum.2014.00748
Crawley, H., & Skleparis, D. (2017). Journal of ethnic and migration studies. *Journal of Ethnic and
   Migration Studies, 44*, 48–64. https://doi.org/10.1080/1369183X.2017.1348224
Dara, M., Solovic, I., Sotgiu, G., D'Ambrosio, L., Centis, R., Tran, R., et al. (2016). Tuberculosis care
   among refugees arriving in Europe: A ERS/WHO Europe Region survey of current practices. *The
   European Respiratory Journal, 48*, 808–817. https://doi.org/10.1183/13993003.00840-2016
Dixon, J. (2017). Thinking ill of others without sufficient warrant?' Transcending the accuracy–
   inaccuracy dualism in prejudice and stereotyping research. *The British Journal of Social
   Psychology, 56*, 4–27. https://doi.org/10.1111/bjso.12181
Doctors of the World. (2017). *Falling through the cracks: The failure of universal healthcare cov-
   erage in Europe*. London: European Network to Reduce Vulnerabilities in Health.
Dutt, A., & Kohfeldt, D. (2018). Towards a liberatory ethics of care framework for organizing
   social change. *Journal of Social and Political Psychology, 6*, 575–590. https://doi.org/10.5964/
   jspp.v6i2.909
Esposito, R. (2008). *Bios: Biopolitics and philosophy*. Minneapolis: University of Minnesota
   Press.
Fassin, D. (2001). The biopolitics of otherness: Undocumented foreigners and racial discrimination in French public debate. *Anthropology Today, 17*, 3–7.
Fassin, D. (2006). La biopolitique n'est pas une politique de la vie. *Sociologie et sociétés, 38*,
   35–48.
Fein, S., & Spencer, S. J. (1997). Prejudice as self-image maintenance: Affirming the self through
   derogating others. *Journal of Personality and Social Psychology, 73*, 31.
Fiske, S. T., Cuddy, A. J. C., Glick, P., & Xu, J. (2002). A model of (often mixed) stereotype
   content: Competence and warmth respectively follow from perceived status and competition.
   Journal of Personality and Social Psychology, 82, 878–902.
Foucault, M. (2003). *Abnormal: Lectures at the Collège de France* (Graham Burchell, Trans.).
   New York: Picador 50 1974-1975 SRC-BaiduScholar FG-0.
Gordon, S., Davey, S., Waa, A., Tiatia, R., & Waaka, T. (2017). *Social inclusion and exclusion,
   stigma and discrimination, and the experience of mental distress*. Auckland: Mental Health
   Foundation of New Zealand.

Hankivsky, O. (2014). Rethinking care ethics: On the promise and potential of an intersectional analysis. *The American Political Science Review, 108*, 252–264. https://doi.org/10.1017/S0003055414000094

Hankivsky, O., Grace, D., Hunting, G., Ferlatte, O., Clark, N., Fridkin, A., & Laviolette, T. (2012). Intersectionality-based policy analysis. In O. Hankivsky (Ed.), *An intersectionality-based policy analysis framework* (pp. 33–45). Vancouver, BC: Institute for Intersectionality Research and Policy, Simon Fraser University.

Harper, I., & Raman, P. (2008). Less than human? Diaspora, disease and the question of citizenship. *International Migration, 46*, 3. https://doi.org/10.1111/j.1468-2435.2008.00486.x

Harvey, D. (2007). *A brief history of neoliberalism*. Oxford: Oxford University Press.

Haslam, N., & Loughnan, S. (2014). Dehumanization and infrahumanization. *Annual Review of Psychology, 65*, 399–423. https://doi.org/10.1146/annurev-psych-010213-115045

Hilton, J. L., & von Hippel, W. (1996). Stereotypes. *Annual Review of Psychology, 47*, 237–271.

Hoppania, H. K., & Vaittinen, T. (2015). A household full of bodies: Neoliberalism, care and "the political". *Global Society, 29*, 70–88. https://doi.org/10.1080/13600826.2014.974515

Huddleston, T., Bilgili, Ö., Joki, A.-L., & Vankova, Z. (2015). *Migrant integration policy index 2015*. Barcelona: CIDOB and MPG.

Hurtado, A. (2018). Intersectional understandings of inequality. In P. L. Hammack (Ed.), *The Oxford handbook of social psychology and social justice* (pp. 157–187). Oxford: Oxford University Press.

Huschke, S. (2014). Performing deservingness. Humanitarian health care provision for migrants in Germany. *Social Science & Medicine, 120*, 352–359. https://doi.org/10.1016/j.socscimed.2014.04.046

Ingleby, D., Petrova-Benedict, R., Huddleston, T., & Sanchez, E. (2018). The MIPEX health strand: A longitudinal, mixed-methods survey of policies on migrant health in 38 countries. *European Journal of Public Health, 29*, 458–462. https://doi.org/10.1093/eurpub/cky233

Kehr, J. (2012). Blind spots and adverse conditions of care: Screening migrants for tuberculosis in France and Germany. *Sociology of Health & Illness, 34*, 251–265. https://doi.org/10.1111/j.1467-9566.2011.01415.x

Lemke, T. (2016). Rethinking biopolitics: The new materialism and the political economy of life. In S. Wilmer & A. Zukauskaite (Eds.), *Resisting biopolitics: Philosophical, political, and performative strategies* (pp. 57–73). New York: Routledge.

Lemke, T., Casper, M. J., & Moore, L. J. (2011). *Biopolitics: An advanced introduction*. New York: NYU Press.

Leyens, J. P., Demoulin, S., Vaes, J., Gaunt, R., & Paladino, M. P. (2007). Infra-humanization: The wall of group differences. *Social Issues and Policy Review, 1*, 139–172. https://doi.org/10.1111/j.1751-2409.2007.00006.x

Liberty. (2018). *A Guide to the Hostile Environment: The border controls dividing our communities – and how we can bring them down.* Retrieved from https://www.libertyhumanrights.org.uk/policy/policy-reports-briefings/guide-hostile-environment-border-controls-dividing-our-communities-%E2%80%93

Mummendey, A., & Wenzel, M. (1999). Social discrimination and tolerance in intergroup relations: Reactions to intergroup difference. *Personality and Social Psychology Review, 3*, 158–174.

Murray, D. R., Kerry, N., & Gervais, W. M. (2017). On disease and deontology: Multiple tests of the influence of disease threat on moral vigilance. *Social Psychological and Personality Science, 10*, 44–52. https://doi.org/10.1177/1948550617733518

Newton, L. (2012). "It is not a question of being anti-immigration": Categories of deservedness in immigration policy making. In A. L. Schneider & H. M. Ingram (Eds.), *Deserving and entitled: Social constructions and public policy*. Albany: SUNY Press.

Nyers, P. (2006). *Rethinking refugees: Beyond states of emergency*. New York: Routledge.

Ong, A. (2006). *Neoliberalism as exception: Mutations in citizenship and sovereignty*. Durham: Duke University Press.

Opotow, S. (1990). Deterring moral exclusion. *Journal of Social Issues, 46*, 173–182.

Pareek, M., Watson, J. P., Ormerod, L. P., Kon, O. M., Woltmann, G., White, P. J., et al. (2011). Screening of immigrants in the UK for imported latent tuberculosis: A multicentre cohort study and cost-effectiveness analysis. *The Lancet Infectious Diseases, 11*, 435–444. https://doi. org/10.1016/S1473-3099(11)70069-X

Pratto, F., Sidanius, J., & Levin, S. (2006). Social dominance theory and the dynamics of intergroup relations: Taking stock and looking forward. *European Review of Social Psychology, 17*, 271–320.

Razum, O., & Bozorgmehr, K. (2016). Restricted entitlements and access to health care for refugees and immigrants: The example of Germany. *Global Social Policy, 16*, 321. https://doi. org/10.1177/1468018116655267

Razum, O., & Wenner, J. (2016). Social and health epidemiology of immigrants in Germany: Past, present and future. *Public Health Reviews, 37*, 4. https://doi.org/10.1186/s40985-016-0019-2

Reicher, S. (2004). The context of social identity: Domination, resistance, and change. *Political Psychology, 25*, 921–945. https://doi.org/10.1111/j.1467-9221.2004.00403.x

Rogers, W. A. (2006). Feminism and public health ethics. *Journal of Medical Ethics, 32*, 351–354. https://doi.org/10.1136/jme.2005.013466

Sandgren, A., Sañé Schepisi, M., Sotgiu, G., Huitric, E., Migliori, G. B., Manissero, D., et al. (2014). Tuberculosis transmission between foreign- and native-born populations in the EU/ EEA: A systematic review. *The European Respiratory Journal, 43*, 1159–1171. https://doi. org/10.1183/09031936.00117213

Schmitt, S., Mutz, G., & Erbe, B. (2018). Care economies—Feminist contributions and debates in economic theory. *Österreichische Zeitschrift für Soziologie, 43*, 7–18. https://doi.org/10.1007/ s11614-018-0282-1

Scott, N. (2018). Anarchism and health. *Cambridge Quarterly of Healthcare Ethics, 27*, 217–227. https://doi.org/10.1017/S0963180117000561

Scott, P., Odukoya, D., & Von Unger, H. (2014). The classification of "migrants" as a discursive practice in public health: A sociology of knowledge approach. *Discussion Paper SP III 2014– 601*. Berlin: Wissenschaftszentrum Berlin für Sozialforschung.

Scott, P., Von Unger, H., & Odukoya, D. (2017). A tale of two diseases: Discourses on TB, HIV/ AIDS and im/migrants and ethnic minorities in the United Kingdom. *Social Theory & Health, 15*, 261. https://doi.org/10.1057/s41285-017-0026-5

Sidanius, J. (1993). The psychology of group conflict and the dynamics of oppression: A social dominance perspective. In S. Iyengar & W. J. McGuire (Eds.), *Explorations in political psychology* (pp. 183–219). Durham, NC: Duke University Press.

Sidanius, J., & Pratto, F. (1999). *Social dominance: An intergroup theory of social oppression and hierarchy*. Cambridge: Cambridge University Press.

Simon, B. (1992). The perception of ingroup and outgroup homogeneity: Reintroducing the intergroup context. *European Review of Social Psychology, 3*, 1–30.

Sindic, D. (2015). Power by the people and for the people: Political power and identity in the separation and integration of national states. In D. Sindic, M. Barreto, & R. Costa-Lopes (Eds.), *Power and identity* (pp. 140–161). Hove: Routledge.

Stephan, W. G., & Stephan, C. W. (2000). An integrated threat theory of prejudice. In *Reducing prejudice and discrimination* (pp. 23–46). Mahwah, NJ: Lawrence Erlbaum Associates. https:// doi.org/10.1002/9780470672532.wbepp139

Stephan, W. G., Ybarra, O., & Bachman, G. (1999). Prejudice toward immigrants. *Journal of Applied Social Psychology, 29*, 2221–2237. https://doi.org/10.1111/j.1559-1816.1999. tb00107.x

Sue, D. W. (2003). *Overcoming our racism: The journey to liberation*. San Francisco: Wiley.

Tajfel, H., & Turner, J. C. (1979). An integrative theory of intergroup relations. In S. Worchel & W. G. Austin (Eds.), *The social psychology of intergroup relations* (pp. 33–47). Monterey: Brooks-Cole.

Taylor, R. C. R. (2013). The politics of securing borders and the identities of disease. *Sociology of Health & Illness, 35*, 241–254. https://doi.org/10.1111/1467-9566.12009

Tronto, J. (2017). There is an alternative: *Homines curans* and the limits of neoliberalism. *International Journal of Care and Caring, 1,* 27–43. https://doi.org/10.1332/2397882 17X14866281687583

Tronto, J. C. (1993). *Moral boundaries: A political argument for an ethic of care.* London: Routledge.

Turner, J. C. (2005). Explaining the nature of power: A three-process theory. *European Journal of Social Psychology, 35,* 1–22. https://doi.org/10.1002/ejsp.244

Turner, J. C., Hogg, M. A., Oakes, P. J., Reicher, S. D., & Wetherell, M. S. (1987). *Rediscovering the social group: A self-categorization theory.* Oxford: Blackwell.

Turner, S. (2015). What is a refugee camp? Explorations of the limits and effects of the camp. *Journal of Refugee Studies, 29,* 139. https://doi.org/10.1093/jrs/fev024

Vaes, J., & Muratore, M. (2013). Defensive dehumanization in the medical practice: A cross-sectional study from a health care worker's perspective. *The British Journal of Social Psychology, 52,* 180–190. https://doi.org/10.1111/bjso.12008

van Ewijk, M., & Grifhorst, P. (1998). Controlling and disciplining the foreign body: A case study of TB treatment among asylum seekers in the Netherlands. In K. Koser & H. Lutz (Eds.), *The new migration in Europe* (pp. 242–259). Basingstoke: Palgrave Macmillan.

Wenner, J., Namer, Y., & Razum, O. (2019). Migrants, refugees, asylum seekers: Use and misuse of labels in Public Health Research. In A. Krämer & F. Fischer (Eds.), *Refugee migration and health. Challenges for Germany and Europe.* Cham: Springer.

Wilkinson, R., Marmot, M., & World Health Organization. (2003). *Social determinants of health: The solid facts* (2nd ed.). Copenhagen: Centre for Urban Health, World Health Organization.

Willen, S. S. (2012). How is health-related "deservingness" reckoned? Perspectives from unauthorized im/migrants in Tel Aviv. *Social Science & Medicine, 74,* 812–821. https://doi.org/10.1016/j.socscimed.2011.06.033

Willen, S. S., & Cook, J. (2016). Health-related deservingness. In F. Thomas (Ed.), *Handbook of migration and health* (pp. 95–118). Cheltenham: Edward Elgar Publishing.

Chapter 12
Health System Responsiveness to the Mental Health Needs of Forcibly Displaced Persons

Daniela C. Fuhr, Bayard Roberts, Aniek Woodward, Egbert Sondorp, Marit Sijbrandij, Anne de Graaff, and Dina Balabanova

Abbreviations

MHPSS	Mental health and psychosocial support
NGOs	Non-governmental organisations
STRENGTHS	Syrian Refugees Mental Health Care Systems
WHO	World Health Organization

In this chapter, we discuss health system responsiveness to the mental health needs of forcibly displaced persons. First, we discuss health system responsiveness as key health system characteristic and introduce a conceptual framework guiding its assessment. We then present the use of rapid appraisal methodology upon which the

D. C. Fuhr (✉) · B. Roberts
Department of Health Services Research and Policy, Faculty of Public Health and Policy, London School of Hygiene and Tropical Medicine, London, UK
e-mail: Daniela.Fuhr@lshtm.ac.uk; Bayard.Roberts@lshtm.ac.uk

A. Woodward · E. Sondorp
KIT Royal Tropical Institute, Amsterdam, The Netherlands
e-mail: A.Woodward@kit.nl; E.Sondorp@kit.nl

M. Sijbrandij · A. de Graaff
Clinical Psychology, Faculty of Behavioural and Movement Sciences, VU Amsterdam, Amsterdam, The Netherlands
e-mail: e.m.sijbrandij@vu.nl; a.m.de.graaff@vu.nl

D. Balabanova
Department of Global Health and Development, Faculty of Public Health and Policy, London School of Hygiene and Tropical Medicine, London, UK
e-mail: Dina.Balabanova@lshtm.ac.uk

© Springer Nature Switzerland AG 2020
K. Bozorgmehr et al. (eds.), *Health Policy and Systems Responses to Forced Migration*, https://doi.org/10.1007/978-3-030-33812-1_12

conceptual framework is based. Finally, we present findings of a case study on mental health care amongst Syrian refugees residing in the Netherlands employing this methodology.

Mental Health Service Provision for Refugees

It is now recognised that refugees have high levels of mental health needs due to the exposure to violence and traumatic events and ongoing exposure to daily stressors during and after the displacement (Silove et al. 2017; Lindert et al. 2009). However, evidence suggests that utilisation of mental health and psychosocial support (MHPSS) services by refugees and other forcibly displaced persons remains low (Norredam et al. 2006). Some of the reasons for this low utilisation include the following: low levels of awareness of mental health and MHPSS services, different cultural perspectives of mental health and associated services, stigma around mental health including discrimination against refugees, linguistic barriers, costs of services, poor quality of services and low trust in health services and service providers (Bartolomei et al. 2016).

MHPSS is defined as any type of local or outside support that aims to protect or promote psychosocial well-being and/or prevent or treat mental disorders (IASC 2007). MHPSS is a composite term that acknowledges the need for continuing and comprehensive care for people who are facing or have faced adversity. Consequently, MHPSS incorporates services for both prevention and treatment provided by multiple providers (specialists and non-specialists). MHPSS services should, overall, provide holistic care: i.e. through community programmes that offer psychosocial support to prevent the onset of mental disorders and to build resilience for persons with mild or moderate mental distress and through health-care platforms offering more targeted health system interventions for persons who are in need of more specialised support (UNHCR 2013).

There are contrasting approaches to delivering MHPSS services for refugees in Europe. In Germany, for example, mental health services are commonly delivered by specialist mental health-care providers such as psychiatrists and psychotherapists. This has caused bottlenecks in accessing care as the demand for services outstrips the supply, with waiting times typically over 6 months (Aida 2018; Bajbouj 2016). In addition, these specialists have limited training on the particular MHPSS needs, experiences and cultural perspectives of refugees and limited funds for interpreters (Bajbouj 2016; Böttche 2016; Priebe et al. 2016). It has been argued that this specialist care may not be required or appropriate for the majority of refugee mental health needs as they relate to more mild and moderate mental disorders that could be addressed through psychosocial support or low-intensity psychological interventions. Some NGOs in Germany have established psychosocial centres, but these only reach around 4% of the estimated number of refugees who likely require MHPSS support (BAfF 2015). A contrasting response has been the dependence on parallel systems of MHPSS care in countries such as Greece and Italy which is predominantly provided by NGOs as well as church and community groups. This type of care has commonly focused more on psychosocial support rather than on more specialist mental health services. These services are essential in the absence of state-provided services. However, they are often short term, fragmented and disjointed (Lionis et al. 2018). Limited staff capacity and language and cultural barriers are also common, and trust of refugees in these services was reported to be low amongst refugees in camps in Greece (Priebe et al. 2016; Satinsky et al. 2019; Ben Farhat et al. 2018). Regulation on the types of MHPSS services being provided and oversight of their quality and effectiveness is also very limited (Priebe et al. 2016). Countries such as Sweden and the Netherlands have taken more balanced approaches through greater provision of MHPSS care at the primary care level, incorporating services provided by more regulated NGOs. However, these have limited coverage, and access challenges remain (Satinsky et al. 2019).

Health system responsiveness is understood as the way in which individuals are treated and the environment in which they are treated in, encompassing the individual's experience of contact and interaction with the health system (Valentine 2003). Responsiveness is therefore not a measure of how the system responds to health but of how the system performs relative to non-health aspects, meeting or not meeting a population's expectations of how it should be treated by providers of prevention, care or services (Darby et al. n.d.; Valentine 2003; Papanicolas and Smith 2013). Health system responsiveness was conceptualised by the World Health Organization (WHO) as a composite measure to grasp both patient satisfaction with treatment and also the interaction of the patient with the health system (Valentine 2003) and was incorporated as measure in the WHO World Health Survey (WHO 2018b). Eight domains related to responsiveness have been identified: (1) autonomy (involvement in decision on health care), (2) choice (of health-care decisions), (3) communication (adequate communication from and with provider), (4) confidentiality (of records and personal information), (5) dignity (respectful treatment by provider), (6) quality of amenities (quality of health-care surroundings/clinics), (7) prompt attention (no treatment delay) and (8) family and community support (building on family and community support in care and treatment) (Papanicolas and Smith 2013). Responsiveness is a complex construct: Its domains are not discrete entities and overlap to some extent with the definition of other health system outcomes such as access, quality, coverage and safety. This has also been recognised by Mirzoev and Kane who argue that not only health system expectations by patients such as availability of services and health system resources which are available for treatment but also access and quality expectations shape patient's judgement of anticipated success or failure of service outcomes including the system's responsiveness (Mirzoev and Kane 2017). Table 12.1 operationalises responsiveness domains according to the conventional definition of the WHO and indicates their relevance to intermediate health system outcomes such as access, coverage, quality and safety (defined further in Box 12.1).

Box 12.1 Key Health System Characteristics: Access, Coverage, Quality and Safety

Access and Coverage

We define access according to the framework of Penchansky and Thomas (1981) which overlap in their definition with measures of coverage:

Availability—the volume (coverage) and type of existing services and whether this is adequate for the volume and needs of service users.

Accessibility—the relationship between the location of the services/supply and the location of the people in need of them. This should take into account transportation, travel time, distance and cost.

Accommodation—the relationship between the organisation of resources (appointment systems, hours of operation, walk-in facilities) and the ability of service users to accommodate to these factors. User perceptions on the appropriateness of these factors should also be taken into account.

Affordability—the prices of services in relation to the income of service users. The user perception of the worth relative to total cost should also be taken into account.

Acceptability—the relationship of attitudes of service users about personal and practice characteristics of services to the actual characteristics of the existing services, as well as to provider attitudes about acceptable personal characteristics of service users.

Quality

We conceive quality according to the control knobs framework (Roberts et al. 2008) which understands quality as follows:

The scope of care (and quantity) which is provided to the patient (conceived as the amount of care necessary to achieve a desired treatment outcome)

The clinical quality of the service provided to the patient (cleanliness of facility, but also skills and decision-making of the provider, in addition to equipment and supplies; the use of an evidence-based intervention)

Service quality and acceptability of the service: convenience (e.g. travel time, waiting time, opening hours, etc.) and interpersonal relations (e.g. whether providers are polite and emotionally supportive and whether patients receive appropriate information and respect)

Safety

Safety is defined as the degree to which health-care processes avoid, prevent and ameliorate adverse outcomes or injuries that stem from the processes of health care itself (Kelley and Hurst 2006).

Table 12.1 Responsiveness domains and linkage with other key health system characteristics adapted from Papanicolas and Smith (2013)

Responsiveness domains	Domain operationalisation: example items for measurement of responsiveness at the individual level	Links to intermediate health system outcomes
1. Autonomy: involvement in decisions on care and services	Involvement in decisions about health care, treatment and services Obtaining information about other possible types of services	Quality and safety
2. Choice: choice of health-care providers and services	Freedom to choose health-care provider Freedom to choose health-care facility or service	Access
3. Communication: clarity of communication	Service conducted in mother tongue of patient (or interpreter available) Health-care provider explains things clearly and listens carefully Allowing patient time to ask questions about treatment and care	Quality
4. Confidentiality: confidentiality of personal information	Personal information about medical history is kept confidential Talks with doctors or nurses are done privately, and other people are not being able to overhear what is being said	Quality
5. Dignity: respectful treatment and communication	Health-care professionals treat patient with respect/talk to patients in a respectful manner	Quality
6. Quality of basic amenities: surroundings	Cleanliness of facility where service is provided Basic quality of waiting room and office where service is provided (space, seating, fresh air)	Quality, access (accommodation)
7. Prompt attention: convenient travel and short waiting times	Travelling time to facility/service Short waiting times for appointments and consultations Getting fast care in emergencies	Access (availability, accessibility), quality and safety
8. Access to family and community support: Contact with family and maintenance of regular activities	Facility/service provider encourages interaction and collaboration with family/friends during course of mental health treatment Facility/service provider encouraged to continue social and religious customs during treatment	Access (availability, accessibility)

Conceptual Framework on Health System Responsiveness and Pathways of Care

We have developed a conceptual framework for health system responsiveness to the mental health needs of refugees (see Fig. 12.1) which is based on key health system's literature (WHO 2000, 2007) and other health system responsiveness frameworks (Mirzoev and Kane 2017). The conceptual framework conceives the health system according to the definition of the WHO (2007) and considers both state-governed mental health services and non-state provision of mental health services as parts of the mental health system for refugees. Examples of non-state provision might be (a network of) non-governmental organisations (NGOs) funded by donors or United Nations agencies providing MHPSS services to refugees.

We conceive the health system as being influenced by the wider socio-economic and cultural environment of the country, which in turn shapes social and public policies formulated by the government (as indicated by the two outer layers of Fig. 12.1). Wider social and public policies are policies, legislation and social protection schemes influencing the health system. They reflect values, principles and objectives of a society, which can influence health outcomes but also broader societal outcomes such as employment (see also Chap. 13). Public attitudes towards mental health, knowledge about mental health and resulting behaviour of individual people will determine stigma towards people with mental illness in a given society (Evans-Lacko et al. 2012). Stigma consists of two components, namely discrimination (being treated unfairly) and prejudice (stigmatising attitudes) (Clement et al. 2013), which negatively influences help-seeking behaviour of the patient (Vistorte et al. 2018) and leads to adverse treatment

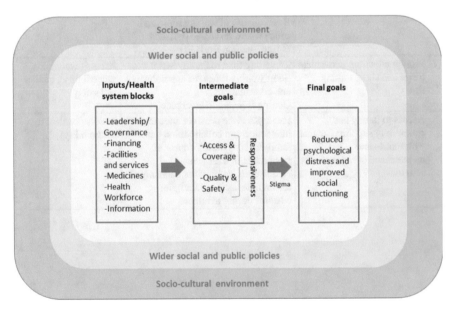

Fig. 12.1 Conceptual framework for assessing the responsiveness of the mental health system for refugees with mental health needs

outcomes (Hatzenbuehler et al. 2013). The importance of context has been recognised in other responsiveness frameworks as well (Mirzoev and Kane 2017).

The health system inputs can be organised around the WHO building blocks (i.e. leadership/governance; financing; facilities and services; medicines, health workforce, information) (WHO 2007). These key health system inputs will vary according to country income group, overall disease burden, needs and priorities of the government to provide treatment for mental disorders.

As in other health system frameworks (WHO 2007), we conceptualise access, coverage, quality and safety as intermediate health system goals (described in Box 12.1) which link health system inputs and the final health system goal such as improved health by ensuring adequate access to and coverage of effective health interventions, without compromising efforts to ensure provider quality and safety (WHO 2000).

In contrast to the conventional health system's framework of the WHO which understands responsiveness as final goal (WHO 2007), we conceptualise responsiveness as intermediate outcome. There is a debate whether responsiveness should be understood as intermediate or final outcome (Kelley and Hurst 2006). For example, the Organisation for Economic Co-operation and Development conceptualises access as a component of responsiveness and due to its overlap with other health system goals (such as quality and safety) as intermediate outcome (Kelley and Hurst 2006). The Commonwealth Fund argues similarly and includes responsiveness in the definition of quality and access (Commonwealth Fund 2016). The WHO refers to responsiveness as respect for persons (health system and health provider's respect for dignity, autonomy and confidentiality) which can be understood as dimensions of quality of care and client orientation (right to prompt attention to health needs, access to patient social support networks and choice of institutions providing care) (WHO 2000, 2007; Papanicolas and Smith 2013) which include components of Penchansky and Thomas access definitions. Due to the overlap between several domains of responsiveness and key intermediate health system goals (as outlined in Box 12.1), we argue that access as defined by Penchansky and Thomas, coverage, quality and safety can be conceived as proxy responsiveness measures. Responsiveness as intermediate outcome may be especially important for mental health as patients may not seek or continue mental health services if the system is not responsive to their needs (e.g. by providing access to family and community support services, delivering services such as psychological therapies in the patient's mother tongue and offering choice of health-care providers and services). Those responsiveness domains are key for mental health and will determine if people with mental disorders seek or continue care. This is supported by evidence of the literature: an unresponsive system which does not provide prompt attention for mental health needs may lead to adverse mental health treatment outcomes and high unmet need at the population level (Wang et al. 2004, 2007).

Therefore, we conceptualised responsiveness as precursor of improved mental health as a patient's initial perception of responsiveness, and subsequent interaction with the health system (Mirzoev and Kane 2017) may determine health-seeking behaviour and treatment outcomes. Demand-side factors influence help-seeking as well and play a key role in the recovery from mental illness. People with mental disorders may not seek care for three reasons: (1) lack of knowledge about evidence-based treatments and the treatability of mental disorders, (2) lack of knowledge about where and how to access treatment and (3) expectations of discrimination and prejudice against people with a mental disorder (Henderson et al. 2013). The latter is important as experience of stigma at the individual or community level (in form of public attitudes and behaviour) or institutional level (reflected in legislation, funding, availability of services) (Corrigan et al. 2004) may prevent patients from accessing services; this is something which needs to be tackled so that the needs of people with mental health can be adequately responded to (e.g. through community anti-stigma campaigns, by educating providers on these sensitivities and by advocating for mental health at the wider policy level) (see also Chap. 11). It is only then when improved population mental health will be achieved (Hatzenbuehler et al. 2013).

The final goal in our conceptual framework is reduced psychological distress and improved social functioning at the level of the population which has been facilitated by a responsive health system. Reduced psychological distress can be operationalised by measures of improvement in symptoms of common mental disorders, such as depression, anxiety and post-traumatic stress disorder, or reduced levels of stress, fear and helplessness. Improved social functioning can be conceived as an individual's ability to perform and fulfil normal social roles without disruption such as domestic responsibilities, interacting with other people, self-care and/or participating in community activities (Hirschfeld et al. 2000).

Pathways of Care

The assessment of the responsiveness of the mental health system is guided by the conceptual framework and key intermediate outcomes. In addition, we also assess pathways of care and how refugees in host countries navigate the mental health system. Our assessments of pathways of care is guided by the literature suggesting main components of a mental health-care model (Thornicroft and Tansella 2004, 2013) and the mhGAP intervention guide (WHO 2010b), suggesting evidence-based treatment steps for a person with common mental disorders (see Fig. 12.2). Figure 12.2 indicates that the gateway into mental health care may be the community or primary health care. Case detection in the community or screening in primary health care is key to identify probable cases of mental disorders and patients who might need help (see also Chap. 10). Low-intensity psychological interventions (such as brief psychological therapies delivered by a trained lay health-care providers) may be offered first. In case of non-response or clinical worsening, patients may be referred to higher-intensity treatment or tertiary care. Ideally, a case manager coordinates the care of the patient including any after care. The mhGAP intervention guide not only identifies essential treatment and services for people with mental disorders but also suggests to follow principles of care (e.g. being respectful, ensuring provider's communication is sensitive to culture and age and urging to protect human rights) which addresses domains of responsiveness. Therefore, we conceive a responsive mental health system as a service structure which facilitates treatment entry, offers evidence-based treatments according to MhGAP and ensures that key domains of responsiveness (Table 12.1) are adhered to during treatment delivery.

A proposed pathway of care is presented in Fig. 12.2.

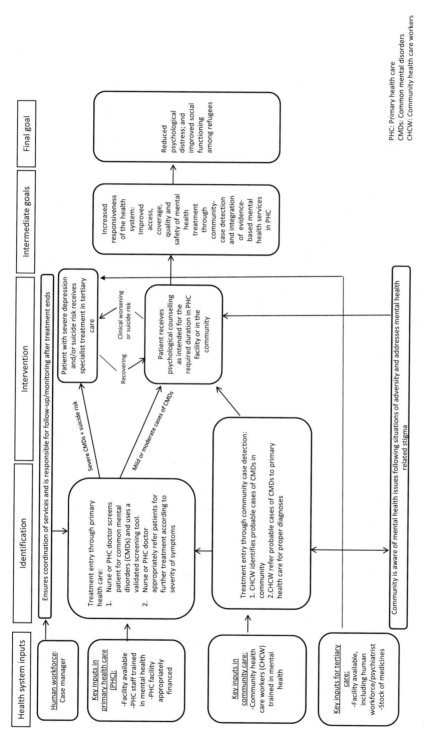

Fig. 12.2 Suggested pathway of care

The Rapid Appraisal Methodology to Investigate Health System Responsiveness

Rapid appraisal methodology employs multiple evaluation techniques to quickly but systematically collect data on a distinct health topic (McNall and Foster-Fishman 2007). By using diverse but interlinked methods (such as interviews, focus groups, mini surveys, community discussions or secondary data analysis), it seeks to produce coherent data. Different information sources are validated by triangulation of data (USAID 2010). It is highly action oriented and iterative: data can be analysed while other data are being collected, and preliminary findings are used to guide decisions about additional data collection until theoretical saturation is achieved (McNall and Foster-Fishman 2007). Rapid appraisals are relatively quick, systematic and cost-effective (USAID 2010) and draw on the perspectives of multiple stakeholders (e.g. patients, health-care providers, key informants such as policymakers and NGO workers) (Kumar 1993). They allow taking a patient-centred approach (Balabanova et al. 2009) assessing how the patient navigates through the health system (which can be used to understand health systems' bottlenecks and inefficiencies). Rapid appraisals have been widely used for different purposes: for example, to assess health system performance for maternal and child health (Anker et al. 1993), for chronic conditions such as diabetes and hypertension (Balabanova et al. 2009; Risso-Gill et al. 2015), for alcohol and substance use in conflict-affected settings (UNHCR and WHO 2008) and for MHPSS in emergencies (WHO/UNHCR 2012). The latter rapid appraisal suggests topics that ought to be addressed in MHPSS; however, it did not consider an assessment of health system responsiveness as such and did not provide a theoretical framework guiding its assessment. For this reason, the MHPSS rapid appraisal presented in this chapter specifically focusing on the health system responsiveness to the mental health needs of forcibly displaced persons presents a valuable new perspective.

Our rapid appraisal is based upon a conceptual framework (Fig. 12.1) and has been developed for the Syrian Refugees Mental Health Care Systems (STRENGTHS) study which explores the health system responsiveness towards the mental health needs of Syrian refugees in Jordan, Lebanon, Turkey, Egypt, Germany, the Netherlands, Sweden, Egypt and Switzerland. The STRENGTHS study explicitly focuses on Syrian refugees as Syrians make up the largest refugee population group in the countries under study. One important aspect of the rapid appraisal is to investigate how Syrian refugees enter the mental health system in these countries and how they navigate it (Fig. 12.2). We predominantly employ three methods in the rapid appraisal. First, desk-based reviews are employed to elicit information on country-specific health system inputs and intermediate health system goals (access, coverage, quality and safety) as suggested by our conceptual framework; second, analyses of existing country-specific qualitative data (where available); and third, collection of primary qualitative data obtained through semi-structured interviews to understand pathways of care for Syrian refugees in host countries. Desk-based reviews were conducted to obtain a better understanding of the structure and components of the different health systems Syrian refugees seek care in. A data extraction sheet has been specifically developed for this purpose, extracting information on health system inputs (described in the first part of this chapter) and processes related to investing these. The review included peer-reviewed literature (quantitative and qualitative studies, primary and secondary sources) and grey literature sources (e.g. documents from international and local NGOs). Validity of the collected information was ensured by using multiple methods and data sources (i.e. triangulating government reports with other research studies) and by seeking expert opinion on major themes and discrepancy in the collected information collected from different sources. In the STRENGTHS study, the desk-based review was complemented by existing qualitative data from partner countries (which were collected as formative work to support the adaptation of a scalable MHPSS interventions developed by WHO for use in low- and middle-income countries and conflict-affected settings).

A core part of our methodology relies on new primary qualitative data collected via semi-structured interviews and focus group discussions to obtain information on intermediate health system goals and other domains of responsiveness. The sampling approach needs to be adapted to local circumstances and should include purposive (including convenience) sampling to select a diverse range of respondents on the basis of their characteristics, roles or experiences and snowball sampling, asking respondents to nominate other people they know. This is important to ensure a mix of respondents (e.g. providers from different tiers of the health system and from diverse specialties) are interviewed, covering a range of perspectives. Respondents should include key informants (with detailed knowledge of how the system(s) for mental health work, such as from government, health system/service managers, donor agencies, NGO, academia); MHPSS providers (such as nurses, social workers, peer support workers, psychologists or psychiatrists); Syrian refugees receiving MHPSS services/care (recruited from primary health-care facilities, community psychosocial support centres); and family members of Syrian refugees receiving MHPSS services/care.

Data obtained from existing country-specific qualitative data were analysed using both deductive and inductive analysis. Deductive analysis involved coding units of data according to key inputs, processes and outcomes specified in the conceptual framework. Inductive analysis (seeking to elicit new themes or unexpected findings) was done through assigning new codes (outside of our conceptual framework) and further refining and categorising these.

Case Study: The Netherlands

We present here some initial findings of a rapid appraisal we conducted in the Netherlands on the responsiveness of the health system to the mental health needs of Syrian refugees. The study was conducted as part of the STRENGTHS study. Data sources were obtained from a desk-based review and transcripts from existing country-specific qualitative data collected by STRENGTHS partners to inform the development and implementation of a trial evaluating a low-intensity psychological intervention for Syrian refugees. We did not collect primary qualitative data ourselves and did not use a topic guide which included specific questions on responsiveness. Therefore, we used access, coverage, quality and safety as proxy responsiveness measures as justified above. Qualitative data were from semi-structured interviews with key informants, such as psychiatrists, general practitioners (GPs), nurses, counsellors ($n = 10$) and MHPSS providers (psychiatrists, family doctors, nurses and counsellors) ($n = 11$), and semi-structured interviews ($n = 10$) and focus group discussions ($n = 4$) with Syrian refugees not using MHPSS services. Data were collected between May and August 2017. Ethics clearance for these interviews was obtained by the Ethics Review Committee of the VU University Medical Center, Amsterdam. The following sections present a summary of key findings.

Wider Health System Environment and Policies

From April 2011 to June 2017, 33,897 Syrians sought asylum in the Netherlands which represents 3.5% of the total Syrian asylum applications in Europe (UNHCR 2017). In 2016, 27,971 Syrian nationals were given a residence permit (61.3% male, 38.7% female, 36.1% below 18 years of age) (CBS 2017). Refugees whose temporary permit expires after 5 years can receive a permanent permit if protection is still required and if refugees have successfully completed the Dutch integration exam (Government of the Netherlands 2017b).

Mental Health System Inputs

Leadership and Governance The Netherlands has a mental health policy and plan (WHO 2011) which is considered fully implemented (WHO 2014). Dedicated mental health legislation exists, and legal provisions for mental health are covered by other laws such as the Health Insurance Act (Kroneman et al. 2016).

Financing and Expenditure In 2014, the Dutch government spent 10.7% of its gross domestic product on health (The World Bank 2017). Of the total expenditure on health, 10.7% was used for mental health in 2011, of which 59.2% was spent on mental health hospitals (WHO 2011). The Dutch mental health system is financed by the following sources: the social support act and youth act (via the city councils), health insurance act (via health insurers), justice (in criminal cases) and the long-term care act (Wlz) (via care offices) (GGZ Netherlands 2018a). Basic health insurance including mental health care is mandatory for all citizens (Kroneman et al. 2016). Insurance covers basic psychological support offered by a psychological well-being practitioner (nurse, community worker or psychologist) located at the general practitioner's (GPs) practices. Specialised mental health care is only covered when a diagnosis complies with the Diagnostic and Statistical Manual of Mental Disorders, 5th Edition. Asylum seekers are insured collectively under the Asylum Seekers Healthcare Scheme and are entitled to nearly all health care, including mental health, provided under the standard package and the Wlz (Government of the Netherlands 2017a). Once refugees receive refugee status and are settled into a municipality, they are required to start paying a monthly insurance premium and a deductible of up to €385 per year out of pocket for most health care except general practitioner consultations and care for children under the age of 18 years (Kroneman et al. 2016). Interpreters are covered by the insurance for refugees residing in asylum seeker centres; however, this is not the case for refugees who obtained a residence permit.

Facilities and Services   In 2011, there were 1.19 mental health outpatient facilities, 260.1 day-treatment facilities and 0.12 community residential facilities per 100,000 population available in the Netherlands (WHO 2011). Mild to moderate mental disorders are treated in basic ambulatory care settings (e.g. primary mental health care offered by a psychological well-being practitioner) (Mossialos et al. 2016). More severe and complicated cases are referred by GPs to specialist mental care providers and/or institutions, also called 'GGZ-instellingen' [mental health-care institutions] which provide care for all people of all ages (Mossialos et al. 2016; GGZ Netherlands 2018b).

Mental Health Workforce   The Netherlands has a high number of psychiatrists (20.2 per 100,000 population) and psychologists (90.76 per 100,000 population) but a low number of nurses working in mental health (2.87 per 100,000 population) (WHO 2014). Larger GP practices are generally supported by a psychological well-being practitioner/mental health-care worker (called POH-GGZ in Dutch; usually a nurse, community health worker or a psychologist working at a GP facility) or social-psychiatric nurse, who are able to diagnose, offer basic treatment and make referrals in consultation with the GPs.

Information and Research   Sources collecting information on mental health care at the national level do not disaggregate data for refugees. NGOs involved in livelihood and provision of social support for asylum seekers and refugees do not consistently publish data on their activities on their websites (except for the Dutch Council for Refugees).

Intermediate Health System Goals and Responsiveness

Care Pathways   The following care pathways were obtained from interviews with key stakeholders: adult asylum seekers receive a medical screening at the GP practice that is linked to the asylum centre they are residing in. However, this medical screening may not always include psychological questions. Early detection and referral can also be conducted by case managers, Dutch Council for Refugees volunteers, Community Health Services and other NGO volunteers. Self-referral is also possible. Asylum seekers are assigned to a GP practice at the asylum centre linked to their community, while refugees in the community can choose their own GP.

Syrian refugees have similar care pathways as the Dutch nationals. The GP can make an initial mental health diagnosis and, if needed, treats or refers to secondary care. GPs are responsible for treating people with milder forms of mental illness (Rijksoverheid 2018). A POH-GGZ worker/psychological well-being practitioner (often available at larger GP practices) may also support a patient, but the GP retains ultimate responsibility for the patient (Rijksoverheid 2018). People suffering from severe and complex mental disorders are generally admitted to mental health-care institutions, either ambulatory or residential (Rijksoverheid 2018).

Availability and Accommodation Findings about the scope of services and workforce that are available were mixed. According to some providers interviewed for this study, there are sufficient resources to provide care for refugees; the scope of services to respond to the needs of refugee children was also seen as appropriate. However, a few other interviewees raised concerns about service availability especially in rural areas and highlighted the lack of culturally appropriate MHPSS care. Training in cultural competence was recommended for all mental health providers. Some interviewees raised availability and accommodation concerns: a MHPSS provider complained that the POH-GGZ worker (a well-being practitioner supporting the GP at their practice) works for 1 day a week only. This was confirmed by another provider who indicated that it is sometimes difficult to have the right amount of care/services available due to fluctuating numbers of asylum seekers arriving in the Netherlands leading to difficulties in planning. A refugee added further that the Dutch Council for refugees was only open 1 day a week (for 2 h) which was not considered to be sufficient.

(Geographic) Accessibility Providers and key informants commented that travel costs, time and logistics of accessing MHPSS services may be a barrier for Syrian refugees. This was also confirmed by the literature (Van Berkum et al. 2016). A provider reported that refugees generally receive social benefits but may have limited financial means. Moving accommodation (which some refugees have to undergo regularly) may lead to dropout during treatment. Several providers were concerned about the accessibility of mental health services for Syrians residing in rural areas specifically where less (culturally appropriate) services are available. In a focus group, Syrian refugees discussed that women may not be allowed to travel or attend appointments without their husbands. This suggests that physical access to services may be particularly problematic for women especially in rural areas. Geographic barriers may be less relevant for asylum seekers, as key informants explained that primary health services for this group are available at the asylum centres.

Affordability   Several barriers to affordability of MHPSS were raised by study participants. Key informants were concerned that Syrian refugees may experience barriers in seeking MHPSS due to the need to pay the health insurance deductible out of pocket (Van Berkum et al. 2016). This deductible applies to settled refugees only, not to asylum seekers. 'Health insurance' may be a foreign concept to Syrian refugees, and some providers felt that this concept is difficult to explain to a refugee, especially the deductible component. Another key informant highlighted that, while refugees on social welfare can get the greater part of their deductible costs refunded, the reimbursement process is complicated. Financial barriers were also raised with regard to professional interpreter services. These services are covered for asylum seekers (Asylum Seekers Healthcare Scheme); however, the health insurance of settled refugees does not cover interpreter services.

Acceptability   A commonly mentioned barrier amongst respondents was related to the acceptability of services. Language was mentioned as a key obstacle for Syrian refugees in seeking support and receiving appropriate MHPSS care in the Netherlands. Both Syrian refugees and health-care providers who were interviewed experienced communication problems. Refugees found it difficult to clearly express their mental health needs to providers in a foreign language or through an interpreter. Similarly, providers perceived it challenging to fully comprehend their patients' psychological complaints, even if interpreters were present. Interviewees suggested to have 'interpreters who are being reimbursed and ideally of Syrian Arabic origin' and to employ primary and specialist care providers who understand mental health issues of Syrian refugees and have some knowledge of the Syrian culture. Employing Syrian mental health providers was considered a good option; however, according to interviewees, their qualifications are usually not recognised in the Netherlands.

Key informants added that stigma may be an important reason why Syrian refugees refuse or delay mental health care. Syrian refugees interviewed for this study expressed a fear of being labelled as 'crazy'. While seeking professional support for mental health issues is becoming socially more acceptable amongst Syrians, particularly for the young and the more educated, most Syrians prefer to keep these issues to themselves or within their families. A few Syrians indicated a concern that their psychological complaints may be reported in their 'file' and that this may negatively affect their citizenship status, child custody and/or work opportunities.

Quality and Safety   Long waiting times in mental health care was the most frequently mentioned quality-related concern. Waiting times were regarded as particularly problematic for larger specialist intercultural services like i-psy (i-psy is a country-wide institution specialised in transcultural mental health care providing treatment to patients from different cultural backgrounds). According to a provider, smaller culturally sensitive centres have shorter waiting times but are less well-known to refugees. Key informants explained that providers commonly refer refugees with mental health needs to i-psy as its facilities as they employ providers from different cultural backgrounds and staff with a range of language abilities.

Another concern raised by study participants was related to continuity of care. The fact that many refugees are forced to move between different locations before being more permanently settled in a community was perceived as challenging. A key informant added that it may be difficult to find a new culturally appropriate provider for a Syrian patient who moved into a new area and that it may take time to build up trust.

The findings from the qualitative work also suggest that Syrians who do seek support may not always receive appropriate treatment. Interviewees mentioned that Syrian refugees commonly express their psychological needs in terms of physical complaints (e.g. headache, fatigue). Health-care workers, according to several interviewees, may be insufficiently trained to recognise that in some cases, mental health symptoms may underlie somatic conditions.

Discussion on Mental Health System Responsiveness in the Context of Forced Migration

The initial findings from our rapid appraisal indicate mixed results in relation to the responsiveness of the mental health system to the mental health needs of Syrian refugees in the Netherlands. Our rapid appraisal shows that the Netherlands has a high number of mental health professionals per population resulting in an adequate service coverage for the general population; this situation is similar to other Western European countries (WHO 2018a). While mental health services may be available for Syrian refugees in urban areas, there seems to be scope to increase coverage of effective services in both urban and rural areas for this specific population group. Effective services are evidence-based treatments recommended for the treatment of mental disorders which have been tailored to the cultural needs of refugees and take account of different thoughts, schemas, beliefs or norms on mental health and mental illness (Dinos 2015).

Acceptability of services and language seem to be key barriers for Syrian refugees hindering help-seeking. It becomes evident that not only providers in primary health care and the community need to be culturally trained but that also services need to be adapted to the specific needs of this population group to facilitate service use. Interpreters may be indispensable during psychological treatment; however, for effective treatment delivery, the cultural background of interpreters themselves needs to be considered. To increase service uptake of culturally appropriate interventions, mental health stigma experienced by Syrian refugees needs to be addressed. Recommendations include policymakers and health-care workers in the community advocating for mental health awareness and providing educational activities to increase demand of mental health services.

While formal care pathways are in place, not all Syrian refugees may be benefiting from this service structure. Specifically, there is a need to improve early detection of psychological problems. This could be achieved by two means: firstly, by training case workers and social workers in mental health (who may interact with refugees on a frequent basis) so that different manifestations of mental health symptoms and acute worsening can be easily recognised in the community. Secondly, by strengthening the gatekeeping function of primary health care, by providing more GP practices with mental health-care workers or social-psychiatric nurses who are culturally competent in working with Syrian refugees. We see that integration of mental health services into primary health may not necessarily provide greater access to care and may fail short for refugees or patients who come from a different cultural background. Syrian refugees may not access primary health care in the Netherlands or any other European host country because of barriers related to language and culture (Bartolomei et al. 2016) and the complexity of the health system which refugees fail to navigate (Langlois et al. 2016). The initial assessment of pathways of care suggests that a collaborative model of care in which lay health-care providers/social workers work together with trained mental health professionals may facilitate treatment entry. For example, a low-intensity psychological intervention (e.g. a brief counselling intervention delivered by trained lay health-care providers) could be made available in centres like i-psy in which a large proportion of Syrian refugees seek help. There is evidence to suggest that choosing lay health-care providers such as peer-refugees trained in the intervention itself may be more acceptable to refugees and contribute to reducing the waiting times and the high workload of mental health specialists in these centres (Patel et al. 2018; van Ginneken et al. 2013). Integration of such an intervention into the public health-care system of the Netherlands would require financial resources, possibly through health insurance. Insurance companies, however, may be unwilling to cover services provided to people who show signs of psychological distress only (as this is considered prevention) and by health workers who are not professionally registered. This means that this intervention may need to be funded by alternative sources such as (inter)national donors or local municipalities (see also Chap. 3). The cost-effectiveness and financial sustainability of such an intervention will therefore be critical.

The responsiveness of the health system in the Netherlands towards the mental health needs of Syrian refugees may be similar to other Western European countries (WHO 2010a), where utilisation of mental health services remains low amongst refugees despite availability of services in the community (Priebe et al. 2013). Quality of services in European countries are usually high as providers are accredited and have undergone years of training. However, there are reports that refugees may not respond well to these treatments because of mistrust in the provider and unfamiliarity with psychological treatments (Mangrio and Sjogren Forss 2017; Bartolomei et al. 2016). There also seems to be a need to strengthen collaboration and coordination between different services in European host countries to increase service use (Priebe et al. 2016). Community outreach by social workers may be necessary to identify refugees in need of mental health services so that case workers can link refugees with culturally appropriate services in the community or primary health care (Priebe et al. 2012). It is the case worker who can provide information about services and the health system and link the patient with the treatment provider. For European host countries, it remains important to overcome poor utilisation of services amongst refugees as those may be a sign of stigma and discrimination (Bartolomei et al. 2016) and may lead to further isolation and exclusion reinforcing mental ill health (Langlois et al. 2016).

Conclusion

In this chapter, we discussed health system responsiveness to the mental health needs of forcibly displaced persons. We have presented a conceptual health system's framework, which guided our rapid appraisal applied to Syrian refugees residing in the Netherlands. Our conceptual framework conceives responsiveness as intermediate outcome and suggests that access, coverage, quality and safety may well act as proxy responsiveness measures if primary data cannot be collected. It thereby allows an initial assessment of the responsiveness of the health system by also taking pathways of care into account. Our rapid appraisal methodology is different to current rapid appraisals in MHPSS amongst conflict-affected populations as it specifically seeks to assess the responsiveness of the health system which is critical for service uptake and planning further investments in the health system. The development and implementation of evidence-based interventions may benefit from conducting a rapid appraisal on responsiveness as it can generate important insights into the functioning of a mental health system before a new intervention is scaled up.

Acknowledgments The STRENGTHS project is funded under Horizon 2020—the Framework Programme for Research and Innovation (2014–2020). The content of this chapter reflects only the authors' views, and the European Community is not liable for any use that may be made of the information contained therein.

References

Aida. (2018). *Asylum information database*. Germany: Health Care. Retrieved from http://www. asylumineurope.org/reports/country/germany/reception-conditions/health-care

Anker, M., Guidotti, R. J., Orzeszyna, S., Sapirie, S. A., & Thuriaux, M. C. (1993). Rapid evaluation methods (REM) of health services performance: Methodological observations. *Bulletin of the World Health Organization, 71*(1), 15–21.

BAfF. (2015). *Aufforderung zur Sicherstellung der gesundheitlichen und psycho-sozialen Versorgung Geflüchteter in Deutschland*. Bundesweite Arbeitsgemeinschaft der Psychosozialen Zentren für Flüchtlinge und Folteropfer.

Bajbouj, M. (2016). Psychosocial health care for refugees in Germany. *Die Psychiatrie, 13*, 187–191.

Balabanova, D., McKee, M., Koroleva, N., Chikovani, I., Goguadze, K., Kobaladze, T., et al. (2009). Navigating the health system: Diabetes care in Georgia. *Health Policy and Planning, 24*(1), 46–54. https://doi.org/10.1093/heapol/czn041

Bartolomei, J., Baeriswyl-Cottin, R., Framorando, D., Kasina, F., Premand, N., Eytan, A., et al. (2016). What are the barriers to access to mental healthcare and the primary needs of asylum seekers? A survey of mental health caregivers and primary care workers. *BMC Psychiatry, 16*(1), 336. https://doi.org/10.1186/s12888-016-1048-6

Ben Farhat, J., Blanchet, K., Juul Bjertrup, P., Veizis, A., Perrin, C., Coulborn, R. M., et al. (2018). Syrian refugees in Greece: Experience with violence, mental health status, and access to information during the journey and while in Greece. *BMC Medicine, 16*(1), 40. https://doi.org/10.1186/s12916-018-1028-4

Böttche, M. (2016). Psychotherapeutic treatment of traumatized refugees in Germany. *Nervenarzt, 87*(11), 1136–1143.

CBS. (2017). *Immi- en emigratie naar geboorteland [Immi- and emigration by country of birth]*. Centraal Bureau voor de Statistiek. Retrieved October 10, 2018, from http://statline.cbs.nl/Statweb/publication/?DM=SLNL&PA=03742&D1=0&D2=0&D3=0&D4=221&D5=0&D6=1&HDR=G3,G2,T&STB=G1,G5,G4&VW=T

Clement, S., Lassman, F., Barley, E., Evans-Lacko, S., Williams, P., Yamaguchi, S., et al. (2013). Mass media interventions for reducing mental health-related stigma. *Cochrane Database of Systematic Reviews*, (7), Cd009453. https://doi.org/10.1002/14651858.CD009453.pub2

Commonwealth Fund. (2016). *Framework for a high performance health system for the United States*. New York: The Commonwealth Fund.

Corrigan, P. W., Watson, A. C., Warpinski, A. C., & Gracia, G. (2004). Stigmatizing attitudes about mental illness and allocation of resources to mental health services. *Community Mental Health Journal, 40*(4), 297–307.

Darby, C., Valentine, N., Murray, C., & de Silva, A. (n.d.). *World Health Organization: Strategy on measuring responsiveness*. Retrieved December 3, 2018, from http://www.who.int/responsiveness/papers/paper23.pdf

Dinos, S. (2015). Culturally adapted mental healthcare: Evidence, problems and recommendations. *BJPsych Bulletin, 39*(4), 153–155. https://doi.org/10.1192/pb.bp.115.050872

Evans-Lacko, S., Brohan, E., Mojtabai, R., & Thornicroft, G. (2012). Association between public views of mental illness and self-stigma among individuals with mental illness in 14 European countries. *Psychological Medicine, 42*(8), 1741–1752. https://doi.org/10.1017/s0033291711002558

GGZ Netherlands. (2018a). *Bekostiging [Financing]*. Retrieved February, 28, from http://www.ggznederland.nl/themas/financiering

GGZ Netherlands. (2018b). *GGZ-Sector [Mental healthcare sector]*. Retrieved March 1, 2018, from http://www.ggznederland.nl/pagina/ggz-sector

Government of the Netherlands. (2017a). *Health insurance and residence permit*. Retrieved October 10, 2018, from https://www.government.nl/topics/health-insurance/health-insurance-and-residence-permit

Government of the Netherlands. (2017b). *Hoe verloopt het aanvragen van asiel? [What is the asylum procedure?]*. Retrieved October 10, 2018, from https://www.rijksoverheid.nl/onderwerpen/asielbeleid/vraag-en-antwoord/procedure-asielzoeker

Hatzenbuehler, M. L., Phelan, J. C., & Link, B. G. (2013). Stigma as a fundamental cause of population health inequalities. *American Journal of Public Health, 103*(5), 813–821. https://doi.org/10.2105/ajph.2012.301069

Henderson, C., Evans-Lacko, S., & Thornicroft, G. (2013). Mental illness stigma, help seeking, and public health programs. *American Journal of Public Health, 103*(5), 777–780. https://doi.org/10.2105/ajph.2012.301056

Hirschfeld, R. M., Montgomery, S. A., Keller, M. B., Kasper, S., Schatzberg, A. F., Moller, H. J., et al. (2000). Social functioning in depression: A review. *The Journal of Clinical Psychiatry, 61*(4), 268–275.

IASC. (2007). *IASC guidelines on mental health and psychosocial support in emergency settings*. Geneva: Author.

Kelley, E., & Hurst, J. (2006). *Health care quality indicators project: Conceptual framework paper*. Paris: OECD.

Kroneman, M., Boerma, W., Van den Berg, M., Groenewegen, P., De Jong, J., & Van Ginneken, E. (2016). Netherlands: Health system review. *Health Systems in Transition, 18*, 1.

Kumar, K. (1993). *Rapid appraisal methods*. Washington, DC: World Bank.

Langlois, E. V., Haines, A., Tomson, G., & Ghaffar, A. (2016). Refugees: Towards better access to health-care services. *Lancet, 387*(10016), 319–321. https://doi.org/10.1016/s0140-6736(16)00101-x

Lindert, J., Ehrenstein, O. S., Priebe, S., Mielck, A., & Brahler, E. (2009). Depression and anxiety in labor migrants and refugees—A systematic review and meta-analysis. *Social Science & Medicine (1982), 69*(2), 246–257. https://doi.org/10.1016/j.socscimed.2009.04.032

Lionis, C., Petelos, E., Mechili, E. A., Sifaki-Pistolla, D., Chatzea, V. E., Angelaki, A., et al. (2018). Assessing refugee healthcare needs in Europe and implementing educational interventions in primary care: A focus on methods. *BMC International Health and Human Rights, 18*(1), 11. https://doi.org/10.1186/s12914-018-0150-x

Mangrio, E., & Sjogren Forss, K. (2017). Refugees' experiences of healthcare in the host country: A scoping review. *BMC Health Services Research, 17*(1), 814. https://doi.org/10.1186/s12913-017-2731-0

McNall, M., & Foster-Fishman, P. G. (2007). Methods of rapid evaluation, assessment and appraisal. *American Journal of Evaluation, 28*(2), 151–168.

Mirzoev, T., & Kane, S. (2017). What is health systems responsiveness? Review of existing knowledge and proposed conceptual framework. *BMJ Global Health, 2*(4), e000486. https://doi.org/10.1136/bmjgh-2017-000486

Mossialos, E., Wenzl, M., Osborn, R., & Sarnak, D. (2016). *2015 international profiles of health care systems*. New York: The Commonwealth Fund.

Norredam, M., Mygind, A., & Krasnik, A. (2006). Access to health care for asylum seekers in the European Union—A comparative study of country policies. *European Journal of Public Health, 16*(3), 286–290. https://doi.org/10.1093/eurpub/cki191

Papanicolas, I., & Smith, P. (2013). *Health systems performance comparison. An agenda for policy, information and research*. Maidenhead: Open University Press.

Patel, V., Saxena, S., Lund, C., Thornicroft, G., Baingana, F., Bolton, P., et al. (2018). The Lancet Commission on global mental health and sustainable development. *Lancet, 392*(10157), 1553–1598. https://doi.org/10.1016/s0140-6736(18)31612-x

Penchansky, R., & Thomas, J. W. (1981). The concept of access: Definition and relationship to consumer satisfaction. *Medical Care, 19*(2), 127–140.

Priebe, S., Giacco, D., & El-Nagib, R. (2016). *Public health aspects of mental health among migrants and refugees: A review of the evidence on mental health care for refugees, asylum seekers and irregular migrants in the WHO European Region*. Copenhagen: World Health Organization Regional Office for Europe.

Priebe, S., Matanov, A., Barros, H., Canavan, R., Gabor, E., Greacen, T., et al. (2013). Mental health-care provision for marginalized groups across Europe: Findings from the PROMO study. *European Journal of Public Health, 23*(1), 97–103. https://doi.org/10.1093/eurpub/ckr214

Priebe, S., Matanov, A., Schor, R., Strassmayr, C., Barros, H., Barry, M. M., et al. (2012). Good practice in mental health care for socially marginalised groups in Europe: A qualitative study of expert views in 14 countries. *BMC Public Health, 12*, 248. https://doi.org/10.1186/1471-2458-12-248

Rijksoverheid.(2018).*Primaryandsecondarymentalhealthcare*.RetrievedApril5,2018,fromhttps://www.government.nl/topics/mental-health-services/primary-and-secondary-mental-health-care

Risso-Gill, I., Balabanova, D., Majid, F., Ng, K. K., Yusoff, K., Mustapha, F., et al. (2015). Understanding the modifiable health systems barriers to hypertension management in Malaysia: A multi-method health systems appraisal approach. *BMC Health Services Research, 15*, 254. https://doi.org/10.1186/s12913-015-0916-y

Roberts, M. J., Hsiao, W., Berman, P., & Reich, M. R. (2008). *Getting health reform right: A guide to improving performance and equity*. Oxford: Oxford University Press.

Satinsky, E. Fuhr, D. C., Woodward, A., Sondorp, E., & Roberts, B. (2019). Mental health care utilisation and access among refugees and asylum seekers in Europe: A systematic review. Health Policy, 123(9):851–863.

Silove, D., Ventevogel, P., & Rees, S. (2017). The contemporary refugee crisis: An overview of mental health challenges. World Psychiatry, 16(2), 130–139. https://doi.org/10.1002/wps.20438

The World Bank. (2017). World Bank Open Data. Retrieved September 19, 2017, from https://data.worldbank.org

Thornicroft, G., & Tansella, M. (2004). Components of a modern mental health service: A pragmatic balance of community and hospital care: Overview of systematic evidence. The British Journal of Psychiatry, 185, 283–290. https://doi.org/10.1192/bjp.185.4.283

Thornicroft, G., & Tansella, M. (2013). The balanced care model: The case for both hospital- and community-based mental healthcare. The British Journal of Psychiatry, 202(4), 246–248. https://doi.org/10.1192/bjp.bp.112.111377

UNHCR. (2013). UNHCR's mental health and psychosocial support for persons of concern. Geneva: Author.

UNHCR. (2017). Syria regional refugee response: Inter-agency information sharing portal. Europe: Syrian Asylum Applications. Retrieved September 19, 2018, from http://data.unhcr.org/syrianrefugees/asylum.php#

UNHCR and WHO. (2008). Rapid assessment of alcohol and other substance use in conflict-affected and displaced populations: A field guide. Geneva: Author.

USAID. (2010). Performance monitoring and evaluation tips: Using rapid appraisal methods. Author. Retrieved October 18, 2018, from https://s3.amazonaws.com/gpei-tk/reference_links/en/2010_USAID_-_Using_rapid_appraisal_methods.pdf?1505707314

Valentine, N. B. (2003). Patients experiences with health services: Population surveys from 16 OECD countries. In C. J. Murray & D. B. Evans (Eds.), Health systems performance assessment: Debates, methods and empiricism. Geneva: WHO.

Van Berkum, M., Smulders, E., Van den Muijsenbergh, M., Haker, F., Bloemen, E., Van Wieringen, J., et al. (2016). Zorg, ondersteuning en preventie voor nieuwkomende vluchtelingen: Wat is er nodig? [Care, support and prevention for newly arrived refugees: What is needed?]. Utrecht: Pharos.

van Ginneken, N., Tharyan, P., Lewin, S., Rao, G. N., Meera, S. M., Pian, J., et al. (2013). Non-specialist health worker interventions for the care of mental, neurological and substance-abuse disorders in low- and middle-income countries. The Cochrane Database of Systematic Reviews (11):Cd009149. https://doi.org/10.1002/14651858.CD009149.pub2

Vistorte, A. O. R., Ribeiro, W. S., Jaen, D., Jorge, M. R., Evans-Lacko, S., & Mari, J. J. (2018). Stigmatizing attitudes of primary care professionals towards people with mental disorders: A systematic review. International Journal of Psychiatry in Medicine, 53(4), 317–338. https://doi.org/10.1177/0091217418778620

Wang, P. S., Angermeyer, M., Borges, G., Bruffaerts, R., Tat Chiu, W., De Girolamo, G., et al. (2007). Delay and failure in treatment seeking after first onset of mental disorders in the World Health Organization's World Mental Health Survey Initiative. World Psychiatry, 6(3), 177–185.

Wang, P. S., Berglund, P. A., Olfson, M., & Kessler, R. C. (2004). Delays in initial treatment contact after first onset of a mental disorder. Health Services Research, 39(2), 393–415. https://doi.org/10.1111/j.1475-6773.2004.00234.x

WHO. (2000). The World health report 2000. Health systems: Improving performance. Geneva: Author.

WHO. (2007). Everybody's business. Strengthening health systems to improve health outcomes. WHO's framework for action. Geneva: Author.

WHO. (2010a). How health systems can address health inequities linked to migration and ethnicity. Copenhagen: WHO Regional Office for Europe.

WHO. (2010b). mhGAP Intervention Guide for mental, neurological and substance use disorders in non-specialized health settings. Retrieved October 10, 2018.

WHO. (2011). *Mental health atlas 2011*. Netherlands. Retrieved October 10, 2018, from http://www.who.int/mental_health/evidence/atlas/profiles/nld_mh_profile.pdf?ua=1

WHO. (2014). *Mental health atlas country profile 2014*. Netherlands. Retrieved October 10, 2018, from http://www.who.int/mental_health/evidence/atlas/profiles-2014/nld.pdf?ua=1

WHO. (2018a). *Mental health atlas 2017*. Geneva: Author.

WHO. (2018b). *World health survey*. Retrieved October 21, 2018, from http://apps.who.int/health-info/systems/surveydata/index.php/catalog/whs/about

WHO/UNHCR. (2012). *Assessing mental health and psychosocial needs resources*. Geneva: Author.

Chapter 13
Global Social Governance and Health Protection for Forced Migrants

Alexandra Kaasch

Abbreviations

CRSR   Convention Relating to the Status of Refugees
GFMD   Global Forum on Migration and Development
HFA   "Health for All"
ICESCR   International Covenant on Economic, Social and Cultural Rights
ILO   International Labour Organisation
IOM   International Organisation on Migration
OECD   Organisation for Economic Cooperation and Development
PHAME   WHO Public Health Aspects of Migration in Europe
PHC   Primary Health Care
R202   ILO's Social Protection Floors Recommendation
SDGs   Sustainable Development Goals
UN   United Nations
UHC   Universal Health Coverage
UNHCR   UN High Commissioner on Refugees
UN GA   United Nations General Assembly
WHA   World Health Assembly
WHO   World Health Organization

Introduction

The distinction between different groups of migrants, though morally or normatively irrelevant, does matter regarding the access to national and local systems of social protection and, thus, also to health services. Migrants entering a host country as family members of national citizens or residents usually face a much more regu-

A. Kaasch (✉)
Faculty of Sociology, Bielefeld University, Bielefeld, Germany
e-mail: Alexandra.kaasch@uni-bielefeld.de

© Springer Nature Switzerland AG 2020   235
K. Bozorgmehr et al. (eds.), *Health Policy and Systems Responses to Forced Migration*, https://doi.org/10.1007/978-3-030-33812-1_13

lated and clearer situation of access. Newly arriving labour migrants are treated under specific immigration regulations that usually also include defining access to social protection and health protection. Forced migrants are those who leave their countries because of conflict; because they are threatened based on their religion, sexual orientation, political opinion and so on; or because of natural disasters. Thus, this group of migrants often does not have the time and opportunity to prepare for migration. They usually do not have a job or work permit of the country they arrive in, nor do they have access to social and health services as relative of a person covered by social protection. What is provided to these groups of people in a situation of forced migration is somewhere between humanitarian aid, asylum rights and rights to health. The right to health is often characterised by restricted entitlements except for particular groups such as women giving births, newborns or unaccompanied minors. This also creates a situation of incomplete and insecure protection in case of illness and injury for forced migrants.

In general, the need for proper health systems to ensure universal access to health care has a long history and is supported by a number of global actors. For migrants without citizenship of the host country, in particular, there are even additional issues in terms of accessing health care. There are specific demands on health systems to make sure everybody can enjoy his or her rights to health and social security. One of the challenges regarding access to health care in the context of migration is that it is often two or more countries' health systems that matter regarding rights to, and levels of, health care. There are numerous and complex situations connected to the place of origin that is usually characterised by a breakdown of existing protection arrangements (be it personal, family, state, religious and the like), in addition to a general destruction of infrastructure, and situations of mental distress and trauma (Gostin and Roberts 2015). Neighbouring countries, the most likely target destination of refugees, often face similar situations or are characterised by limited resources and infrastructure to provide health care for large numbers of additional people. The risk of epidemics as well as of other health and social risks increases for people living in refugee camps under uncertain conditions. Moreover, the affected people often also lack knowledge of their rights in the respective host country (Gostin and Roberts 2015).

This chapter discusses issues of social and health policy for people in a situation of forced migration from a global social policy and governance perspective. It draws on global social policy scholarship that is positioned between international, comparative social policy analysis and development studies. It also engages with transnational forms of regulation and human rights, international relations and global governance. Such a global perspective to tackling health issues of migrants is important as the scope of national regulation and legislation to solve global problems is limited. Furthermore, drawing on global social policy literature is particularly useful in this context as it allows combining analytical with normative positions on appropriate and transformative social policies.

Global Social Policy, Social Rights and Migrants' Rights to Health

Social policymaking, including health policymaking, happens at multiple levels of governance. This is even more true when it concerns groups of people migrating between countries. It is relevant with regard to rights to health and social security in home, transit and host countries alike.

"Global social policies" describe ideas, processes and provisions of social policy that happen at global scales. Their making includes intergovernmental negotiations, the involvement and interactions of international and supranational agencies and the formulation and enforcement of transnational norms and rules (Kaasch and Martens 2015). Global social policy literature commonly distinguishes two main types: one being social policy prescriptions to national governments by international actors. This may include policy recommendations not only on appropriate health system reform but also appropriate treatment of non-nationals in a host country. The other one is a "truly" global social policy in the sense of global social redistribution, regulation and rights (Deacon 2007). Here, we can think about the emergence of human rights on social protection, responding to different social needs, as well as the human right to health. At the same time, regulation on migration, trade and labour may also form transnational systems of social and health policy. Global redistribution, though of a different form and quality to what we know from national welfare states, includes not only development aid and emergency aid but also remittances all of which with an impact on people migrating.

Looking at global social rights more specifically, we think of those rights associated with what a person needs to live her or his life and take part in society (Dean 2007). Furthermore, they relate to situations in which a person cannot fully care for her- or himself and thus needs financial support, personal care, health care and the like (Maciejczyk Jaron 2009). We can distinguish between social rights that are connected to a particular group of (vulnerable) people, the so-called rights *of*, and those related to a specific social need or problem, the so-called rights *to* (for a discussion, see Kaasch 2016). Understanding the specific situation and social needs of migrants in a context of health requires a combination between the two forms, namely, the right to health and the (social) rights of people under forced migration. Regarding the right to health, various international agreements and treaties formulate that, at the very minimum, primary and basic health care should be free and accessible to every human being. This is based on Article 25 of the Universal Declaration of Human Rights. The Alma-Ata Declaration (1978) and Article 12 of the International Covenant on Economic, Social and Cultural Rights (ICESCR) are more specific and concrete of what this right is supposed to include and imply, but there is no internationally common understanding of what is required to realise the right to health (see also Chap. 7). Looking at the "rights of" migrants, in the case of this chapter, we can see that particularly refugee rights are dealt with in the Convention Relating to the Status of Refugees (CRSR) from 1951. In general, group-related rights also include the right to health, applied to a specific group. The idea and reasoning behind is one of equal treatment and non-discrimination. These rights often "represent an advocacy and adjustment tool for claiming and improving the situation of particular groups of people" (Kaasch 2016, p. 79).

The meaning of the human right to health, as included in the Universal Declaration of Human Rights, provides a set of standards regarding health systems (and beyond). Looking from the individual's level, when we think about the right to health, we associate the right of everybody to enjoy the highest attainable standard of health, which is part of many international treaties dealing with specific groups and social problems. As all countries have ratified one or more international treaty that is binding, we can indeed speak of a global social right representing an internationally shared norm and connected to certain mechanisms to enforce it. Nevertheless, it is basically the responsibility of national governments to realise the right to health through functioning health systems (Backman et al. 2008; Tarantola 2008).

Health systems are, at the same time, considered to be part of systems of social protection and, therefore, also matter in the context of rights to social security and global concepts of social protection floors (most prominently the ILO's Social Protection Floors Recommendation (R202) from 2012). The right to social security as such is subject to the ICESCR's Article 9, saying that "The State Parties to represent the Covenant recognize the right of everyone to social security, including health insurance". The ILO's social security standards go more into detail with this right by setting social security standards and recommendations on the establishment of social security systems. Most comprehensively, this has been tackled in the ILO Social Protection Floors Recommendation (R202) from 2012 (Hujo et al. 2017). Scheil-Adlung (2013, p. 147) emphasises how that is important making health policies more effective and efficient and for coordinating them with socio-economic policies. That would facilitate progress on universal health coverage. She further explains that R202 provides guidance to states in setting up social protection floors in the sense of basic social security guarantees to ensure that—including other provisions—access to essential health care and basic income is provided over the life cycle. This includes the expectation for national governments to create systems that combine preventive, promotional and active measures; that establish appropriate benefits and social services; and that promote economic activity and formal employment. It should also be coordinated with other relevant policies (Scheil-Adlung 2013, p. 161). Accordingly, social protection in the field of health care implies guarantees for "essential health benefits", which includes preventive and maternal care, provided to everybody and with adequate quality (universal health care) (Scheil-Adlung 2013, p. 162).

When it concerns coverage regarding at least basic health services, the problems are usually at the level of inequities in access to health care, caused by a variety of factors, including affordability and availability (Scheil-Adlung 2013, p. 167). Underlying factors contributing to inequitable access to health care are commonly related to poverty, work status and formal lack of access to institutions, services and benefits of social security. When we look at the specific group of migrants under forced migration, many of these determinants are structurally linked with citizenship status and the right to work (and by that way get access to national systems of social protection). As Hennebry (2014) says, social protection floors initiatives are often focused on national strategies and models to protect a country's citizens, with a particular emphasis on poor countries. Initiatives for migrants, even formal migrant workers, have not been in focus (Hennebry 2014, p. 381). At the same time, there is no unified system that regulates or governs migration from a transnational level. Migrants thus lack strong national agencies to secure their human rights in many countries (Ratel et al. 2013, pp. 2–3).

Overall, while there has been significant advancement at the level of global norms and recommendations on social health protection, setting up appropriate protection in health for people under forced migration remains a major challenge. In the following sections, the focus is on what international agencies are key players with regard to this specific issue, as well as on ideational and discursive developments in global social and health policies since the so-called refugee crisis.

Global Social Policy Actors in the Field of Health Systems and Migration

Global social policy and governance in general is characterised by multiple actors, overlapping agencies and competing ideas on appropriate social policies. This also applies to the field of health systems. There are several international organisations claiming to have a say on appropriate health systems (as well as a broad range of specific public health issues) and at the same time a rather small group of global health experts within these international organisations coming with an encompassing, systems view. The field is broad and complex, and it is characterised by deficiencies. More concretely, when we look at the global governance of health-care systems, we can identify a multilayered, polyarchic and pluralistic institutional architecture. The positions of specific organisations change over time and new actors emerge, which leads to varying configurations of relevant actors (Kaasch 2015, p. 3).

Looking at the issue of the social situation and needs of migrants in their host countries, we focus on a combination of social policy prescriptions by international organisations to national governments in issues of providing at least basic social protection to migrants and global social rights. We do not focus on a particular country or world region but rather turn our view to the global social policy arena in terms of mandates, positions and discourse on the subject matter. The emerging picture may be used as a frame for social and health policymaking on migrants at other policy levels.

The international community, including a number of international organisations inside and outside the UN system, holds implicit and explicit mandates to engage with issues of social rights, the right to health and migrants and refugees. Regarding the field of health systems with a focus on the social health protection of people under forced migration, we can distinguish those actors with a focus on migration issues and those concerned with health policies. Common actors—here with a focus on international (governmental) organisations—in the field of global health governance are the World Health Organization (WHO) and the World Bank. To a lesser degree, also, the International Labour Organisation (ILO) and the Organisation for Economic Cooperation and Development (OECD) come into the picture (Kaasch 2015). Looking at migration governance, the picture is more diverse (for a discussion on the character and shape of migration governance, see, for example, Betts (2010), but the major international organisations include not only the International Migration Organisation (IOM) and the UN High Commissioner on Refugees (UNHCR) but also organisations like the ILO.

The UN High Commissioner for Refugees (UNHCR) office was established in 1950, in a context of large-scale migration from and within the European region following the World War II. It supports states and migrants in situations of major migration streams. It aims at ensuring that all refugees have access to life-saving and essential health care. The focus is less on health systems in a comprehensive sense but more on the identification of specific health issues (e.g. HIV/AIDS-related health care and prevention, reproductive health or specific communicable diseases like measles) and health determinants (e.g. food, nutrition, water, sanitation, hygiene). According to its website, UNHCR provides assistance in refugee camps and other places where forced migrants stay. The mandate is connected to the 1951 Refugee Convention and requests access to health services for refugees equivalent to that of the host population (UNHCR 1951). Whatever goes beyond emergency care, the emphasis is on primary health care (PHC) and secondary hospital care. UNHCR provides a number of guidance documents that relate to health care and associated issues of migrants and refugees in particular. In 2012, UNHCR issued "A Guidance Note on Health Insurance Schemes for Refugees and other Persons of Concern to UNHCR" (UNHCR 2012). While making recommendations and stating to provide guidance, this document does not demonstrate a profound understanding of how health systems work and what are mechanisms of integrating groups of populations into different types of health systems in order to ensure or improve their health care. The document advocates for basic primary health care and emergency services to be provided to refugees in emergency situations. It also refers to specific vaccinations and preventive measures related to what is considered to be the major life threats in the context of forced migration. The recommendations also claim not to make differences between national and non-nationals in the provision of health care. Overall, the guidance is not really coherent but rather reflects considerations from different sources that do not necessarily speak a common language. Nevertheless, the UNHCR is committed and also to some extent resourced to support migrants and refugees to access health care in different ways: claiming inclusion (though not speaking a right-based language), providing resources for paying insurance fees and reflecting upon different health systems and the challenges to include refugees. It advocates public health systems in a more general way; other documents and guiding principles are rather focused on specific diseases or health risks. Furthermore, the Principles and Guidance for Referral Health Care for Refugees and Other Persons of Concern (UNHCR 2009) reflects the organisation's emergency focus and Primary Health Care approach.

The International Organisation on Migration (IOM) was established around the same time and has over 170 member states. The IOM's website describes its mandate as to promote humane and orderly migration for the benefit of all by providing services and advices to governments and migrants alike. Its mandate comprises migration and development, regulating migration and forced migration, as well as the promotion of protection of migrants' rights and migration health. The IOM includes a Migration Health Division through which it provides comprehensive, preventive and curative health programmes to address migrants' needs. One focus of its work—though in collaboration with WHO—is on migrant sensitive health systems. Similar to the UNHCR, the focus of IOM is on supporting migrants and countries to improve health coverage for migrants through technical support, information and promotion. Activities include the strengthening of national health systems—with the aim of "the strengthening of migrant-friendly and migrant inclusive health systems which benefit migrants and the communities in which they live" (IOM 2019).

WHO is the UN agency mandated with health issues of all kinds. This includes ensuring appropriate structure and functioning of health system, so that they cover different vulnerable groups, different countries and world regions and different sorts of health problems, illnesses or diseases. WHO's work on refugee and migrant health links prominently and explicitly to the right to health while describing the problem as a lack of access to health services and protection for refugees and migrants. Furthermore, WHO's work on the issue is guided by the aim to achieve universal health coverage (UHC) and equitable access to quality health services (WHO 2019). Compared to the other two actors, WHO has produced "soft law" on the issue of migrants' health. In 2017, the World Health Assembly endorsed the Resolution "Promoting the Health of Refugees and Migrants", setting plans for international engagement for improving refugees' situations (WHA 2017). It lists guiding principles including the right to health, the principles of equality and non-discrimination, equitable access to health services, people-centred and refugee- and migrant-sensitive health systems, and whole of government approaches (see also WHO 2015).

In conclusion, there are three main actors involved in global health policy and governance for forced migrants. It is striking that WHO has the leading role, while the financial means to support migrants is rather with the two other actors. Furthermore, WHO does not have a migrant health division except for WHO EURO. In the following section, the focus will be on the general global policy development with regard to migrants and refugee health, which commonly brings these three actors (with other actors) together on pushing the agenda on social protection in health and migration.

Evolving Global Health Governance on Social Health Protection for Migrants

The Alma-Ata Declaration of the 1970s provided a framework of Primary Health Care (PHC) and "Health for All" (HFA). Since then, international organisations have provided reports providing more in-depth analysis and understanding on the meanings and functions of health systems in different types of countries. There has been increasing consensus emerging about the general importance of health-care systems. Nevertheless, there are differences on priorities and strategies of different global actors on how to develop and improve health-care systems. The need for universal health care, meanwhile, is increasingly acknowledged in the global health community (Kaasch 2015).

There are several international organisations engaging with issues of global migration governance. However, in contrast to global health governance, for a long time, there has not been a UN migration organization (Betts 2011, p. 1). In the meantime, the IOM has been given such a status. Nevertheless, we cannot speak of a truly international migration regime. However, asylum seekers are supported by the 1951 Convention on the Status of Refugees and the UNHCR. The Global Forum on Migration and Development (GFMD) has met on a regular basis since 2007; it also has an important role as a forum to discuss issues of migration. Even more than for health systems, though, decisions on the regulation of migration and the local rights of migrants are taken by national policymaking.

Nevertheless, combining key components of global migration and health governance, the normative claim would be straightforward: as human beings, forced migrants do have a right to health, and therefore, national governments have to do their best to guarantee this right, regardless of migration status. That was also part of the 1951 Refugee Convention and its 1967 Protocol that obliges national governments to provide appropriate social security and health care for injuries, maternity, sickness and disability (Gostin and Roberts 2015).

In response to the significant increases in refugees/migrants, particularly into European and other high-income countries, there were additional human-right-focused measures taken at the UN level. In September 2016, the UN General Assembly adopted the New York Declaration for Refugees and Migrants (UN GA 2016). This called upon member states to take international cooperation seriously, as well as the protection of migrants. Regarding health, it alerts states to "address the vulnerabilities to HIV and the specific health-care needs experienced by [...] refugees and crisis-affected populations" (section 30). Furthermore, the states commit themselves to provide access to sexual and reproductive health-care services (section 31). More generally, in section 39, the states announce to "take measures to improve [refugees] [...] integration and inclusion, as appropriate, and with particular reference to access to [...], health care, ...". Regarding migrant children, the commitment to provide access to basic health care is also emphasised (section 59). With regard to refugees, in particular, the Declaration states the commitment to humanitarian assistance, including in the field of health care (section 80). But most explicitly, section 83 says "We will work to ensure that the basic health needs of refugee communities are met and that women and girls have access to essential health-care services. We commit to providing host countries with support in this regard. We will also develop national strategies for the protection of refugees within the framework of national social protection systems, as appropriate".

The New York Declaration for Refugees and Migrants was also meant to start a process towards two separate global compacts: one to deal with refugees in particular and the other one on the so-called "safe, orderly and regular" migration. The idea driving the process of setting up the compacts was not to invent new international policies on migrants but to "improve how the world responds to the needs of refugees as defined in the 1951 Refugee Convention and its 1967 Protocol" (Thomas and Yarnell 2018). In this context, the focus is on the refugee compact and within that on its health component. Within the programme of action, there are defined areas in need of support, including a section on health (section III B 2.3). The statement on health system basically says that resources and expertise will be provided to whatever health system is in place at the place where refugees need to be supported. This should help to facilitate inclusion or refugees into national health systems. Furthermore, it hints at particularly vulnerable groups and lists some of the principles to be met, e.g. "affordable and equitable access to adequate quantities of medicines, medical supplies, vaccines, diagnostics, and preventive commodities".

The UNHCR was the responsible global agency for the compact, holding numerous consultations with various stakeholders, including the so-called High Commissioner's Dialogue on Protection Challenges. In 2018, the process of drafting the compact took place; formal consultation happened in summer 2018; the final draft was then presented at the UN General Assembly in September 2018. Despite a number of states opting out in advance of the conference, in December 2018, both compacts got adopted. The Global Compact on Refugees got more support (perhaps because of the humanitarian aspect of refugee crises). It was adopted by the UN General Assembly by a recorded vote of 181 in favour to 2 against (United States and Hungary), with three abstentions (Eritrea, Libya, Dominican Republic). Seven countries did not vote: Democratic People's Republic of Korea, Israel, Micronesia, Nauru, Poland, Tonga and Turkmenistan.

WHO, in cooperation with IOM and UNHCR, also engaged with the required health component as part of the Global Compact for Safe, Orderly and Regular Migration (WHO and IOM 2016). The reason is that, looking beyond the concrete plans for such a compact and considering the common vision of the Sustainable Development Goals (SDGs), health rights and needs of migrants need to be adequately addressed. It is argued that global and national health policies, strategies and plans have not sufficiently considered the implications of large-scale migration. That concerns not only information and data systems but also health policies and public health interventions. The emphasis in the report is on the right to the enjoyment of the highest attainable standard of physical and mental health for all; equality and non-discrimination through comprehensive laws and health policies and practices; equitable access to people-centred, migrant- and gender-sensitive, and age-responsive health services; non-restrictive health practices based on health conditions; and whole-of-government and whole-of-society approaches. This implies the goals of realising health rights as part of international human rights, addressing the social determinants of health and improving migrants' access to health services. Among the actionable commitments and means of implementation, point 5 is on providing UHC and right-based and inclusive health services and more specifically "ensuring that the necessary health services are delivered to migrants in line with human rights standards and in a people-centred, gender-responsive, culturally and linguistically appropriate way, without any kind of discrimination and stigmatization; providing access to quality health services to migrants, …; identifying and/or developing sustainable models of health care financing to cover migrant health". There is now the need to develop, reinforce and implement occupational, primary health and safety services and health insurance as social protection for migrant workers and their families in response to WHA resolutions (WHA60.26 and WHA70.15) and ILO conventions and protocols.

The WHO Regional Office for Europe came up with considerations on how to handle health issues in the context of migration and the increase in refugees to Europe. Their report calls for "evidence-based public health interventions to address the health needs of migrants that could save a significant number of lives and reduce suffering and ill health" (WHO Regional Office for Europe 2016, p. v). The WHO Public Health Aspects of Migration in Europe (PHAME) project focused on migrant health and host populations with the aim to "assist Member States in responding adequately to the public health challenges of migration" (WHO Regional Office for Europe 2016, p. v), applying the Health 2020 strategy. This could be "a basis for the preparation of migrant-sensitive health systems and makes a strong case for investment and action through whole-of-governments and whole-of-society approaches. It gives national ministries of health the opportunity to lead a multisectoral collaboration to optimize their health system preparedness and capacity" (WHO Regional Office for Europe 2016, p. v). "Migrant-sensitive health systems" is a concept that at a more general level, and already in 2008, the WHA had called upon member states to adopt (WHA 2008). In 2010, a Global Consultation on Migrant Health followed, "which asks Member States to take action on migrant-sensitive health policies and practices, and directs WHO to promote migrant health on the international agenda, in collaboration with other relevant organizations and sectors" (WHO 2010, p. 4). The considerations here are primarily on the implementation of national health policies for equal access to health services for migrants, inclusion in social protection schemes in the field of health and the general improvement of social security for migrants (WHO 2010, p. 4). Among the arguments reflected in the report are that the main responsibility for setting up institutions to facilitate access to health facilities, goods and services for migrants is with the member states' governments. If required, multilateral cooperation could assist government in attempts to including migrants (WHO 2010, p. 12–13). Explicit connections to human rights are also made (WHO 2010, p. 13).

Meanwhile, the Declaration on Primary Health Care (WHO and UNICEF 2018) attempts to revive the PHC spirit of Alma-Ata (1978) and links to the 2030 Agenda for Sustainable Development and health for all. The vision is on strong and accessible health systems and links to the right to health "without distinction of any kind". There are also explicit links to migrants but mostly to health personnel migrating and the risk of brain drain to developing countries. A civil society document to the Astana conference, though, called for "inclusive access and utilization of health services as well as prevent discrimination, addressing first those most in need, including … refugees and migrants …" (Civil Society Engagement Mechanism for UCH2030 2018, p. 4). Furthermore, at a side event at the Global Conference on

Primary Health Care (Astana, Kazakhstan, October 2018), the IOM's Migration Health Division Director, Jacqueline Weekers, said: "High costs are often cited by governments as the main reason to not include migrants in health systems. Meanwhile, migrants contribute more in taxes than they receive in benefits, send remittances to home communities and fill labour market gaps in host societies. Equitable access for migrants to low cost primary health care can reduce health expenditures, improve social cohesion and enable migrants to contribute substantially towards the development" (IOM 2018).

Conclusions

This chapter discussed some of the roles and activities of global social policy and governance actors on the issue of social health protection for people in the situation of forced migration. Despite a group of international organisations mandated to act on migration and health, what has developed in terms of global regulations is fairly limited (see also Chap. 2).

Addressing the needs of forced migrants is complex and increasingly politicised. This has made it difficult to implement meaningful transnational mechanisms to support their needs. As a result, major developments in the definition and promotion of human rights including the right to health, and developments on health systems, social protection floors and UHC, have not yet sufficiently benefited forced migrants in transit or in a host country. Regional, rather than global, efforts may offer means of improving transnational social policies, including the social protection in health for migrant populations (see also Chap. 5). Particularly for WHO, this would require, though, even greater leadership and investment on health and migration.

As long as international processes primarily happen as intergovernmental struggles on how to distribute irregular migrants, the potential for global social policy and governance to strengthen the right to health remains underdeveloped. Particularly regarding forced migrants, the critical issues are more about the weakness of international organisations than about a lack of knowledge or already formulated global rights.

References

Backman, G., Hunt, P., Khosla, R., Jaramillo-Strouss, C., Mekuria Fikre, B., Rumble, C., et al. (2008). Health systems and the right to health: An assessment of 194 countries. *Lancet, 372,* 2047.

Betts, A. (2010). *Global migration governance - The emergence of a new debate. Briefing Paper. G. E. G. Programme.* Oxford: Department of Politics and International Relations, University of Oxford.

Betts, A. (Ed.). (2011). *Global migration governance.* Oxford: Oxford University Press.

Civil Society Engagement Mechanism for UCH2030. (2018). Civil society statement. In *Global conference on primary health care.* Astana: Author.

Deacon, B. (2007). *Global social policy and governance*. London: Sage.

Dean, H. (2007). Social policy and human rights: Re-thinking the engagement. *Social Policy and Society, 7*(1), 1–12.

Gostin, L. O., & Roberts, A. E. (2015). Forced migration: The human face of a health crisis. *JAMA, 314*, 2125. https://doi.org/10.1001/jama.2015.14906

Hennebry, J. (2014). Falling through the cracks? Migrant workers and the Global Social Protection Floor. *Global Social Policy, 14*(3), 369–388.

Hujo, K., Behrendt, C., & McKinnon, R. (2017). Introduction: Reflecting on the human right to social security. *International Social Security Review, 70*, 5–12.

IOM. (2018). *Evidence shows primary healthcare for migrants is cost-saving*. Retrieved from https://www.iom.int/news/evidence-shows-primary-healthcare-migrants-cost-saving

IOM. (2019). *Health promotion and assistance for migrants*. Retrieved from https://www.iom.int/health-promotion-and-assistance-migrants

Kaasch, A. (2015). *Shaping global health policy. Global social policy actors and ideas about health care systems*. Basingstoke: Palgrave Macmillan.

Kaasch, A. (2016). Conceptualising transnational social rights: Developments and forms. In A. Fischer-Lescano & K. Möller (Eds.), *Transnationalisation of social rights* (pp. 67–84). Cambridge: Intersentia.

Kaasch, A., & Martens, K. (Eds.). (2015). *Actors and agency in global social governance*. Oxford: Oxford University Press.

Maciejczyk Jaron, A. (2009). *Constitutional courts as actors in fundamental social rights. EUI Working Paper LAW 2009/05. European University Institute Social Law Working Group*. San Domenico di Fiesole: EUI.

Ratel, M.-H., Williams, G., & Williams, K. (2013). *Inserting migrants into the global social protection floor*. Waterloo, ON: The Centre for International Governance Innovation.

Scheil-Adlung, X. (2013). Revisiting policies to achieve progress towards universal health coverage in low-income countries: Realizing the pay-offs of national social protection floors. *International Social Security Review, 66*(3–4), 145–170.

Tarantola, D. (2008). Global justice and human rights: Health and human rights in practice. *Global Justice: Theory Practice Rhetoric, 1*, 11–26.

Thomas, A., & Yarnell, M. (2018). *Ensuring that the global compacts on refugees and migration deliver*. Refugees International: Washington, DC.

UN GA. (2016). *New York declaration for refugees and migrants. A/Res/71/1*. New York: Author.

UNHCR. (2012). *A guidance note on health insurance schemes for refugees and other persons of concern to UNHCR*. Geneva: Author.

UNHCR. (1951). *Convention and protocol relating to the status of refugees*. Author.

UNHCR. (2009). *UNHCR's principles and guidance for referral health care for refugees and other persons of concern*. Geneva: Author.

WHA. (2008). *Health of migrants. WHA61.17*. Geneva: WHO.

WHA. (2017). *Promoting the health of refugees and migrants: Draft framework of priorities and guiding principles to promote the health of refugees and migrants: Report by the Secretariat*. Geneva: WHO. A70/24.

WHO. (2010). *Health of migrants - The way forward. Report of a global consultation*. Geneva: Author.

WHO. (2015). *Contributing to social and economic development: Sustainable action across sectors to improve health and health equity (follow-up of the 8th global conference on health promotion). Report of the Secretariat*. Geneva: Author.

WHO. (2019). *The guiding principles of WHO's work*. Retrieved from https://www.who.int/migrants/about/guiding-principles/en/

WHO and IOM. (2016). *Proposed health component. Global compact for safe, orderly and regular migration*. Author.

WHO and UNICEF. (2018). *Declaration of Astana. Global conference on primary health care*. Astana: Author.

WHO Regional Office for Europe. (2016). *Toolkit for assessing health system capacity to manage large influxes of refugees, asylum-seekers and migrants*. Copenhagen: Author.

Index

Printed in the United States
By Bookmasters